Organizational Structure, Problem Solving, and Effectiveness

A Comparative Study of Hospital Emergency Services

Basil S. Georgopoulos

Organizational Structure, Problem Solving, and Effectiveness

A Comparative Study of Hospital Emergency Services

Jossey-Bass Publishers

San Francisco   •   London   •   1986

ORGANIZATIONAL STRUCTURE, PROBLEM SOLVING, AND EFFECTIVENESS
A Comparative Study of Hospital Emergency Services
by Basil S. Georgopoulos

Copyright © 1986 by: Jossey-Bass Inc., Publishers
433 California Street
San Francisco, California 94104

&

Jossey-Bass Limited
28 Banner Street
London EC1Y 8QE

Library of Congress Cataloging-in-Publication Data

Georgopoulos, Basil Spyros (date)
   Organizational structure, problem solving, and
effectiveness.

   (The Jossey-Bass social and behavioral science
series)
   Includes bibliographies and index.
   1. Hospitals—Emergency service-Quality control.
2. Hospitals—Emergency service—Cost effectiveness.
I. Title. II. Series. [DNLM: 1. Emergency Service,
Hospital—economics.   2. Emergency Service, Hospital—
organization and administration. WX 215 G352o].
RA975.5.E5G47   1986   362.1'8   86-81398
ISBN 1-55542-021-4 (alk. paper)

Manufactured in the United States of America

The paper in this book meets the guidelines for
permanence and durability of the Committee on
Production Guidelines for Book Longevity of the
Council on Library Resources.

JACKET DESIGN BY WILLI BAUM

FIRST EDITION

Code 8640

A joint publication in
The Jossey-Bass Health Series
and
The Jossey-Bass Management Series

Contents

Preface

Despite the continuing burden of enormous health care expenditures, increased cost-consciousness, and mounting pressures for cost containment in the United States, efforts to resolve the problem of costs without lowering the quality of services have been only marginally successful at best. The explosive and almost chaotic proliferation in the mid 1980s of payment, provider, and care-delivery modalities—some motivated by self-interest, others by the desire to provide better service, and still others by competition—exemplifies the great and continuing difficulties being experienced throughout the health services system. Many of these organizational efforts represent trial-and-error approaches that are also likely to fail, partly because little dependable knowledge on which they could usefully draw actually exists about the effectiveness of differently organized health service systems. Moreover, organizational research efforts that might have generated the necessary knowledge have not yet been undertaken to any significant extent, partly because problems of organization (unlike problems of financing, quality, and costs) have received insufficient attention by all concerned, and partly because of meager funding by the government and the private sector alike.

Regardless of which particular organizational modalities for health care delivery prevail eventually, some will inevitably turn out to be more effective than others in terms of such criteria as quality, cost, access, patient satisfaction, and so on. Only through organizational research such as that reported here can the effectiveness of particular care-delivery systems be adequately assessed, compared, or demonstrated. A great deal of systematic, high-quality organizational research is needed now and in the future, if the basic problems of our health services system and its various subsystems and components are to be properly analyzed and understood. Until more and better organizational knowledge becomes available, many cost-containment efforts will falter, and the system's major problems will probably remain difficult to resolve.

Seeking to add to the existing organizational knowledge base, this book discusses the results of a major comparative study of one important type of health care delivery organization—the emergency unit, or department, of general hospitals. This familiar yet complex health care facility, which constitutes both the principal source of emergency care and a major source of nonemergency outpatient care in this country, has received little research attention as an organizational system. The present research focuses on the organization and effectiveness of hospital emergency units (EUs), using an open-system theory perspective and an extensive array of data from a scientific sample of thirty institutions and nearly 1,500 individuals (physicians, nurses, patients, administrators, and others) associated with them. It attempts to narrow the gap in our understanding of these organizations in at least two important ways: (1) by providing and testing a better methodology than heretofore available for assessing the effectiveness of hospital emergency services and ascertaining existing interinstitutional differences in effectiveness and (2) by making available some important new knowledge about the major organizational factors, both structural and social-psychological, which account for such differences.

Two different but carefully integrated sets of results are presented here: one about the concept, criteria, and measurement of effectiveness and differences in effectiveness among hospitals (Chapters Four through Eight), and the other about the organization of hospital EUs, and specifically the basic structural features and internal organizational problem solving of the system, and the relationship between organization and effectiveness (Chapters Three, Nine, and Ten). EU effectiveness was measured at the institutional level, using economic and clinical performance, or efficiency, as the primary criteria, and supplementing these with measures of promptness of medical attention (patient waiting time), patient satisfaction, staff satisfaction or "social efficiency," and other secondary criteria.

Obviously, this book is neither a text nor a practice manual. It is a scholarly and theory-based but problem-oriented research contribution. The book is addressed primarily to an academic audience—researchers, scholars, teachers, and graduate students in the fields of complex organizations, health services research, organizational psychology and sociology, medical care organization, and health care planning, management, and policy. At the same time, however, the research findings it discusses should be of considerable interest to practitioners in hospital and health services administration, emergency medicine, health care planning, and organization development, and to others who may be concerned with the problems and performance of our health services.

Practitioners who want to understand the organizational bases of effective performance by health service systems such as the hospital EU or learn what structural and social-psychological variables make a difference with regard to system performance should find the results useful and instructive. Graduate students wishing to learn how to design and conduct comparative organizational research should find the methodology, theory, and results of the study equally valuable. Social scientists and researchers will be especially interested in the rigorous methodology used for comparative organizational analysis, the integration of this methodology with open-system theory, and the new approaches used to assess effectiveness at the institutional level, particularly the quasitracer patient conditions approach (Chapter Five) and the patient visit staging approach (Chapter Six). Finally, all readers will probably find the results about the separate and combined effects of organizational structure and problem solving on the effectiveness of the system illuminating.

Organization of the Book

The first three chapters discuss the theoretical, methodological, and substantive foundations of the research. The next four chapters are devoted to the concept, criteria, and measurement of EU effectiveness, and the question of interinstitutional differences on the various criteria of effectiveness. The interrelationships found among the different criteria are discussed next, followed by the presentation of results about the relationships between organization structure variables and effectiveness and between organizational problem solving and effectiveness.

Discussed in Chapter One are the context, rationale, and conceptual-theoretical framework of the research. The research design, study sample, sources of data used and response rates attained, and related issues are considered in Chapter Two, which presents the general methodology of the study. (More specific aspects of method and procedure, including analytical and statistical issues, are discussed throughout the book in the appropriate chapters.) Substantive information about the organizations studied is presented in Chapter Three, which summarizes descriptive data and findings concerning some of the basic organizational characteristics of hospital EUs. These include staffing patterns and resources, institutional goal priorities, perceived weaknesses and strengths by organizational members and other relevant respondents, organizational structure characteristics, and the composition of patient inputs. This descriptive overview provides the reader with the necessary background for considering the research problem investigated—the relationship between the organization and effectiveness of hospital EUs—in proper empirical context.

The issues and difficulties encountered in assessing the effectiveness of hospital EUs at the institutional, or system, level are considered in Chapter Four. After the concept of effectiveness is defined and analyzed in relation to the organizational rationality of the system, various approaches to evaluating the quality of patient care, or clinical efficiency of the system, are reviewed. Then, the economic efficiency criterion is considered, followed by several secondary criteria of effectiveness.

The approach, data, and measures used to evaluate clinical efficiency are discussed in Chapter Five. This chapter describes in detail both the research procedures used, including the quasitracer patient conditions approach, and the measures and indices developed to assess the quality of medical and nursing care provided to patients at the EUs studied. Observed interinstitutional differences in the quality of medical and nursing care are also discussed in this chapter. Perhaps some readers, possibly among practitioners, will find part of the material in this chapter to be too technical. If so, they may wish to skip Chapter Six, which presents more technical details about the measures of patient care quality, and go to Chapter Seven, particularly if they are satisfied with the measures of quality discussed in Chapter Five.

Presented in Chapter Six is a rich array of detailed findings concerning the validation and validity of the quality of care indices. More specifically, these findings concern the relationships of the developed indices to such additional variables as promptness of medical attention, patient satisfaction, patient death rates, the appropriateness of clinical procedures and staff performance of particular care activities (along the patient management continuum), ratings of the quality of patient care by knowledgeable non-EU physicians and by selected community respondents, and certain other measures based on data from patient records reviewed ("audited") by two physician researchers. On theoretical as well as pragmatic grounds, these particular variables could be regarded as indicators of clinical efficiency in addition to the principal measures and indices discussed in Chapter Five.

The economic efficiency of hospital EUs, which constitutes another primary criterion of institutional effectiveness, is discussed in Chapter Seven, along with the observed interinstitutional differences in economic efficiency. Readers should note, incidentally, that the specific financial figures shown represent costs and charges at the time of data collection in the late 1970s and not current dollar figures, which would be much higher. The empirical relationships among all of the primary and secondary criteria of effectiveness examined in this research are shown in Chapter Eight.

One of the basic hypotheses of the study concerns the relationship between organizational structure and effectiveness. Aspects of the system's structure that were expected to account for a significant part of the difference in EU effectiveness across institutions are discussed in Chapter Nine. This chapter begins with a consideration of the significance of organizational structure to the effectiveness of organizations. Presented next is a brief empirical exploration of the likely significance to effectiveness of certain structural aspects of the system's environment, followed by the results testing the relationship between staff-linked aspects of EU organization (for example, medical staffing patterns) and EU effectiveness. Then, the hypothesized relationships between size and size-related aspects of EU organization and the various criteria of effectiveness are tested. The chapter concludes with a discussion of the combined and individual effects of selected structural variables on the clinical and economic efficiency of hospital EUs, and also on the secondary criteria of institutional effectiveness that were included in the research.

The second major hypothesis of the research—that concerning the relationship of organizational problem solving to effectiveness—is tested in Chapter Ten, in the form of a series of more specific hypotheses involving the adequacy or relative success of organizational problem solving in the areas of organizational strain, resource allocation, organizational coordination, integration, and organizational adaptation to the environment. The measures and indicators of problem solving in these important areas, and their interrelationships, are presented in this chapter, as are certain findings concerning the relationship between organizational structure and problem solving. The principal findings on the relationship between the adequacy of organizational problem solving and the effectiveness of hospital EUs are presented next. Then, results showing the relative importance and joint contribution of selected aspects of organizational problem solving to effectiveness are discussed. The chapter concludes with a consideration of the joint effects of organizational structure and problem solving on effectiveness.

The concluding chapter of the book, Chapter Eleven, briefly reviews some of the major findings, considers some of the scientific and practical implications of the results, and suggests directions for future organizational research. The three appendixes that follow Chapter Eleven discuss the underlying conceptual-theoretical framework of the research, the sample of organizations studied, and the characteristics of respondents and local populations involved.

Acknowledgments

The study of hospital emergency services on which this book is based, and for which I was the principal investigator, was supported by Research Grant Number 3 RO1 HS 02538 from the National Center for Health Services Research, U.S. Department of Health and Human Services. Initiated in the summer of 1976, the study proper was funded for a four-year period. The data were collected during this period. I am very thankful to the National Center for its financial support.

The research was conducted in the Organizational Behavior Program of the Survey Research Center, Institute for Social Research, under my direction. The project could not have been carried out, however, without the participation and services of a diligent research staff whose work efforts and contributions I value highly. Staff members who worked on the project in various capacities and for varying periods of time included Robert A. Cooke, associate research scientist; Barry A. Macy, assistant research scientist; and graduate student research assistants Linda M. Argote, Mark F. Peterson, Lorraine M. Uhlaner, and N. Eser Uzun (all four of the research assistants completed their doctoral dissertations using data from the project). In addition, Carl R. Goble and Pamela E. O'Connor were the project's computer specialists, and Cheryl J. Peck served as secretary and administrative assistant. It is with both thanks and friendship that I acknowledge the individual and collective participation of all these associates.

Several units of the Institute, including its personnel and data-processing facilities, and the Sampling Section, Field Section, and Coding Section of the Survey Research Center also provided important services to the project in the areas of their expertise.

Within the University of Michigan, the project also benefited from the advice of health economists Sylvester E. Berki and Paul J. Feldstein, concerning economic efficiency issues, and physicians Beverly C. Payne and Paul Y. Ertel, concerning medical care issues. I am very appreciative of their inputs.

I also want to thank Alvin H. Novak, W. Richard Scott, and Stephen M. Shortell. At my request, these colleagues from other universities reviewed the original research proposal, shortly after the project had been funded, and made a number of useful suggestions.

Early contacts informing relevant professional associations about the research, including the American College of Emergency Physicians, the American College of Surgeons, the American Medical Association, the Catholic Hospital Association, the American Osteopathic Hospital Association, and the American Hospital Association, also facilitated implementation of the project.

I am indebted to all of the above individuals and organizations for their support and contributions. They should all share part of the credit for the success of the project, while responsibility for any shortcomings must be mine. In addition, I want to thank Arnold Tannenbaum for his thoughtful comments on an earlier draft, Thomas D'Aunno and Richard Saavedra for reading and commenting on the manuscript, and Wendy Lanum for typing it. It is also important, but probably self-evident, to acknowledge that the research would not have been possible without the generous cooperation of the many hospitals, emergency departments, and individuals who provided the data. To all of them, I express my gratitude.

Finally, I wish to thank the *Annals of Emergency Medicine* for permission to use in this book Tables 9-2 and 9-4 and related material, *Emergency Medical Services* for permission to incorporate Figure 1-1 (as modified), and the Institute for Social Research for permission to use material included in Appendix A and Appendix C of the book.

Ann Arbor, Michigan   Basil S. Georgopoulos
March 1986

The Author

Basil S. Georgopoulos is a research scientist at the Institute for Social Research and professor of psychology at the University of Michigan. In recent years, he has also been chairman of the university's Doctoral Program in Organizational Psychology. He received his B.A. degree (1952), *magna cum laude,* in sociology and psychology from Bowling Green State University, his M.A. degree (1953) in sociology from the University of California at Los Angeles, and his Ph.D. degree (1957) in social psychology from the University of Michigan.

The author's main interests have been in the social psychology of complex organizations, in organizational psychology and open-system theory, and in comparative organizational analysis. At the Institute for Social Research, Georgopoulos has been directing a research program concerned with the organization, social-psychological problems, and performance of health service systems, particularly hospitals. He has written extensively in this area over the years, and his previous books include: *The Community General Hospital* (1962, with F. C. Mann), *Organization Research on Health Institutions* (1972), and *Hospital Organization Research: Review and Source Book* (1975). He has twice (in 1964 and in 1974) received the best book of the year award—the James A. Hamilton Hospital Administrators' Book Award—from the

American College of (Hospital Administrators) Healthcare Executives.

Georgopoulos has lectured at many institutions, professional meetings, and conferences and has served as consultant to various professional and academic organizations, government agencies, journals and publishers, and researchers. He is a member or fellow of a number of scientific and professional associations and has been listed in *American Men and Women of Science, Contemporary Authors,* and *Who's Who in America.*

Organizational Structure, Problem Solving, and Effectiveness

A Comparative Study of Hospital Emergency Services

Chapter One

Introduction and Overview

Occasionally, organizational researchers can study a sizable number of organizations simultaneously and at a relatively intensive level using the same approach and research design. They can use an explicit theoretical framework, or research model, and identical methods and procedures to investigate in considerable depth and detail some important substantive problem across organizations. In this volume, I discuss one such unusual study—a problem-oriented as well as theory-based study—and its principal findings. This is a comparative study of the organization and performance of emergency departments (often called "emergency rooms") in general hospitals. In this book, these health service organizations are referred to as hospital emergency units (EUs).

Thirty outpatient emergency care facilities and nearly 1,500 individuals associated with them provided data. The study was partly descriptive and partly analytical, or explanatory, relying heavily on quantitative data analysis. Its main purpose was to investigate the relationship between the organization of hospital EUs and their institutional performance or effectiveness. The underlying question was "What organizational factors and social-psychological conditions contribute to an efficient and effective emergency unit?" In addressing this question, the study made use of multiple sources of data and measurement procedures, including a new method—the "quasitracer patient conditions approach"—for evaluating the quality of patient care provided by the EUs studied.

The research had three specific objectives: (1) to describe and analyze the organization, structure, and problem-solving

1

practices of hospital EUs; (2) to assess the effectiveness of EUs at the institutional (or system) level in terms of several major criteria, and ascertain the nature and magnitude of differences in EU effectiveness among hospitals; and (3) to identify some of the major organizational and social-psychological sources and correlates of interinstitutional differences in effectiveness—that is, to study the relationship between EU organization and EU effectiveness. This book is primarily concerned with the second and third objectives; the first objective has been the subject of other publications (see, for example, Argote, 1979, 1982; D'Aunno, 1984; Georgopoulos, 1978; Georgopoulos, Cooke, and Associates, 1980; Peterson, 1979, 1985; Uhlaner, 1980; Uzun, 1980).

In this research, effectiveness was assessed at the institutional, or system, level in terms of both clinical and economic performance. It was evaluated with data from several different sources, so as to take into account a number of legitimate perspectives, using multiple criteria and methods of measurement. The primary criteria employed, respectively representing clinical performance and economic performance, were the EU's quality of patient care (clinical efficiency) and the costs of care (economic efficiency). Quality was evaluated separately for the care provided by the medical and nursing staff.

Each primary criterion was assessed using several different measures, which, after careful analysis of their methodological properties (including discriminability, reliability, and validity), were combined into a composite measure or index. Each index was then examined for methodological adequacy and validated against various specific measures that were expected (on substantive, theoretical, or methodological grounds) to correlate with the criterion being measured by the index.

The study also examined several secondary criteria: promptness of medical attention to incoming patients, patient satisfaction, staff satisfaction or "social efficiency," EU responsiveness to community needs and expectations, and institutional reputation. The different criteria of effectiveness were not necessarily expected to correlate highly, or even significantly, with one another in all cases; in fact, a supplemental purpose of the research was to ascertain the relationships among the various criteria.

Although the research focused on the above substantive objectives, it was also designed to increase our theoretical understanding of organizations by using an open-system theory model. This model views hospitals and hospital EUs as specialized service delivery systems that fit neither a "mechanistic" nor an "organic" view of organizations but, rather, a combination of the two. Theoretically, hospital EUs were viewed as complex work-performing and problem-solving systems that function partly on the basis of programmed activity, authority relations, and bureaucratic procedures and partly on the basis of professional autonomy and discretion, nonprogrammed communication and coordination, and voluntary staff adjustments. In short, they were viewed as *mechan-organic* systems.

It was assumed that, controlling for the nature of the external environment as it bears upon the resources and patient inputs of hospital EUs, the overall effectiveness of these systems would mainly depend on two basic aspects of their organization: (1) the nature of their organizational structure, including size-related aspects, medical staffing pattern, teaching affiliation, training programs, service complexity and specialization, the breadth or scope of service, and other structural variables; and (2) the adequacy of their internal problem solving in such key areas as organizational resources, coordination, strain, and integration. Therefore, different aspects of organizational structure and problem solving constituted the principal independent variables in the research while EU effectiveness was the dependent variable.

One general hypothesis of the study was that differences among EUs on each criterion of institutional effectiveness would be associated with corresponding differences in the organizational structure variables studied; that is, each of these independent variables would be found to affect, or at least correlate significantly with, either the clinical or the economic efficiency of hospital EUs. Further, it was hypothesized that differences among EUs on the major criteria of effectiveness would be significantly related to the adequacy of organizational problem solving within EUs.

Another goal of the study was to make available a considerable array of measures and corresponding organizational norms that depicted the distribution of the EUs studied on the variables measured (together with the research instruments developed and used to collect the data). Such norms (which were included in a special report of descriptive findings that was sent to the participating institutions in return for their cooperation*) could be used by individual EUs as empirical standards against which to compare and evaluate their own organizational performance. They could also serve as a useful data base for further research.

Achievement of the above objectives obviously required data from a considerable number of institutions and a research design relying on cross-hospital comparisons. The proper unit of description and analysis in this research, therefore, was the hospital EU as an organizational system. For this reason, the study sample consisted not of individuals but of organizations—the emergency departments of the thirty hospitals that participated in the research. A probability sample of general hospitals was selected randomly (using a "controlled selection technique") from a population of 436 such institutions that was stratified according to location, institutional control, and organizational size.

The data were obtained in several ways from several independent sources: (1) interviews and questionnaires completed by seven different groups of respondents associated with each institution, including EU nurses and physicians, top administrators and selected key physicians from the parent hospital, a group of recent patients, and certain individuals from the community; (2) organizational and administrative records from each institution containing information about financial, staffing, and patient characteristics; (3) the emergency-visit medical records of recent patients, who also completed a mailed questionnaire shortly after visiting the EU; and (4) certain supplementary sources, such as the American Hospital Association's annual *Guide to the Health Care Field* and U.S. Census reports. Most of the required data were obtained from the first two of these sources. The study sample,

*The results presented in this report were subsequently incorporated into a more extensive report of the descriptive findings of the study (Georgopoulos, Cooke, and Associates, 1980), which also included the research instruments developed to collect the data.

respondents, and data collection instruments are discussed in detail in Chapter Two.

Research Context and Rationale

The empirical data base about the organization and effectiveness of the dominant source of emergency (and much nonemergency) care in this country—the hospital EU—is still in a primitive state. Although many of the operating problems experienced by hospital EUs are widely appreciated from a practical standpoint, they are inadequately understood in terms of their causes and correlates and even more poorly understood in terms of their interrelationships and likely solution requirements.

Particularly lacking is dependable knowledge about the organizational and social-psychological factors that facilitate or hinder the effectiveness of hospital EUs in its major aspects— quality of care, economic efficiency, and other desirable outcomes, such as patient and staff satisfaction. Also lacking is knowledge about the cross-hospital differences in EU effectiveness. For the most part, the magnitude, sources, and determinants of such important differences remain unknown, partly because of the paucity of studies assessing EU effectiveness at the institutional/ system level and partly because of the paucity of comparative organizational research in the more general field of emergency medical services.

With few exceptions, the research literature has little to offer on EU organization and effectiveness; this applies not only to the quantity and quality of available findings but also to the state of associated methodology. Not long ago, for example, Gibson and his associates (Gibson, 1976, 1977; Gibson, Pickar, and Wagner, 1977) reviewed the problems of evaluating emergency medical systems. They described many research deficiencies and the need to develop methodology, improve measurement capabilities, and achieve conceptual progress. They also discussed the problems of "categorization" and specialization of emergency medical systems.

Similarly, when the present research was undertaken, the literature contained only a handful of comparative organizational studies of hospital EUs—those by Lawrence (1969), Gibson,

Bugbee, and Anderson (1970), and Gunter and Ricci (1974). None of these investigations, however, focused on organizational effectiveness or on the analysis of differences in clinical performance and economic efficiency among EUs.

Generally, research in the emergency medical services field has concentrated on four principal concerns: (1) the demography of users and related utilization trends in hospital EUs (see, for example, Weinerman and Edwards, 1964; Alpert and others, 1969; Stoddard, 1969; Roth, 1971); (2) the level of "severity" or "urgency" of condition of EU patients, usually examined in conjunction with utilization questions and at the individual patient level (see, for example, Lavenhar and others, 1968; Robinson and others, 1969; Richardson, 1970); (3) financial considerations, especially ambulatory care costs, again mainly in relation to utilization issues (for example, see Richardson, 1970; Lave and Leinhardt, 1972; L. Lave, 1973); and (4) case studies of certain other aspects, such as clinical decision making for some types of patient problems (for example, myocardial infarctions or burns), medical protocols or "algorithms" for particular diagnoses, such as lacerations or chest pain (see, for example, Frazier and Brand, 1979; Greenfield and others, 1981), and individual performance by selected personnel (for example, emergency medical technicians) in some institutions—usually one or two hospitals at a time. (For illustrative studies, see *Emergency Medical Services Research Methodology Workshop 2*, Research Proceedings Series, National Center for Health Services Research, 1979; and *Emergency Medical Services Systems Research Project Abstracts, 1979*, Research Management Series, National Center for Health Services Research, 1980.)

Some attention has also been given to staffing needs and trends, but the research to date has not investigated rigorously, or even systematically, the complex problems of EU organization and effectiveness in a substantial number of institutions simultaneously. In the absence of such comparative organizational analysis, progress in this area has been understandably slow, despite the fact that the familiar hospital EU is not only socially important as a health care facility but is also highly interesting from an organization theory standpoint. The EU is both a vital component of our contemporary health services system and a challenging type of organization to analyze and understand.

Though relatively small in size, organizationally the hospital EU constitutes one of the most complex and most problematic departments of a hospital. It is one of the hospital's major care-delivery units and a semiautonomous organizational entity which, in order to do its work, must be able to deal with a variety of difficult problems—internally, in relation to the parent hospital, and even in relation to the external environment. These include problems of input and output, as well as problems associated with internal structure and process. Moreover, in order to carry out its patient care functions, the EU must use a highly specialized, intensive work technology, much of which is under the control of other hospital services and departments. In terms of the scope and complexity of its functions, which also require staff readiness for prompt response to the health problems of individual patients under conditions of relatively high uncertainty, the emergency department could well be regarded as a mini-hospital or a microcosm of its parent hospital.

Compared to other outpatient services and most of the inpatient care units of a hospital, the EU is a unique and complex system. First, it handles a significant portion of the parent hospital's work; for example, the present study found that for each inpatient admission to a hospital there were 2.4 patient visits to its EU. In the process, the EU must deal directly not only with the rest of the hospital but also with the external environment (various health care organizations, community agencies, and patients from the community). In other words, the EU is an adaptive as well as a production "subsystem" of the hospital, with the responsibility to perform a dual set of organizational functions and meet requirements associated with both. (For a discussion of the characteristics of these and other subsystems of organizations, see Katz and Kahn, 1966, 1978.)

Second, the EU must provide individualized care services on a twenty-four-hour basis while simultaneously processing a workflow that is highly variable and involves both a great deal of uncertainty in patient inputs and rapid patient turnover. In addition, an EU must rely heavily on the timely cooperation, services, and support of other clinical, ancillary, and administrative departments, and at the same time "compete" with these other units for needed resources from the parent hospital.

Unlike these other units, however, EUs are like hospitals within hospitals, for they are called upon to treat a large number of patients who present a great diversity of medical problems. Further, their patients typically require immediate action, or at least rapid response, by those who do the work. EU cases may not all be acute or true emergencies, but they are generally nonuniform and unpredictable (at least in the short run and at the individual hospital level). Moreover, the work cycle in these care facilities is unusually short, for EU patients "turn over" very rapidly, within a matter of hours if not faster. In such a work setting, the performers must continually deal with uncertainty, tolerate ambiguity while being intolerant of error, and be prepared to act promptly and properly in both planned and spontaneous ways.

The staff of hospital EUs, which includes a variety of professional workers often augmented by "on-call" medical specialists from the parent hospital, as well as technicians and clerical and administrative personnel, may also be organizationally unstable, adding to the complexity and difficulties that apparently characterize EUs as organizational systems. The medical staffing patterns of EUs, for example, vary from having individual physicians on contract (in some cases only on a part-time basis), through rotating staff arrangements, to non-hospital-based group practices. Frequently, a hospital has little or no direct control over the medical staff of its emergency unit. The nursing staff, on the other hand, is typically provided by the parent hospital and is under direct control of the hospital's nursing department. Nevertheless, at times there is considerable turnover in many EUs among their clinical staff.

Finally, the autonomy of an EU within the hospital is limited, not only in terms of organizational accountability but also in terms of dependence. An EU must rely on its parent hospital for many of its human resources, including nonmedical personnel, and for its physical plant and equipment. Accordingly, in carrying out its functions, an EU must observe not only constraints imposed by the nature of its work but also constraints imposed by the parent hospital and even by conditions in the external environment or by the larger health services system. (Additional characteristics of the organizational situation of hospital EUs are considered in Chapter Three, which summarizes a variety of descriptive data from the present study.)

For these and other reasons, a hospital EU must have an unusually flexible internal organization. Obviously, it cannot be highly bureaucratized because it is staffed by professionals who require a certain amount of autonomy and freedom to exercise professional discretion and judgment; yet it must follow the policies and rules of its parent institution and be accountable to it. In addition, it must adhere to particular treatment protocols and maintain acceptable professional standards in carrying out its clinical activities and procedures. For effective performance, both organizational order and flexibility seem to be required, along with professional discipline and a high level of cooperation and voluntary adjustment among the staff.

To understand the organization and effectiveness of hospital EUs, therefore, one must carefully study and analyze the above problems. In general, there is need for high-quality organizational research that focuses on these and other important problems and issues. Particularly desirable are theoretically grounded and methodologically rigorous studies that focus on a number of institutions simultaneously. (See, for example, Flood, Scott, Ewy, and Forrest, 1982; Georgopoulos and Mann, 1962; Forrest, Scott, and Brown, 1976.) In principle, such investigations are capable of going well beyond single case studies and addressing these problems on a scale commensurate with their magnitude and complexity. Comparative designs such as the one used in the present research, therefore, would seem especially promising to develop and implement, particularly when coupled with explicit theoretical frameworks and carefully specified research models.

Conceptual-Theoretical Considerations: The Research Model

Available organization theory is not too enlightening, either as a guide to organizing and managing systems such as the hospital EU in ways that would facilitate problem solving and promote organizational effectiveness, or as a means for explaining differences in staff attitudes and actions in relation to effectiveness. Neither the so-called organic models, with their emphasis on participative decision making and supportive human relations in the work setting, nor the mechanistic models of organizations, with their emphasis on job prescriptions, bureaucratic rules, and centralized-hierarchical control, seem to fit the case of the hospital EU, which is a mechan-organic system. A more adequate theoretical model and a better empirical data base than heretofore available must be developed in order to understand the relationship between EU organization and EU effectiveness. The present research was designed and carried out with both of these goals in mind.

The conceptual-theoretical framework of this study draws heavily on the organizational research model developed by the author in previous hospital studies (see, especially, Georgopoulos, 1972, 1975; Georgopoulos and Mann, 1962; Georgopoulos and Matejko, 1967) and is more fully described in Appendix A and earlier publications (Georgopoulos, 1978; Georgopoulos and Cooke, 1979). Conceptually, in this framework, hospitals and hospital EUs are viewed as complex work-performing and problem-solving systems that are rationally structured and organized to provide certain medical and nursing services to the public. Theoretically and analytically, the hospital EU is treated as a specialized organizational system, while the parent hospital is viewed as the relevant suprasystem. Structurally and functionally, however, the EU is neither a free-standing system nor a self-contained organization.

Empirically, and from the standpoint of organizational operation, the EU functions as a major *sub*system of the hospital. As such, the EU shares with its parent organization certain structural characteristics and depends upon the hospital for a variety of resources, services, and supports, as well as for its maintenance and survival as an organization; conversely, the hospital also depends on the EU—for patients, for meeting legal obligations, and for adaptation to the environment (D'Aunno, 1984). The EU is also interdependent with other hospital subsystems, with which it both competes for resources and cooperates in providing services to patients. Accordingly, the organization and effectiveness of hospital EUs cannot be fully understood without some knowledge of the larger organizational context within which they function, especially knowledge of their linkages to the hospital and relationships with other hospital subsystems. The major independent variables on which the study focuses— organizational structure and organizational problem solving— were chosen with these considerations in mind. (For more detailed discussion, see Chapters Nine and Ten.)

Organizational Effectiveness

In a generic sense, organizational effectiveness* concerns the ability of the system to achieve and maintain high levels of output (in the form of a product, service, or information, or some combination of these) in terms of quantity, quality, cost, acceptability, and related criteria (not all of which are positively interrelated), given the human and nonhuman resources at its disposal (Georgopoulos, 1972, 1975, 1978). Generally, it involves (1) the achievement of efficient and reliable performance by organizational units, groups (staffs), and members at all levels, without undue strain for the participants or dissipation of the system's resources, and (2) the provision of adequate solutions to certain enduring problems of the system, including the problems of adaptation to the environment, resource allocation, internal strain, coordination of efforts, and social-psychological integration.

The accomplishment of these outcomes implies successful social as well as technical performance, which, in turn, depends

*For useful discussions and critiques of this concept, as used in organizational research in various settings, see Becker and Neuhauser (1975); Cameron and Whetten (1983); Etzioni (1964); Evan (1976); Georgopoulos (1972, 1975); Georgopoulos and Mann (1962); Georgopoulos and Matejko (1967); Georgopoulos and Tannenbaum (1957); Ghorpade (1971); Goodman, Pennings, and Associates (1977); Johnson (1981); Kanter (1981); Katz and Kahn (1966, 1978); Mott (1972); Neuhauser (1971); Perrow (1972); Pickle and Friedlander (1967); Price (1968, 1972); Scott and Shortell (1983); Seashore (1983); Shortell and Kaluzny (1983); Steers (1975, 1976); Yuchtman and Seashore (1967); Zey-Ferrell (1979).

upon the organization's providing opportunities for its members to participate meaningfully in the decision-making processes of the system and to satisfy individual needs. In the specific case of hospitals and hospital EUs, organizational effectiveness can be viewed as the joint (though not equally weighted) outcome of three essential but very different kinds of efficiency—clinical, economic, and social. Roughly, these correspond to the quality of patient care, the quantity of services provided at a given cost, and the quality of working life in the organization.

Clinical efficiency, which may be defined in terms of the quality of medical and nursing inputs and patient care outputs of the system, reflects the clinical performance of the system, that is, the performance of physicians, nurses, and others who carry out the patient care activities. It requires and depends upon the achievement of clinical rationality. *Economic efficiency,* which may be defined in terms of the financial investments or inputs of the system and the costs of services provided, reflects the economic performance, or productivity, of the system. It depends on and requires the achievement of economic rationality. *Social efficiency,* which may be defined in terms of the personal, or social-psychological, investment of participants and the satisfaction of their individual needs through membership and work in the system, reflects the social or social-psychological performance of the system and depends on the achievement of social rationality.

Briefly, then, EU effectiveness is a joint function (or outcome) of clinical, economic, and social efficiency. The levels of these three kinds of efficiency, in turn, depend upon the following distinct but interrelated classes of key variables: (1) organizational rationality; (2) the structural arrangements of the system, that is, organization structure variables; and (3) organizational problem solving in certain critical areas, particularly adaptation to the environment and coordination of internal efforts. For the most part, according to the research model employed, it is differences in these three major aspects of organization that determine both the level of institutional effectiveness for a hospital EU and interinstitutional differences in EU effectiveness. The concept of effectiveness is further elaborated in Chapter Four.

Organizational Rationality

Hospital EUs, like other complex organizations, are purposeful associations of people that are more or less rationally designed to perform particular tasks and to pursue specific types of goals, such as high-quality patient care at reasonable cost, through collaborative activity and concerted effort. They are work-performing and problem-solving systems, organized so as to perform special functions and achieve particular objectives. Rationality is critical to the functioning and effectiveness of such systems.

Organizational rationality represents the extent to which decisions in the system are made on the basis of available knowledge about cause-and-effect relationships and on the basis of means-ends considerations that are likely to promote particular outcomes. Other things being equal, the higher the rationality, the greater the congruence between decisions and actions, the greater the predictability of outcomes, and the greater the chances for successful problem solving and organizational effectiveness.

Hospitals, however, face many obstacles and difficulties as they strive toward greater rationality (see Georgopoulos, 1982). Unlike industrial or manufacturing organizations, for example, hospitals and hospital EUs are constantly faced with the problem of balancing and integrating the three very different components of organizational rationality—clinical, economic, and social rationality. Clinical rationality is based on professional-technical knowledge, mainly specialized biomedical knowledge; economic rationality is based on knowledge of economics, marketing, finance, and the like; and social rationality is mostly based on knowledge from the social and behavioral sciences, especially psychology and sociology, and the humanities.

The main objective of clinical rationality is to generate and implement decisions that will meet the clinical needs of patients, as defined by the doctors, or facilitate professional-clinical performance and high performance standards—that is, to achieve clinical efficiency, regardless of the financial costs involved. Economic rationality, on the other hand, is mainly concerned with decisions and controls that are likely to minimize costs, that is, with the achievement of economic efficiency, in both clinical and nonclinical areas. Thus, while clinical rationality may promote the quality of patient care, it may interfere with economic efficiency, and economic rationality may promote economic efficiency but interfere with clinical efficiency. The picture becomes further complicated with the addition of social rationality, which is mainly concerned with decisions that are likely to promote the social-psychological well-being and the quality of work life of organizational members, such as the physicians, nurses, and administrators who make the decisions in this system. Such decisions may promote social efficiency but are not always compatible with the requirements of clinical or economic efficiency.

Because of differences in the knowledge base associated with the three components of rationality, differences in the objectives that are emphasized by each, and differences in the professional orientations and values of the decision makers (physicians, administrators, nurses, trustees, and so on), it is extremely difficult for a hospital or hospital EU to integrate fully the three components or take them all properly into account when formulating goals, setting priorities, or solving problems. Basically, the three components of rationality and the three kinds of efficiency that they promote cannot be simultaneously maximized by the system. Nor can efficiency in one area significantly compensate for (or substitute for) deficiency in another on a long-term basis. The relationship of organizational rationality to effectiveness is further discussed in Chapter Four (see also Georgopoulos, 1982).

Organizational Structure

In the generic sense, organizational structure refers to the relatively stable arrangement of the component parts that make up an organization. The components may be either concrete or abstract (for example, either persons and organizational members or organizational roles and positions). Moreover, an organization encompasses not one but a variety of structures. The following discussion will focus only on the theoretical significance of organizational structure; the concept of organizational structure adopted in this research and the specific structural variables studied are discussed in greater detail in Chapter Nine.

According to the research model employed in this study, the major organizational structures of hospital EUs (including the role and task structure, the control and authority structure, the communication and coordination structure, and the normative structure) constitute the basic problem-solving framework of the system. In a sense, they constitute the system's multipurpose problem-solving apparatus. The nature of these and other structures is determined in large part by the character and qualifications of the system's components (for example, its staff), the organization of the parent hospital and the nature of the work to be done, and such basic system properties as those of differentiation, interdependence, patterning, and continuity (see Appendix A; Georgopoulos, 1972; Georgopoulos and Cooke, 1979). Whatever their specific determinants, existing structures serve as the primary base for organizational problem solving, the base on which the various organizational members and groups can rely to perform their assigned roles and tasks and to solve related work problems. Thus, structures promote operational continuity and predictability of behavior on a system-wide basis.

The same structures provide the participants with a framework for elaborating existing performance programs and for initiating or developing new ones for the solution of system problems and the attainment of system objectives. In addition, they facilitate selecting among available means and mechanisms of problem solving those that are appropriate for dealing with the specific problems and are consistent with the character of the system. In short, the system's basic structures enable an EU to maintain organizational continuity and regulate the behavior of members, to control task performance, and to solve work problems on an organization-wide basis. Structure variables, therefore, are expected to affect both problem solving and the effectiveness of the system.

Structure and Problem Solving. Generally, system problems can be approached in terms of either programmed or nonprogrammed solutions (March and Simon, 1958; Georgopoulos and Mann, 1962). Programmed solutions are normally based on existing organizational structures and programs that specify the appropriate means for action or both the means and ends of action; they normally rely on existing rules, regulations, and procedures that are dictated by the formal structures of the system. Nonprogrammed solutions are generally associated with performance programs that usually specify the objectives to be achieved but not the particular means of action; they are generally left to the professional judgment and discretion of the performers (physicians and nurses, for example, in the case of the EU). Nonprogrammed solutions also require a great deal of informal communication, coordination, and feedback, and frequent and spontaneous adjustments among the participants.

The specific types of problem solving that are appropriate in a given situation also relate to the system's structures and performance programs. Corrective and regulatory problem solving, for example, are the likely types when both the objectives and means of organizational performance are specified. In contrast to these mainly mechanical or computational types of problem solving, only nonprogrammed problem solving of the preventive or promotive type is possible (apart from trial-and-error behavior or by-default solutions) when both means and objectives are unspecified or uncertain.

In effect, the programmed mode and corrective and regulatory types of problem solving are more prevalent in bureaucratic organizations and mechanistic systems, in which structures (particularly the role and authority structures) are well specified and prescribed in detail. The nonprogrammed mode and preventive and promotive types of problem solving, on the other hand, are relatively more prevalent in organic systems and organizations, where basic structures are more flexible and less fully prescribed (for example, in professional organizations, which tend to rely a great deal on member participation in both decision making and problem solving). Hospital EUs appear to be a hybrid case, a mixture of mechanistic and organic systems.

The picture is even more complicated, however, because of the structural inconsistencies that characterize social systems. The basic organizational structures involved, all of which have both formal and informal components, are juxtaposed and coexist in the system, but they are not necessarily well coordinated or mutually supportive and reinforcing. At best, they are only partially matched and imperfectly integrated. Therefore, associated inconsistencies, which are fairly common both within and between organizational structures, often constrain the solution of work problems and depress the performance potential of the system, while also generating strain for the system and the participants.

At any rate, organization structure variables, such as those examined in the present study, have direct and important implications for organizational problem solving at institutions such as hospital EUs and thus for the overall effectiveness of these organizational systems—the subject of the present study. Organizational structure and problem solving, in short, are both expected to affect institutional effectiveness: Differences in the effectiveness of hospital EUs are expected to relate significantly and systematically to corresponding differences in their organizational structures and internal problem solving. In other words, a substantial portion of the observed interinstitutional variability in the clinical and economic efficiency of hospital EUs can be accounted for by interinstitutional differences in the structural and problem-solving variables studied.

Organizational Problem Solving

Hospitals and hospital EUs, like other complex organizations, may be viewed as work-performing and problem-solving systems. From this perspective, their organizational effectiveness depends on the ability of the system to provide adequate solutions to certain major problems. These problems are encountered all along the input-transformation-output work cycle of the system and include problems of input and output, problems of internal structure and process, and even external affairs problems. The problems relate to the basic properties of the system, to each other, and to the effectiveness with which the system accomplishes its work and objectives (see Appendix A; Georgopoulos, 1972; Georgopoulos and Cooke, 1979).

The significance of problem solving for system effectiveness has been recognized in the literature on organizations and other social systems, beginning with the work of Parsons and his associates (for example, see Parsons, Bales, and Shils, 1953). Parsons proposed and discussed four major "functional problems" that are encountered by all social systems—adaptation to the environment, internal integration, tension management, and goal attainment. Bales (1953) analyzed the performance of groups in terms of these same system problems. Bakke (1959) similarly viewed organizations as problem-solving entities. Thompson (1967), following the distinction initially made by Parsons (1958), discussed the problems of organizations at three levels of decision making: (1) the institutional (concerned with problems of adaptation), (2) the technical (concerned mainly with problems associated with the "core" or "production" activities of the system), and (3) the managerial (concerned with problems of control, resource allocation, and conflict resolution). Similarly, contemporary open-system theorists Katz and Kahn (1966, 1978) have distinguished a number of specialized organization "subsystems" (including the managerial, production, maintenance, and adaptive subsystems) whose main functions correspond to the basic system problems considered by Parsons, Bakke, and Thompson.

Research on organizational problem solving has increased considerably since the early work of Parsons. Over the past twenty years, for example, the author of this book and his associates have systematically developed and refined this perspective, both conceptually and theoretically. This work has evolved into the development of a carefully specified organizational research model or conceptual-theoretical framework for organizational analysis (see Appendix A; Georgopoulos, 1972, 1975, 1978; Georgopoulos and Cooke, 1979). In the process, the resulting model, which views organizations as complex work-performing and problem-solving systems, has also been "tested" in considerable empirical research (see, for example, Argote, 1982; Cheng, 1977; Cooke and Rousseau, 1981; D'Aunno, 1984; Georgopoulos, 1975; Georgopoulos and Mann, 1962; Georgopoulos and Matejko, 1967; Georgopoulos and Wieland, 1964; Longest, 1974; Perkins, 1983; Peterson, 1985; Sutton and Ford, 1982). The findings of these studies have in turn contributed to the refinement of the model. The present study is now added to these efforts.

According to the research model employed, a hospital EU is a complex organizational system that must be able to "solve" certain basic system problems in order to do its work. These generic problems, common to all organizations, are related to the system properties of organizations as well as to one another (see Appendix A). They are major ongoing and multifaceted problems that are not amenable to permanent or complete solution. In dealing with these open-ended problems, an organization can be more or less successful but not completely successful. It can provide only imperfect solutions, that is, solutions that are partial or temporary, or both. Further, the adequacy of solutions may vary a great deal from organization to organization and from one time to another, as well as from one problem to another. In large measure, however, organizational effectiveness depends on the system's ability to provide satisfactory solutions to these important problems, taking the particular problems into account not only individually but also as a set, because of the pervasive structural and functional interdependence that characterizes the system. (In turn, the ability of the system to do so mainly depends upon the structures and resources of the system, especially its human resources, and on environmental conditions.)

More specifically, the institutional effectiveness of hospital EUs, which is viewed as a joint outcome of clinical, economic, and social efficiency, depends on the ability of the system to:

1. Preserve its integrity and continuity; that is, ensure structural stability and orderly behavior patterns, consistent with its norms and values and with the functional interdependence of work participants, while also retaining sufficient flexibility to cope with unanticipated uncertainty and complexity—the problem of *system maintenance* (see also Georgopoulos, 1975, p. 130).

2. Deploy and properly allocate the human and other resources (including available staff, funds, information, technology) that it possesses, or acquires, and uses to accomplish its objectives—the problem of *organizational allocation* (see also Georgopoulos, 1975, p. 144).

3. Link and functionally articulate the diverse yet interdependent activities of the staff so that they converge toward the solution of work problems and the attainment of system objectives, and so that the participants act in concert as they carry out their respective roles—the problem of *organizational coordination* (see also Georgopoulos, 1975, p. 163).

4. Maximize congruence between member expectations and organizational objectives, promote internalization of the system's norms and values, ensure member involvement, cooperation, and compliance with system requirements, and facilitate mutual understanding and adjustment among its various groups and members—the problem of social-psychological *integration* (see also Georgopoulos, 1975, p. 163).

5. Deal with the tensions and strain that arise from inadequate solutions to the other problems, and also from system errors and ambiguities, from inconsistencies among existing structures, and from deficient role performance—the problem of *organizational strain* (see also Georgopoulos, 1975, p. 144).

6. Engage in satisfactory relationships and exchange with the external environment within which it operates; for example, by responding promptly and successfully to relevant exogenous pressures or changes (especially to environmental uncertainty and instability), not only reactively through internal adjustments but also proactively by continually acting to influence the environment in ways that are advantageous to the system and its purposes—the problem of *organizational adaptation* (see also Georgopoulos, 1975, p. 130).

Obviously, these are complex and multifaceted problems. Moreover, these problems have their origins in the basic properties of the system (for example, the properties of internal differentiation, interdependence, patterning, continuity, equifinality), the nature of the work to be done, and the characteristics and qualifications of the performers (see Georgopoulos, 1972; Georgopoulos and Cooke, 1979). As a consequence, their resolution is critical to the functioning and well-being of the system. The different problems are all interrelated, of course, both at the point of their origin and at the point of their resolution, but not in a simple manner (see Appendix A). Generally, in terms of the adequacy or relative success of problem solving, their interrelationships are likely to be positive and mutually reinforcing, at least in the long run. It is also true, however, that resolutions of one type of problem can either facilitate or hinder resolutions of another type of problem, at least in the short run. For example, resolution of the coordination problem may lead to the reduction of strain; on the other hand, in its efforts to resolve the adaptation problem the system could generate internal strain at the same time.*

Of the problems listed above, system maintenance is basically a long-term problem that presupposes satisfactory solutions on a continuing basis to all of the other problems (the result of failure, in this connection, would be dissolution, transformation, or major restructuring of the system). For this reason, the problem of system maintenance was not examined empirically in the present study. The other five problems, however, received a good deal of attention in terms of the system's problem-solving performance and of the relationship of problem solving to institutional effectiveness (see Chapter Ten).†

Summary

Hospital EUs function under a variety of requirements and constraints imposed by the nature of their task and work inputs, their relations with the parent hospitals, and the character of the

---

*For a more extensive discussion concerning the relationships of the various problems to one another and to certain system properties, and the consequences of problem solving for the structures, properties, and effectiveness of the system, see Appendix A; Georgopoulos, 1972; Georgopoulos and Cooke, 1979; Georgopoulos and Matejko, 1967; Katz and Georgopoulos, 1971.

†Certain results from various analyses involving the different problem areas have been reported elsewhere (see Argote, 1982; D'Aunno, 1984; Peterson, 1985; Uhlaner, 1980; Uzun, 1980). The main findings of the study concerning the relationship between EU organization (that is, organizational structure and problem solving) and EU effectiveness, however, are discussed in the present volume.

external environment. The nature of the task, for example, requires certain levels of technical and professional skills and work arrangements without which the objectives of the system could not be attained. The complexity of the task, the specialization of services to be offered, and the diversity, severity, and uncertainty of patient condition pose difficult performance requirements and constraints on the work participants. In addition, the limited organizational autonomy of EUs and their dependence on the parent hospitals for certain resources entail institutional constraints and organizational problem-solving requirements (some of which relate to accountability and control and to the nature of exchange between the EU and the hospital) that affect the behavior of the staff and the performance of the system.

The external environment and community may also affect the work and problems of the system in terms of such elements as the composition of the patient population, interaction with health care agencies or regulatory bodies, and interinstitutional arrangements for the provision of emergency medical services.

According to the research model employed, the institutional effectiveness of hospital EUs is a joint outcome of the clinical, economic, and social efficiency of the system—an outcome that mainly depends upon the organization of EUs, and especially upon the structural and problem-solving aspects of the system. In theory, controlling for the nature of the environment (for example, community and population characteristics) as it bears upon the resources and patient inputs of hospital EUs, institutional differences in EU effectiveness (the dependent variable) should be associated with differences in such independent variables as: organizational size and complexity; medical staffing pattern; staff skills and resources in relation to workload; organizational and staff specialization; the institution's definition or scope of "emergency service"; the nature of relationships between the EU and its parent hospital (for example, the cooperation and support provided by other relevant units); and especially the organization's problem-solving practices, particularly its success in dealing with the basic problems of organizational coordination and control, resource allocation, staff integration and involvement, intraorganizational strain, and organizational adaptation or external affairs.

Figure 1-1. Suggested Relationship Patterns Between Organizational Structure and Problem Solving and the Effectiveness of Hospital EUs.

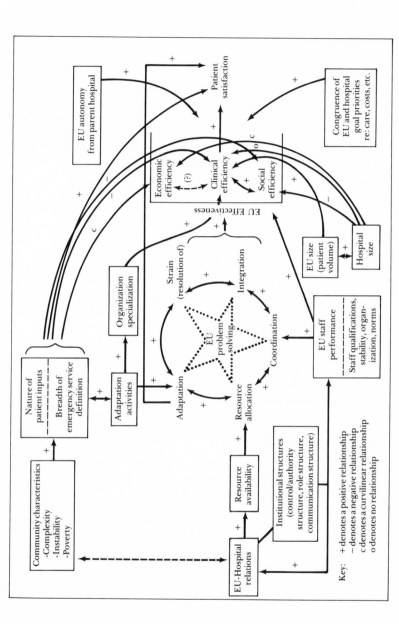

Source: Adapted, with minor revisions, and used with permission, from "An Open-System Approach to Evaluating the Effectiveness of Hospital Emergency Departments" by Basil S. Georgopoulos, *Emergency Medical Services,* 7 (6), Nov./Dec. 1978.

Data were therefore obtained to measure a number of these important independent variables as well as to assess EU effectiveness at the institutional level, and then ascertain the relationship between organization and effectiveness. Figure 1-1 depicts the kinds of relationships that are considered important by the research model employed; those examined empirically in this research are discussed mainly in Chapters Eight, Nine, and Ten.

Chapter Two

Research Methodology: General Considerations

Before discussing the assessment of emergency unit effectiveness or any of the specific measures used, pertinent aspects of the study's overall methodology will be considered. These include (1) important features of the research design, (2) the study sample, (3) sources of data and respondents, and (4) certain aspects of statistical treatment. The methods and procedures used to measure economic efficiency and the quality of patient care, or clinical efficiency, at the EU level are discussed in subsequent chapters.

Important Features of the Research Design

First, as will become apparent from examining its sample, measures, and analysis design, this organizational inquiry focuses on the structure, functioning, and output of hospital EUs rather than on the behavior of any particular group or individuals associated with them. It is a comparative study at the system level, in which the main unit of analysis is the hospital EU as an organizational or institutional entity. Among other things, the research seeks to ascertain interinstitutional differences in EU effectiveness, using both clinical and economic performance as primary criteria, and to determine some of the major sources and correlates of such differences. The achievement of these objectives requires analyses in which a substantial number of EUs are carefully compared and contrasted on characteristics, variables, and relationships that are measured at the system level. In short, this is a *comparative organizational study* of hospital emergency units.

The variables of research interest were selected for their relevance and anticipated importance, both on pragmatic grounds and on the basis of organization theory considerations.* In this regard, a particular conceptual-theoretical framework that views organizations as work-performing and problem-solving systems (see Georgopoulos, 1972, 1975; Georgopoulos and Cooke, 1979) and an identical research methodology were explicitly employed to study the thirty participating EUs. In addition to being a *theory-based* study, and unlike most survey-type organizational investigations, this research aimed at analytical depth approaching that of field-type studies which encompass considerably fewer organizations than it does. In other words, it was also designed as an *intensive* comparative study.

Within the broad class of comparative organizational investigations, the study employs what Przeworski and Teune (1970) call a "most similar systems" design because it deals with one type of system—emergency units (which, as organizations, are alike in many of their major characteristics) operated by community general hospitals. In fact, the study sample was drawn from an even more "restricted" subpopulation of such hospitals.

Deliberate restriction of a natural population/universe, which assumes that substantial variability in the phenomena of research interest will still be found in the obtained sample, is enormously useful when the population is expected to show so much variance that a prohibitively large sample would be required to yield statistical estimates within acceptable levels of confidence. In such circumstances, definitional restriction based on such

---

*For a discussion of the importance of organization theory in the health care institutions field, along with a summary of major organizational variables investigated in nineteen comparative studies of hospitals, see Shortell (1976). For a review of organization research in the same field during the 1960s, which includes propositional (or theory-based) and comparative as well as noncomparative studies, see Georgopoulos (1975). More recent contributions may be found in Shortell and Kaluzny (1983). For a number of organization theory applications in comparative organizational (including international) studies in other fields, see Lammers and Hickson (1979).

characteristics as organizational size and location makes the use of sampling more manageable and economical than would be the case when dealing with the corresponding unrestricted and, therefore, larger and more heterogeneous population. It makes for a relatively "efficient" sample design, while also reducing the range of extraneous variables to permit more rigorous investigation of those variables and relationships in which the research is interested.

Lastly, as in all comparative organizational studies, the research design required that the measures used in the analysis be comparable across sampling units (see Przeworski and Teune, 1970), in this case across hospital EUs. Intentionally and systematically, therefore, the variables of interest, and especially the criterion variables, were defined and operationalized so as to yield measures of high comparability from one EU to another. The principle followed was that, to the greatest extent possible, the measures should have both "validity" *within* each EU (have equivalent meaning to each institution in the sample) and "reliability" *across* EUs (apply consistently across sampling units). In short, the measures should be equally appropriate to all institutions in the sample.

The Study Sample

The research was designed to compare and contrast, in a methodologically rigorous manner, a cross-sectional sample of hospital EUs in order to ascertain the relationship between EU organization and EU effectiveness. Therefore, the sample consisted not of individuals but of institutions, namely the emergency units (departments) of thirty community general hospitals. Technically, it was a stratified random sample of organizations selected with equal probability and without replacement (of hospitals unable to participate), using a "controlled selection" technique.

Particular institutions were selected to represent the nongovernment, not-for-profit, short-stay general hospitals located in the states of Illinois, Indiana, Michigan, Minnesota, Ohio, and Wisconsin, that is, in Health and Human Services (HHS) Region V, formerly Health, Education, and Welfare (HEW) Region V.

Hospitals whose size fell outside the 100–499 beds range, and a few institutions that did not have an emergency department, were excluded. The population of interest turned out to encompass a total of 436 institutions.

The population was restricted in order to (1) reduce heterogeneity to a level that could be adequately represented with a relatively small sample and (2) eliminate both very small hospitals (which would account for only a very small proportion of emergency patients) and hospitals of unusual size and organizational complexity (which would account for only a very small proportion of hospitals).

The sample was designed to represent, in proportion to their numbers in this population, all of the following important subgroups of hospitals: (1) "small" (100–199 beds), "medium" (200–299 beds), and "large" (300–499 beds) hospitals; (2) hospitals in Standard Metropolitan Statistical Areas (SMSA) (urban areas), and in non-SMSA (nonurban) areas; and (3) church-operated as well as non-church-operated hospitals. Ideally, a minimum of ten sample hospitals were desired for each of these strata. Additionally, hospitals were to be selected for the sample in proportion to the number of eligible institutions located in each of the six states involved. Finally, eligible hospitals within each stratum were to have an equal probability of being selected.

Accordingly, before the sample was selected by computer, the eligible population was stratified by organizational size, geographical (state) location, SMSA class, and type of institutional control. Church affiliation, representing type of institutional control, was used as a secondary stratification variable, while size, location, and SMSA class were used as the primary stratification variables. Stratification was used both to ensure representation in the sample of institutions from the different subgroups and to maximize sample efficiency. The objective was to achieve reasonably adequate coverage of both the total population and important subgroups of hospitals with a modest sample size and maximum economy, and to make possible statistical generalization of the relationships found among the variables studied to the population of institutions represented by the sample.

Because of the requirements of the study, including statistical needs, expected sample attrition due to nonparticipation, limited funds and resources, and technical sampling considerations, it was decided that a sample of 40–44 institutions (or about 10 percent of the eligible population) should be drawn. The actual sample selection procedures were carried out by the Sampling Section of the Survey Research Center, using the above criteria and the list of hospitals in the American Hospital Association's 1976 *Guide to the Health Care Field*. The specific procedures used are described in detail in Appendix B.

Table 2-1 shows the selected sample, in relation to the population and strata from which it was drawn, along with the corresponding hospital cooperation rates. Clearly, the distribution of the 44 hospitals in the sample reflects very closely the distribution of the 436 hospitals in the population. The number of hospitals selected from the different strata is proportionate to the total number of institutions in the strata, approximately 10 percent of the population from each stratum having been selected into the sample as intended. By state (not shown in Table 2-1), 14 of the sample hospitals are located in Illinois, 10 in Ohio, 7 in Michigan, 6 in Wisconsin, 4 in Indiana, and 3 in Minnesota. The corresponding numbers of hospitals in the eligible population from the same states were 130, 99, 76, 63, 36, and 32, respectively. Again, the distribution of the sample hospitals across states satisfactorily reflects the distribution of the population.

Eventually, after intensive efforts and persistent negotiations, a total of 33 of the hospitals in the original sample agreed to participate in the research. Four other hospitals were willing to cooperate but were unable to do so (because of other special programs or commitments) until the spring of the next year. Because the project's schedule could not accommodate such a long delay and the data would not have been fully comparable to those obtained from the other hospitals in the sample anyway, these four institutions were not included in the research. The remaining 7 hospitals belonging to the original sample declined to participate, even after every legitimate effort had been exerted to secure their cooperation. Reasons given for nonparticipation included "an ongoing multimillion dollar construction project," "saturation

Table 2-1. The Study Sample: Hospitals Whose Emergency Units Were Studied and the Population from Which They Were Selected.

Hospital Groups (Strata) Used for Sample Selection	Hospitals in Eligible Population	Number of Hospitals Selected into Sample	Hospitals That Cooperated in Study	Sample Hospital Cooperation Rate
All Groupings Combined:	436	44	30	68%
Size strata				
Small hospitals (100–199 beds)	165	17	14	82%
Medium-sized hospitals (200–299 beds)	129	13	9	69%
Large hospitals (300–499 beds)	142	14	7	50%
Location strata				
Hospitals in SMSA (urban) areas	312	31	21	68%
Hospitals in non-SMSA areas	124	13	9	69%
Control strata				
Church-operated hospitals	140	16	9	56%
Non-church-operated hospitals	296	28	21	75%

Notes: The hospitals in the population are all nongovernment, nonprofit institutions. They are short-stay general hospitals located in HHS Region V (Illinois, Indiana, Michigan, Minnesota, Ohio, Wisconsin), and their size falls within the 100–499 bed range. The listing of the eligible population of hospitals from which the sample was drawn was obtained from the 1976 AHA *Guide to the Health Care Field.*

In the sampling process, hospitals were selected separately by state in which located as well as on the basis of SMSA versus non-SMSA location. See Appendix B.

with all kinds of requests for surveys," the source of the research funds, illness of the chief executive officer of a hospital, and refusal by the contracting physicians' group in one case.

Shortly before fieldwork was to begin, two of the institutions that had agreed to participate retracted with apologies, one because of a forthcoming visit by the Joint Commission on Accreditation of Hospitals and the other because of litigation problems; a third hospital withdrew, also with apologies, after the field team arrived (as previously scheduled and agreed) to collect the data. The reason, according to its chief executive officer, was a "gigantic misunderstanding among key people within the institution due to poor internal communication and mishandling of the matter by some, so that it became impossible to honor the previous agreement to participate." Thus, ultimately, 30 of the initially selected institutions, or 68 percent, participated in the study and provided the necessary data.* These constitute the *effective sample* of the study. The distribution of the effective sample, also shown in Table 2-1, is quite satisfactory and, for some of the strata, closer to the distribution of the population than is the original sample.

Given the nature of the sample and organizations involved, the decision to accept only hospitals whose administration, medical staff, and nursing staff all agreed to participate, and the study's heavy data requirements, the attained hospital cooperation rate of 68 percent may be regarded as very good. Moreover, this rate is considerably higher than that of other recent hospital studies with probability sample designs and data requirements approaching those of the present study (for example, see Coffee, 1983; Scott, Forrest, and Brown, 1976). Likewise, the size of the effective sample (N = 30 hospital EUs) is respectable and quite adequate for most analytical purposes.

*Of the participating institutions, 14, 9, and 7, respectively, are small, medium, and large hospitals; 21 are from SMSA (or urban) areas while 9 are from non-SMSA communities; and 9 are church-operated while 21 are not (of the latter, 3 are osteopathic institutions). As it turns out, moreover, 17 of the 30 hospitals involved have some form of medical teaching affiliation (and 13 do not), and 15 have emergency personnel training programs of one kind or another while the other 15 do not.

For the particular strata specified, the cooperation rates ranged from a high of 82 percent in the case of "small" hospitals to a low of 50 percent in the case of "large" hospitals; the second lowest rate, 56 percent, was attained for the church-operated hospitals. Proportionately, more of the small and fewer of the large hospitals in the original sample cooperated. Similarly, fewer of the church-operated than of the non-church-operated institutions participated.

With the exception of the large hospitals (especially the large church-operated hospitals), the effective sample of the study represents the population and most of the stratification groupings quite well. (The effect of the one underrepresentation noted upon the relationships found among the variables studied is probably negligible because these relationships do not require determination of population parameters or strata characteristics.) Most of the relationships, moreover, are based on data from the total sample, and careful analysis of sampling error in the data collected lends further confidence in the sample.

Sampling errors were calculated by the Sampling Section of the Survey Research Center, using actual data from the 30 institutions in the effective sample, with two different procedures: One assumed a probability sample of 44 hospitals with means of zero assigned to the nonparticipating institutions, and the other assumed a probability sample of 30 hospitals. They were calculated for a heterogeneous collection of 19 variables, which had been measured in various ways with data from several different sources, as appropriate. The results show that the precision of estimates is higher than would be obtained from a simple random sample of the same size in 14 of these 19 "test cases," and of about the same level in the remaining five cases. This outcome, which is obtained regardless of which of the two procedures is used, obviously reflects a gain from stratification over simple random sampling. For a more detailed technical discussion of the character of the study sample and related statistical issues, see Appendix B.

Sources of Data and Respondents

One of the study's important methodological principles was to develop measures, particularly for the criterion variables, that would (1) take into account several legitimate perspectives (for example, those of EU doctors and nurses, their medical colleagues within the parent hospital, and patients) and (2) rely as much as possible on independent data sources. Accordingly, relevant data were obtained from the following sources, with most of the data coming from the first two:

1. Personal interviews and questionnaires completed by seven different groups of respondents associated with the hospitals and emergency units studied.

2. Organizational and administrative records of financial, staffing, and patient census characteristics (provided by the chief executive officer of each hospital using a special form constructed by the research staff).

3. The emergency visit records of recent patients, who also completed a mailed questionnaire for the study shortly after their visits.

4. Certain supplementary sources, including U.S. Census reports on community population characteristics and the annual issues of the American Hospital Association's *Guide to the Health Care Field.*

Twelve coordinated data collection instruments (forms) had to be developed in order to obtain the required information.* The instruments were first constructed and then pretested and revised. The relevant data from the participating hospitals and EUs were then collected on location by specially trained professional interviewers from the Institute for Social Research, under research staff supervision. Each of the thirty institutions in the sample was

*All of these instruments have been incorporated in their entirety in a previous publication from the project (Georgopoulos, Cooke, and Associates, 1980). There, they are discussed in detail, along with the manner in which they were administered. The respondents, the groups which they represent, and their background characteristics are also described in that report.

scheduled for a seven-day period during which the fieldwork was carried out.

Identical data collection instruments and procedures were used in all of the hospitals, and each participating group of respondents completed the same instrument (personal interview and/or questionnaire form). The seven groups of respondents were:

1. *Emergency unit physicians* (MDs): all physicians (doctors of medicine or osteopathy), including the medical director of the unit, working in the EU during the seven-day period in which the data were collected from each particular hospital.

2. *Emergency unit registered nurses* (RNs): all full-time and part-time registered nurses working in the EU during the seven-day data collection period, including the head nurse(s) or supervising nurses (SRNs) involved.

3. *Emergency unit licensed practical nurses* (LPNs): all licensed practical nurses working full time in the EU during the same period.

4. *Selected hospital physicians* (HMDs): key physicians in the parent hospital who had knowledge of, but did not work in, the EU, including: the chief or president of the medical staff and chairman of the medical executive committee; the chairman of the emergency department/room committee (if any); the chief pathologist and chief radiologist of the hospital; the chairman of the trauma committee (if any); intensive care unit physicians; the chairman of the medical audit, quality assurance, or peer review committee; the hospital's director of medical education; and the heads of the four major inpatient services—medicine, surgery, pediatrics, and obstetrics/gynecology. (One individual respondent often held more than one of the specified positions.)

5. *Hospital administrators* (HAs): the chief executive officer of each hospital, the next highest administrative official (if any) of the hospital responsible for the emergency unit, and the hospital's director of nursing.

6. *Selected community respondents* (CRs): certain individuals from the community having work contacts with, or special

knowledge about, each hospital's EU, including the local health department director or designate; sheriff's department, police department, and fire department representatives; the coroner or medical examiner; health systems agency (HSA) and emergency medical system (EMS) representatives (if any); ambulance company personnel (for example, emergency medical technicians); and up to three additional individuals named by the chief executive officer of each hospital (when interviewed) as the "most knowledgeable individuals in the community outside the hospital concerning the emergency unit" (these often overlapped with other specified community respondents).

7. *Emergency unit patients* (PATs): all patients over fifteen years of age visiting the EU for care at any time from 8:00 A.M. Friday until 12:00 P.M. Saturday of the week during which fieldwork was carried out, excluding those who were unable to, or who preferred not to, sign a consent form to participate in the research. Subsequently, within approximately three weeks after their emergency visits, these patients were contacted by the research staff and asked to complete a mail questionnaire for the study. Copies of their emergency visit medical records already had been obtained, with their consent, from each participating institution.

The individual respondents, with the notable exception of patients, were treated mainly as "observers" (that is, as informants or evaluators of the EU) rather than as "subjects" (that is, individuals reporting on their own personal, job, or organizational situations or on their own satisfaction or dissatisfaction and other personal concerns). The hospital administrators (HAs), EU physicians (MDs), and registered nurses (RNs) completed both personal interviews and questionnaires for the study. The supervising nurses (SRNs) from the various EUs completed a special questionnaire-type instrument in addition to the forms completed by the RNs. The licensed practical nurses (LPNs) completed a personal interview only. The selected physicians (HMDs) from the parent hospitals completed personal interviews, as did the selected community respondents (CRs) associated with each institution.

Finally, the patients (PATs) completed a mailed questionnaire. The numbers of respondents from each group who provided data for the study are presented in Table 2-2, along with the corresponding response rates (averaged for the thirty EUs in the study).

A grand total of 1,446 persons associated with the thirty hospitals/emergency units studied provided data. Included were 248 MDs, 278 RNs, 47 LPNs (nine of the hospitals had no full-time LPNs working in their EUs), 215 HMDs, 68 HAs, 202 CRs, and 388 PATs (two of the hospitals did not allow patient participation in the study). Thus, on the average, a total of nearly 50 persons per hospital participated as respondents. The specific numbers of respondents associated with the various hospital strata discussed earlier and an additional grouping of institutions according to the annual number of patient visits to the EU also are shown in Table 2-2.

The overall *response rate* for all groups combined, other than patients, who were eligible to participate as respondents from the thirty hospitals combined turned out to be an exceptionally high 94.4 percent. If patients are included with the other groups, the corresponding rate is lower, 87.5 percent, but still high. In the case of EU patients (PATs), from whom data were collected by mailed questionnaire, the overall response rate for the twenty-eight institutions that allowed patient participation averages 73 percent. Though lower than that of the other participating groups, this too is a good response rate, particularly when compared to response rates usually achieved by mailed questionnaire surveys of adult populations or other studies in the health services field involving former hospital patients. The corresponding response rates attained for the other groups of respondents (for all study hospitals combined) are as follows: for MDs, 90 percent; for RNs, 97 percent; for LPNs, 100 percent; for HMDs, 92 percent; for HAs, 100 percent; and for CRs, 95 percent. Obviously, these are all excellent response rates.

Finally, across individual hospitals, the overall response rate achieved for the various groups of respondents combined, but exclusive of the patients, ranges from 79 to 100 percent, with ten of the study hospitals showing a rate of 100 percent. The 79 percent figure signifies the lowest attained response rate for any one

Table 2-2. Number of Individual Respondents Who Provided Data, Shown Separately for the Various Groups of Respondents and Selected Institutional Groupings.

Hospital/Emergency Units (EUs) Involved		Number of Respondents, by Group							
		MDs	RNs	LPNs	HMDs	HAs	CRs	PATs	Total
All Institutions in Study Sample (N = 30 hospital EUs)		248	278	47	215	68	202	388	1,446
Average Response Rate:		90%	97%	100%	92%	100%	95%	73%	88%
Hospitals of:									
Small size (100–199 beds)	(N = 14)	106	111	17	80	28	95	182	619
Medium size (200–299 beds)	(N = 9)	79	92	13	71	20	59	122	456
Large size (300–499 beds)	(N = 7)	63	75	17	64	20	48	84	371
Hospitals/EUs located in:									
SMSA/urban areas	(N = 21)	176	203	39	158	50	135	256	1,017
Non-SMSA areas	(N = 9)	72	75	8	57	18	67	132	429
Hospitals/EUs that are:									
Church-operated	(N = 9)	94	80	9	48	20	60	53	364
Non-church-operated/osteopathic	(N = 3)	18	28	7	25	6	17	45	146
Non-church-operated/other	(N = 18)	136	170	31	142	42	125	290	936
Hospitals with EUs having:									
Low patient volume (under 10,000 visits)	(N = 10)	97	83	8	47	21	70	79	405
Medium patient volume (10,000–20,000 visits)	(N = 10)	72	77	17	85	21	57	112	441
High patient volume (over 20,000 patient visits a year)	(N = 10)	79	118	22	83	26	75	197	600

Notes: MDs, RNs, and LPNs, respectively, designate the physicians, registered nurses, and full-time licensed practical nurses working in the various emergency units. HMDs designates selected physicians from each parent hospital, and HAs designates hospital administrators. CRs designates selected community respondents, and PATs designates patient respondents. (Two institutions did not allow patient participation, and nine of them had no full-time LPNs in their emergency units.)

The overall response rate for all groups combined except patients is 94.4 percent. Response rates were computed by dividing the number of respondents shown for each group by the number of individuals eligible to participate, that is, by the number of potential respondents.

hospital (the next lowest rate was 86 percent). In fact, for twenty-seven of the thirty cooperating hospitals the attained response rate reached or exceeded the 90 percent level. Therefore, considering both the overall hospital cooperation rate achieved and the response rates attained (not only for each of the respondent groups but also for each of the individual hospitals in the sample), the study was very successful in meeting sampling design requirements and obtaining the necessary data. The background characteristics of respondents are described in Appendix C.

Data Aggregation and Statistical Treatment Issues

Analytical and statistical possibilities generally are dictated by the objectives and design of the research and limited by such factors as the nature and size of the sample, (non)response rates, the relevance and quality of the data, and the character of the measures. The preceding discussion suggests that in these important respects the present study is not particularly problematic. Although precluding certain kinds of analysis, for example, the size of the sample (N = 30 EUs) is adequate for the main statistical-analytical requirements of the research (for example, for testing the relationships among the principal independent and dependent variables studied). In general, these requirements can be satisfactorily met using t tests, correlation and regression techniques, and analysis of variance.

Given the nature of the sample and the research questions addressed, simple random sample statistics can be confidently used, at least when the total sample is involved in the testing. Further, the high response rates achieved greatly facilitate the task of statistical treatment while also being indicative of the quality of the data. Finally, as will be shown in subsequent chapters, the large majority of the measures developed and used by the study also are satisfactory from a methodological standpoint.

Because the main unit of analysis in the research is the hospital EU, the principal variables of interest had to be measured at the organizational or institutional level. For some of these variables (for example, EU size or number of patient visits, teaching affiliation, payroll expenditures per patient visit, or percentage of minority population in the community), the data directly represent organizational properties or collectivity-level phenomena. Typically, these data are from sources other than individual respondents, so that the measures based on them did not involve special aggregation problems. The measurement of other variables, however, necessitated the aggregation of question-naire or interview data from individuals to the institutional level (usually in the form of means computed on five-point scales). Such aggregation, which constitutes a dominant type of measurement in contemporary organizational research, raises certain methodological issues.*

For immediate purposes, the single most important aggregation issue involves the question of whether the measures thus derived are in fact meaningful beyond the individual respondent level, that is, whether they represent organizational-level properties or variables as intended. Because of this issue, individuals who provided data for the measurement of organizational variables were basically required to respond as observers (informants) of the EU situation and not from a personal standpoint. In addition, each of the questions to which they responded explicitly and directly had the EU, some other organization or group, or some system characteristic as its referent. Further, for the principal measures constructed by aggregating individual responses, a dual statistical test of appropriateness was used to check on whether they represented organizational-level phenomena.

First, for each of the measures, a one-way analysis of variance was performed with the unaggregated data at the individual level, stratifying by hospital EU and treating the measure as the "dependent variable," to determine whether the between-EU variance was greater than the within-EU variance. (The analysis was performed separately on the data provided by each group of respondents involved.) If the EUs as organizational

---

*For a discussion of some of these issues, along with relevant evidence supportive of measurement approaches such as the one used in the present study, see Lincoln and Zeitz (1980). See also Holt and Turner (1970), Przeworski and Teune (1970), and Scheuch (1970) for more extended discussions.

entities, and not the individuals within them, did indeed constitute the main source of variability (as was assumed for each measure in question), this would be the case and the obtained F ratio should be larger than 1.0.

Second, the eta-squared (η^2) statistic was computed to ascertain the level of agreement/similarity within EUs among the responses of the individuals who actually provided the data that were subsequently aggregated (separately for each group of respondents and each of the thirty EUs in the study) to construct the measure at the institutional level. The extent of such agreement would indicate what portion of the variance in the individual responses could be explained by "cluster" (see Campbell, Converse, and Rodgers, 1976, p. 232; Peterson, 1979, pp. 128–139). Such agreement would be both indicative of intra-EU (or "intra-class") correlation among the responses of the individual participants (who, in effect, were serving as "observers") and suggestive of interrespondent or "interrater" reliability. In effect, it too would support the conclusion that the measure intended to represent differences among EUs, that is, the "criterion" used for defining differences between these organizations, is a meaningful one at this aggregation level.

The particular rule followed in interpreting the results from the above pair of tests may be stated as follows: if, for a given measure, the η^2 was at least .16 (and preferably .20 or more) *and* the F ratio was larger than 1.0 (and preferably significantly larger, with $p \leq .05$), the measure was regarded as meaningful and appropriate at the EU level, that is, at the organizational or system level. All of the key measures of this research which are based on the responses of individuals were subjected to this twofold test.

Summary

This chapter presented an overview of the research methodology employed to study the relationship between the organization and effectiveness of hospital emergency units. Briefly, the methodology can be described as that of an intensive comparative organizational study that is both theory based and problem oriented. The discussion was limited to the general features of the research design, however, leaving the more specific aspects of methodology and measurement for consideration in subsequent chapters, along with the concepts and substantive problems to which they pertain. As additional background for these discussions, Chapter Three describes some of the basic organizational characteristics of the EUs studied.

Organizational Characteristics of Emergency Units

This chapter presents a descriptive overview of the organizations studied, for the purpose of highlighting some of their basic characteristics and for providing general background for subsequent analyses of EU effectiveness and its relationship to organizational structure and problem solving. More specifically, the data and findings summarized in this chapter cover five major areas: (1) selected aspects of organizational structure, (2) institutional goal priorities, (3) the composition of patient inputs, (4) staff resources and staffing patterns, and (5) perceived institutional strengths and weaknesses. (For more detailed documentation concerning most of the descriptive findings discussed in this chapter, see Georgopoulos, Cooke, and Associates, 1980.)

The relevant data were obtained from organizational records and from interviews and questionnaires completed by the various groups of respondents. Descriptive findings concerning the effectiveness of hospital EUs, including economic efficiency and the quality of patient care (clinical efficiency), are presented in subsequent chapters.

Selected Aspects of Organizational Structure

This section is concerned with the gross anatomy of hospital EUs in terms of institutional links to the parent hospitals, medical teaching affiliation, and emergency personnel training programs; patient volume and the breadth of "emergency service"

42

definition prevailing at the various institutions; and the nature of available facilities and services.

Institutional Links and Programs

Twenty-three of the thirty hospitals that participated in the study have an emergency department/room committee for administrative, planning, and institutional control purposes. The same number also have some formal mechanism for "monitoring the performance or the quality of work of their emergency unit." Links such as these presumably facilitate organizational effectiveness. Administratively, the parent hospitals are represented at the various EUs by a supervising nurse who is in charge of the unit and who reports to the hospital's director of nursing, or by an administrative official of the hospital. The medical leadership of the units, on the other hand, depends upon their medical staffing patterns (see later section in this chapter on staffing patterns).

Concerning financial matters, twenty-eight of the thirty EUs are considered separate "cost centers" by their respective parent hospitals. For the most recent quarter prior to fieldwork, the operating budgets of these emergency care facilities averaged 2.54 percent of the total budget of their parent hospitals (the figure ranging from 0.79 percent to 5.92 percent across institutions). The EUs' payroll budgets, which cover all personnel except physicians, on the average amounted to 2.94 percent of the total payroll budget of the parent hospitals (the range in this case being 1.30 percent to 8.19 percent). Apparently, EUs differ considerably in their total and payroll budgets, both of which involve substantial funds. It is also interesting to note that, for the same quarter, the ratio of total EU revenues (exclusive of physician fees) from all patient visits to total EU expenditures averaged 1.89 (for twenty-nine of the thirty EUs in the study for which these data were available). This ratio also varies greatly across institutions, however, ranging from a low of 0.97 to a high of 5.68. On the average, it is highest (2.41) for EUs with a high patient volume—the ten units with the largest number of patient visits.

Additional data show that seventeen of the thirty institutions in the sample have some form of medical teaching affiliation.

Such affiliation is more prevalent among hospitals whose EUs have a medium or high, as opposed to low, patient volume, hospitals which are not church-operated, and hospitals located in SMSA/urban areas, compared to other institutions. Similarly, exactly half of the hospitals in the study have some kind of emergency personnel training program. Most such programs are for technicians; only three institutions reported similar training programs for either emergency nurses or emergency physicians. Training programs for emergency technicians are most often found in hospitals whose EUs have a high patient volume. Both training programs and teaching affiliations are believed by many in the field to correlate positively with patient care quality (concerning this hypothesis, see Chapter Nine).

Patient Volume and "Emergency Service" Definition

In terms of physical capacity, the thirty EUs in the study have an average of 4.4 treatment rooms each, the specific number ranging from a low of 1 to a high of 15. In addition, they have an average of 2.2 "other" rooms (for individual EUs this number ranges from 0 to 10). The mean number of beds per EU turns out to be 6.9, ranging across institutions from 0 to a maximum of 25. As might be expected, the number of treatment rooms, other rooms, and beds in the various EUs increases as the size of the parent hospitals increases. Furthermore, EUs in SMSA/urban areas generally have more treatment rooms, other rooms, and beds than those in non-SMSA areas. The same is true for EUs operated by hospitals having medical teaching affiliations and/or training programs for emergency personnel, compared to their counterparts in hospitals lacking such programs and affiliations.

The average number of patient visits to the thirty EUs in the sample during the most recent quarter prior to fieldwork was close to 5,000 per EU, ranging across institutions from a low of 655 to a high of 11,847 visits. This number increases as the size of the parent hospitals increases, and it is larger for institutions in SMSA/urban compared to nonurban areas and institutions with either teaching affiliations or training programs compared to institutions without these links and programs.

Two EUs, of course, may have an identical number of patient visits but vastly different work requirements. For example, one may have an unusually high proportion of patients who require immediate admission to the hospital as inpatients, while the other may have an unusually high proportion of "primary care" patients who could have been treated in a doctor's office instead of the EU (see section on patient inputs below). Work requirements would be less complex and less demanding in the latter unit, which would probably have a broader institutional definition of "emergency service" than the former. In this research, the relative breadth or scope of emergency service at the different institutions was expected to have implications not only for required resources but also for staff performance and institutional effectiveness (see Chapter Nine).

For these reasons, patient visits to the EUs were examined in relation to a number of other variables of interest, including each hospital's inpatient admissions and inpatient days. In this connection, the institution's most recent quarterly data at the time of the fieldwork showed that, on the average, for every inpatient admission to the thirty hospitals in the sample there were 2.36 patient visits to the institutions' EUs. On the average, moreover, the ratio of EU visits to the parent hospital's inpatient days (which is used in this study to indicate each institution's breadth of "emergency service" definition) was 0.37, ranging across hospitals from a low of 0.09 to a high of 0.94. The higher this ratio, the broader is the *de facto* definition, or scope, of "emergency service" prevailing at an institution.

Available Special Facilities and the Nature of Services Provided

Concerning special emergency care facilities, half of the institutions in the sample report having a poison control or substance abuse center or unit. These facilities are more likely to be found in hospitals whose EUs have a high patient volume and in non-church-operated hospitals. They are also more prevalent in hospitals having emergency personnel training programs than in other hospitals. Similarly, nearly half of the institutions (fourteen of the thirty) report having a trauma center or unit. The likelihood of this kind of center increases as the EU's patient volume increases. It is also greater for hospitals with medical teaching affiliations than for hospitals without such affiliations. Finally, one-third of the institutions in the sample, but half of those whose emergency units have a high patient volume, report having a mental health center or unit.

With respect to the nature of patient services provided, the physicians (MDs) and registered nurses (RNs) working in the various EUs were asked whether their respective units "specialize in, or concentrate on, the treatment of any particular kinds of patients." Only 12 percent of the MDs, from all institutions combined, responded affirmatively to this question, and those who did respond are scattered among twenty-two different EUs. In fact, only one of the thirty EUs is considered to specialize in the treatment of some particular kind of patients by at least half of the MDs who work there. Similarly, only 17 percent of all the RNs report that their EUs concentrate on some particular types of patients. These relatively few respondents again are scattered among twenty-one different EUs, and only one unit is considered to specialize by half or more of its RNs.

Overall, therefore, the data indicate no "specialization in treating particular kinds of patients" on the part of the emergency units studied. Apparently, EUs are like a microcosm of their parent hospitals in this respect, reflecting a great variety of patient types and conditions treated and focusing more on comprehensiveness of service than on special treatment capabilities.

Regarding the comprehensiveness of services offered by the various EUs, information was obtained from the chief executive officer of each hospital. According to this information, only six of the thirty EUs in the sample offer "comprehensive" services. An additional fourteen EUs, however, offer "nearly comprehensive" services. The ten remaining units offer less comprehensive services or just "basic" services. Hospitals with medical teaching affiliations and large hospitals are more likely to have an EU offering comprehensive or nearly comprehensive services than are other hospitals.

Institutional Goal Priorities

For many hospital EUs, comprehensiveness of services also constitutes a top institutional priority. The current goal priorities of EUs, as seen by several key groups of respondents—emergency unit doctors (MDs) and nurses (RNs), selected hospital physicians (HMDs), and community respondents (CRs)—are discussed in this section.

Emergency unit MDs and RNs were asked to rank seven goal priorities intended to reflect the major organizational concerns associated with the clinical, economic, or social efficiency of EUs "in order of their importance to the emergency unit." The specific priorities, in the sequence presented to the respondents, were: "maintaining a good reputation in the community," "improving working conditions for the staff," "minimizing patient waiting time," "keeping the costs of the emergency service down," "maintaining high standards of patient care," "providing comprehensive emergency services," and "maintaining a high level of patient satisfaction."

On the average, these goal priorities were ranked very similarly by both MDs and RNs. Overall, both groups ranked "maintaining high standards of patient care" as the most important priority of all, and "providing comprehensive emergency services" as second most important, followed by "maintaining a high level of patient satisfaction" in third place. At the other extreme, they both ranked "improving working conditions for the staff" in last place (seventh) and "keeping the costs of the emergency service down" next to last (sixth) in overall importance. "Minimizing patient waiting time" was ranked fourth by RNs but fifth by MDs (though the mean-rank score is identical, specifically 4.4, according to the data from both groups), while "maintaining a good reputation in the community" was ranked fourth by MDs but fifth by RNs.

Thus, apart from the minor differences noted, the importance of the seven goal priorities is basically the same for MDs and RNs. Moreover, the above rank-order of priorities based on the data from RNs remains the same even when the several major subgroupings of EUs (that is, subgroupings based on size, location, affiliation, and the like) are considered separately. Thus, when the different subgroups of EUs on each specific goal priority are compared, the mean-rank scores are very similar, with only a few exceptions.*

Generally, then, those goal priorities most directly related to patient care (maintaining high standards, providing comprehensive services, and maintaining a high level of patient satisfaction, in that order) are, on the average, more important to the EUs studied than are other priorities, according to the RNs and MDs who work there. Minimizing patient waiting time and maintaining a good reputation in the community are generally emphasized less. Finally, keeping the costs of service down and improving working conditions for the staff are the least emphasized of the seven goal priorities considered.

It must be pointed out, however, that the situation of individual emergency units may differ from the above patterns, and differ markedly for particular goal priorities. The range of EU mean-rank scores for each priority is considerable for all the priorities except one—maintaining high standards of care (this priority is ranked high at all EUs). In contrast, interunit variability is very high for maintaining a good reputation in the community, and high for keeping the costs of service down. For the remaining goal priorities, the variability across EUs is moderately low based on the data from RNs but moderately high based on the data from MDs.

The HMDs were also asked to indicate *which three* of the same seven goal priorities "are emphasized the most" by the EUs of their respective hospitals. With reference to all thirty EUs in the

---

*In the case of the data from MDs, the exceptions are as follows: Keeping costs down is emphasized more by EUs with a low compared to a medium patient volume; minimizing patient waiting time is emphasized more by EUs in SMSA/urban compared to other areas, while the reverse is true of improving working conditions; the latter is also emphasized less by the EUs of hospitals which have medical teaching affiliations than those which do not. In the case of the data from RNs, the exceptions are as follows: Minimizing patient waiting time is emphasized more by EUs with a high compared to a low patient volume, while the reverse is true of keeping costs down; the latter goal priority is also less emphasized by EUs with a high compared to a medium or a low patient volume.

study combined, the HMDs also indicated the following as the most important goal priorities: (1) maintaining high standards of patient care, (2) providing comprehensive emergency services, (3) maintaining a high level of patient satisfaction, and (4) maintaining a good reputation in the community. This pattern of results is practically the same, moreover, for every major subgrouping of EUs examined.

In short, the pattern of findings concerning the relative importance of the seven goal priorities is remarkably consistent, both when the total sample and when each of several different subgroupings of EUs are examined, and regardless of the specific source of the data—the selected hospital physicians and the emergency unit physicians and registered nurses are all in agreement in this area. In fact, even the selected community respondents (CRs) included among their top three goal priorities the two that were emphasized the most by the other groups of respondents—maintaining high standards of care and providing comprehensive emergency services. Unlike the other respondents, however, the CRs also included "patient waiting time" among the top three goal priorities.

Overall, then, the data show remarkable agreement among the various groups of respondents on the relative importance of the goal priorities specified. Other things being equal, such a high level of consensus should facilitate performance and problem solving in these organizations.

Composition of Patient Inputs

Generally, hospital EUs have little control over their patient inputs (see Chapter One). To a certain extent, however, the nature of a unit's patient inputs over the long run might be affected by the performance of the unit. An EU that is doing consistently excellent work, for example, may come to be "preferred" by referring agencies and individuals in the community or by a particular population of patients. Similarly, an EU that has developed explicit collaborative arrangements, such as patient transfer and referral agreements, with other institutions or agencies in the community in effect exercises some control over the

variability of its patient workload. Still, overall, the patient inputs
of hospital EUs are difficult to control and largely unpredictable.
Yet the work and performance requirements of these organizations
are in large measure dictated by the composition of their respective
patient inputs.

The present study examined the composition of patient
inputs partly in terms of diagnostic categories (see Chapter Five)
but mainly in terms of the proportion of incoming patients having
certain important characteristics, including severity of condition.
More specifically, the investigation considered the proportion of
patients who (1) arrived by ambulance, in life-threatening
condition, and in nonemergency condition; (2) were scheduled in
advance or were transfers from other institutions; and (3) were sent
by the EU to the intensive care unit (ICU), the operating room
(OR), or some other part of the parent hospital, or were transferred
to a different hospital for treatment.

In addition, data concerning the proportion of incoming
patients who were seen by a doctor within fifteen minutes of their
arrival at each EU and the average length of patient visits were
also examined. These latter kinds of data are indicative not only of
patient workload but also of the promptness of medical response
to the patient's problems and of the promptness with which
patient inputs were processed at the various EUs. (Promptness of
medical response was found to correlate with the quality of medical
care provided by hospital EUs; see Chapter Eight.)

Patients Arriving by Ambulance or in Life-Threatening
Condition and Nonemergency Cases

It is probably fair to assume that, other things being equal,
the higher the proportion of EU patients who arrived by ambulance,
the greater the average severity of patient condition, with corresponding implications for staff response and treatment requirements. Data about ambulance arrivals, therefore, were obtained
from the doctors and registered nurses working at each EU in the
sample and, when available, from institutional records as well.

The MDs estimated that, on the average, 15 percent of the
patients visiting their respective units "over the past four weeks"

(preceding data collection) arrived by ambulance. Across EUs, this figure ranges from 5 percent to 41 percent, indicating great variability. The corresponding figures from the data provided by RNs (whose estimates are slightly but consistently higher than those of MDs) are similar, the average figure in this case being 17.5 percent and the range 6 to 32 percent. The estimates provided by RNs, incidentally, correlate significantly with those provided by MDs (r = .44, p < .01, N = 29 EUs). According to similar data from hospital records, the percentage of patients arriving by ambulance "during the most recent month" is smaller than that estimated by either the RNs or the MDs, but still substantial, averaging 9.4 percent and ranging across EUs from 1.5 percent to 29.4 percent. These data from records, available for only nineteen of the thirty EUs in the sample, correlate positively with the corresponding estimates provided by either the MDs (r = .37, p >.05, N = 19 EUs) or the RNs (r = .34, p > .05, N = 19 EUs), but the correlation is statistically significant only at the .10 level.

Regardless of the specific source of data, the findings about ambulance arrivals show considerable interinstitutional variability, but the pattern of results is substantially the same, according to the data from both MDs and RNs. Briefly, the EUs of large hospitals and hospitals in SMSA areas show the highest rates of ambulance arrivals. The data from hospital records are also consistent with this pattern. For discussion of the relationship between the proportion of patients arriving by ambulance and the quality of medical care in the EUs studied, see Chapter Five.

Another indicator of the relative severity of patient condition is based on the responses of MDs, RNs, and hospital administrators (HAs) to the following question: "Over the past four weeks, about what percentage of the patients visiting this emergency unit arrived in what you would judge to be a 'life-threatening' condition?" The estimates provided by MDs are generally smaller than those provided by RNs, which in turn are somewhat smaller than those provided by HAs. According to the MDs, an average of 6.4 percent of the patients at their respective EUs arrived in a "life-threatening" condition; across institutions, this figure ranges from 2.7 percent to 16.7 percent, indicating substantial variability. According to the data from RNs, the average for the thirty EUs is 8.8 percent, and the range is 3.2 percent to 16.1 percent. And based on the data from HAs, the corresponding figures are 9.5 percent, and 2.0 percent to 25.0 percent, respectively.

The data also show that a larger proportion of the patients visiting EUs with a high patient volume arrived in "life-threatening" condition, compared to those visiting EUs with a low or medium patient volume. MDs, RNs, and HAs are all in agreement in this respect. The data from MDs indicate that the EUs of hospitals with medical teaching affiliations and emergency personnel training programs received a somewhat higher proportion of patients in life-threatening condition than did their counterparts in hospitals without such programs and affiliations.

At the opposite end of the spectrum from patients arriving in life-threatening condition are those patients whose medical problems might have been handled in a doctor's office instead of the EU. Data about the proportion of these "primary care" patients were obtained from MDs working in each EU and the selected physician respondents (HMDs) from the parent hospital. The findings are very similar regardless of the source of data. According to both MDs and HMDs, the *majority* of patients visiting the various EUs (over the previous four weeks) "should have gone to a private physician or had a problem that could have been handled in a doctor's office instead of the emergency unit." The average percentage of such patients for the thirty EUs turns out to be 56 percent based on the estimates given by MDs and 52 percent based on the estimates given by HMDs. Across EUs, MDs' estimates range from a low of only 36 percent to a high of 77 percent and HMDs' from 28 percent to 75 percent. The percentage in question is higher for EUs located in non-SMSA compared to SMSA areas, according to the data from both groups of respondents. Apparently, physicians do not regard a very large proportion of the patients who visit hospital EUs as true "emergency" cases.

Patients Scheduled in Advance and Transfer Patients

Certain additional data obtained from institutional records (referred to in this book as RECs) are also useful for describing the nature of patient inputs. Some of these data, for example, show that, on the average, nearly 6 percent of all patient visits to the EUs during the most recent quarter were "scheduled in advance." Across EUs, this figure ranges from 0 percent to 38 percent, indicating major interinstitutional differences in this respect. Interestingly, however, the EUs of the large hospitals in the study had no patient visits scheduled in advance. At the other extreme, the EUs of medium-sized hospitals had 10 percent of their patient visits scheduled in advance (for the EUs of small hospitals the figure was about half as large). The groupings of institutions by location, teaching affiliation, and training programs, on the other hand, show no substantial differences on this variable.

Other data from records show that the percentage of patient visits to the various EUs that were transfers from outside the parent hospital (for example, from other hospitals) in each case was extremely small, averaging less than 1 percent for the thirty EUs. In contrast, transfers into the EU from other parts of the parent hospitals were much more frequent. On the average, during the most recent quarter, 4.2 percent of the patient visits to each EU were transfers of this kind. Such transfers were most prevalent among the EUs of small hospitals and hospitals that do not have medical teaching affiliations or emergency personnel training programs.

Patients Sent to an ICU or OR

The composition of patient inputs can be further described in terms of certain variables that may reflect institutional practices as well as the relative seriousness of condition of the patients. Results from four relevant measures obtained from RECs are available in this connection, showing the percentage of EU patients who were sent for treatment to (1) one of the parent hospital's intensive care units (ICUs), (2) the operating room (OR), (3) another inpatient service of the parent hospital, or (4) another hospital.

First, on the average, for those institutions for which information was available, the results show that 2.2 percent of all the patients visiting the EUs during the most recent quarter were sent (by each EU) to one of the parent hospital's ICUs for treatment. The interhospital range on this measure is considerable, from 0.3 percent to 12.6 percent. Proportionately, more of the patients visiting the EUs of large than of either small or medium-sized hospitals were sent to an ICU. A similar pattern was found for institutions located in SMSA compared to non-SMSA areas, and institutions with medical teaching affiliations compared to those without such affiliations. However, a reverse pattern was characteristic of institutions having emergency personnel training programs compared to those not having such programs.

Second, the percentage of patients who were sent to an OR of the parent hospital by the EU is very small, only 0.6 percent on the average. And the range across institutions is also small (0 percent to 2.4 percent).

In contrast, the percentage of patients who were sent to a part of the parent hospital other than an ICU or the OR for treatment is rather substantial, 17 percent on the average; and the interinstitutional range in this case is very great (4 percent to 79 percent). Thus, the apparent capability and/or desire of EUs to treat their patients without having to send them to another part of the hospital varies widely from one EU to another. Differences in patient composition, in staff practices, and possibly even in hospital admission procedures that increase inpatient occupancy might also be responsible for this variability.

Finally, the percentage of EU patients sent to another hospital for treatment is rather small, averaging 1.1 percent for all the EUs in the study for which data were available. The interinstitutional range on this variable is moderate—specifically, 0 percent to 5.6 percent. The higher the figure, the lower the probability that an EU or its parent hospital can treat EU patients without having to refer them elsewhere. It is also possible, of course, that EUs refer patients elsewhere in the best interests of the patient or because superior treatment facilities are available at the other institutions.

Patients Seen by a Doctor Within Fifteen Minutes
of Arrival and Length of Visits

The final series of patient input findings involves two important aspects of the processing of patient inputs, which probably reflect both the condition of patients and the promptness of medical attention received by the patients at the EUs studied.

Whatever their condition, more than half of the patients visiting the various EUs (59.6 percent, on the average, according to estimates by MDs; 53.2 percent according to estimates by RNs) were seen by a doctor within fifteen minutes after arriving. This would indicate relatively prompt response by EU physicians. The data also show, however, great differences among EUs—specifically, a range of 30.3 percent to 95.5 percent based on the data from MDs and one of 10.2 percent to 97.0 percent based on the data from RNs. In some EUs nearly all of the patients were seen by a doctor within fifteen minutes of their arrival; in others fewer than one-third of them were.

Further, the average length of patient visits also ranged widely across institutions, from 35 to 109 minutes (the mean for the thirty EUs being 51 minutes) based on estimates by the MDs and from 42 to 121 minutes (with a mean of exactly 60 minutes) based on estimates by RNs. The corresponding range based on reports by the patients (PATs) who participated in the study as respondents was 30–120 minutes (with a mean of 67 minutes).

Perhaps the MDs underestimate and the PATs overestimate the length of patient visits to some extent, while the RNs give estimates midway between those provided by these two groups (and probably also more realistic estimates). Still, the three groups show good agreement. More important, it is obvious that interinstitutional variability in medical response, as reflected in the above findings, is very great. Some of the likely implications of this variability for the quality of patient care provided at the various EUs are considered in Chapter Eight.

Staffing Patterns and Staff Resources

The staff resources available to an EU are essential to effective organizational functioning. The size, qualifications, and stability of the medical and nursing staff in particular can greatly affect the clinical, economic, and social efficiency of the system. This section considers the following aspects of institutional resources: (1) basic medical staffing pattern, (2) access to clinical staff and medical specialists, (3) the sufficiency and stability of resources, (4) clinical staff size and hours worked by MDs and RNs, (5) clinical staff hours in relation to workload (patient volume), and (6) staff capability for different levels of patient volume. Some of the findings are based on data from hospital records (RECs) and some are based on questionnaire or interview data.

Medical Staffing Patterns

The medical staff resources of hospital EUs are probably among the most important determinants of institutional effectiveness in these health service delivery systems. The present study, therefore, paid considerable attention to these resources and their organization and utilization.

Data about the basic staffing pattern of EUs were obtained from the chief executive officer of each participating hospital. These data show that nine of the thirty EUs in the sample have a contractual arrangement with some non-hospital-based group of physicians or medical corporation. Five units have a contractual arrangement with a hospital-based group of physicians, that is, a group of physicians associated with the parent hospitals in each case. Seven units are staffed by rotating medical staff from their parent hospitals. Four units are staffed with individual doctors (full or part time) on contract. The remaining five EUs report some other basic staffing pattern, usually a variation of one or another of the preceding patterns.

A number of interesting differences in medical staffing patterns emerge when one compares various subgroups of EUs. Half of the units with a low patient volume, for example, rely on rotation of their parent hospital's attending staff for their medical staffing, while none of the high-volume units uses this type of arrangement. The latter units tend to rely on contractual arrangements with either some hospital-based group (none of the low-volume or medium-volume units uses this arrangement) or, less frequently, a non-hospital-based group or corporation. The medium-volume units use all of the staffing patterns (except the one noted) about equally. The EUs of church-operated institutions use hospital staff rotation (but no contractual arrangements with non-hospital-based groups—the most common pattern for the total sample) more than do the EUs of other institutions.

The EUs of hospitals with teaching affiliations most commonly use contractual arrangements, either with non-hospital-based or with hospital-based groups. Their counterparts in hospitals with no teaching affiliations, on the other hand, use attending staff rotation more than any of the other staffing patterns. The EUs of hospitals that have emergency personnel training programs also predominantly use contractual group arrangements. The relationships between the various medical staffing patterns and the clinical and economic efficiency of hospital EUs are discussed in Chapter Nine.

Whatever their basic staffing patterns might be, most of the EUs report having a doctor physically present in the unit at all times. Specifically, of the thirty EUs in the study, eighteen report that a doctor is physically present in the unit during the day, nineteen report a doctor present on the evening shift, and twenty report a doctor present on the night shift. Apparently, the night shift is as well staffed in this respect as the other two shifts.

The patterns of physician presence in relation to the various groupings of EUs are essentially the same as the patterns concerning the presence of an RN. Exactly two-thirds of the EUs report having at least one RN physically present in the unit for each of the three shifts. Nearly all EUs with a high patient volume report this to be the case, compared to slightly more than half of those with a medium patient volume and fewer than half of those with a low patient volume. The large majority of institutions with medical teaching affiliations, and also emergency personnel training programs, likewise report having an RN physically present in the unit at all times, compared to just less than half of the institutions which do not have such affiliations and training programs. Finally, proportionately more of the institutions located in SMSA/urban areas, compared to other areas, report twenty-four-hour RN presence.

Access to Clinical Staff and Medical Specialists

Whatever the staffing pattern of an EU may be at any particular time, it is also important for the unit to be able to

obtain particular kinds of staff when needed. Accordingly, certain
data concerning the success of EUs in obtaining requested clinical
staff resources from their parent hospitals were collected from the
registered nurses working in the various EUs. The resources in
question included "doctors to work in the EU," "doctors on call to
the EU," and "registered nurses for the EU."

The results show that, on the average, EUs are "*usually* able
to obtain most of what they request" concerning each of these
three kinds of staff resources. Average overall success, in this
respect, is about equal for doctors to work in the unit, doctors on
call, and registered nurses. The results also show, however, that
success varies considerably among individual EUs. Regarding
doctors to work in the unit, for example, some EUs are able to
obtain "all or nearly all" of what they request while others are able
to obtain only "about half" of what they request; the same pattern
holds true for requests for RNs to work on the unit. For doctors on
call, interinstitutional differences are even more pronounced, some
of the EUs managing to obtain only "less than half" of what they
request.

Although individual EUs report different levels of success in
obtaining each of these clinical staff resources, the differences from
one *grouping* of EUs to another (based on location, parent
hospital size, and so on) are not substantial. The data concerning
requests for RNs, in particular, show virtually no differences. Only
the data about doctors on call show some differences, as follows:
the EUs of large hospitals are usually more successful than those
of small hospitals (those of medium-sized hospitals occupy an
intermediate position) in their requests for doctors on call; and the
same is true for the EUs of hospitals with medical teaching
affiliations compared to those without such affiliations.

Access to Particular Medical Specialists

In addition to their regular medical and nursing staff, EUs
typically have access, on an on-call basis, to a variety of medical
specialists who are on the staff of the parent hospitals. A complete
picture of EU staff resources, therefore, also requires information
about each unit's access to such specialists.

Information was obtained about ten different specialists. A cardiologist from the parent hospital is available to the emergency unit on call in twenty of the thirty EUs studied (in one case the cardiologist is working within the unit). Similarly, an obstetrician or gynecologist is available on call to sixteen EUs. Fourteen of the thirty EUs (not necessarily the same ones) have similar access to a pediatrician, to a psychiatrist (in one case a psychiatrist is working within the unit), and to an oral surgeon (again, in one case an oral surgeon is working within the unit). And thirteen have access to an ophthalmologist and to an orthopedist (in one case an orthopedist is working within the unit). At the other extreme, only two EUs have access to a specialist in burn medicine, five to a plastic surgeon, and seven to a neurosurgeon.

The rest of the units in each of the above cases apparently have no access, on an on-call basis, to the designated medical specialist within their parent hospital. Overall, access to the designated specialists is more scarce for EUs with a low patient volume, and for the EUs of hospitals that do not have medical teaching affiliations compared to those that do.

Sufficiency and Stability of Resources

Among other things, the hospital administrators (HAs) from the various institutions and the physicians (MDs) working in the EUs were asked to appraise the *sufficiency* of the following resources available to the EUs: (1) medical staffing, (2) RN staffing, (3) the budget allocated to the EUs, and (4) the physical facilities of these units. The respondents were asked to appraise sufficiency "considering what the unit needs to provide high-quality care to its patients at reasonable cost."

The results show that both HAs and MDs regard the *quantity* of each of the four resources as at least "fairly sufficient" on the average, approaching the "very sufficient" level for some of them. Least sufficient of all, according to both HAs and MDs, are the physical facilities of EUs. The two groups also agree that second among the four resources in overall sufficiency is the RN staffing, which is regarded as close to "very sufficient" by the HAs (the grand mean score of the thirty EUs for this variable is 2.33 on a five-point scale in which 1.00 corresponds to "completely sufficient") and almost midway between "very" and "fairly" sufficient by the MDs (the grand mean in this case is 2.43 on the same five-point scale).

The other two resources, however, are appraised differently by the two groups. According to the data from HAs, the budget allocated to EUs is the most sufficient of all four resources, being regarded as almost "very sufficient" (with grand mean score of 2.26). According to MDs, on the other hand, the budget is much less adequate, being regarded as only "fairly sufficient" (with a score of 2.82) and at about the same level as physical facilities. In contrast, the medical staffing of EUs is the most sufficient of the four resources, according to the MDs, who regard it as "very sufficient" (with a score of 2.15). The HAs, on the other hand, regard medical staffing as less sufficient than do the MDs, and also less sufficient than either the budget or the RN staffing of EUs.

These are average patterns, of course, and do not necessarily describe individual EUs. In fact, the data indicate great variability across EUs concerning the sufficiency of each of the resources involved. This is particularly the case in the data from HAs, but even the data from MDs show sizable differences among EUs. Interestingly, the smallest variability according to the data from both HAs and MDs involves the sufficiency of the budget, which apparently differs less from one unit to another than does the sufficiency of each of the other resources. On the other hand, variability is very substantial for both medical and RN staffing, particularly for the former, according to the data from the same two groups.

The quantity of medical staff is generally seen as more sufficient by both HAs and MDs of hospitals that are not church-operated compared to those that are. Similarly, on the average, the EUs of hospitals with medical teaching affiliations are seen, by both MDs and HAs (especially the latter), to have more sufficient medical staffing than the EUs of hospitals lacking such affiliations. Interestingly, however, institutions without medical teaching affiliations have more sufficient RN staffing than institutions with such affiliations, according to the data from HAs (the difference is in the same direction but minimal, according to the data from MDs). The same pattern emerges with respect to both medical and RN staffing, which are seen as more sufficient for EUs located in SMSA/urban areas compared to other communities. Finally, on the average, medical staffing is regarded as least sufficient, by both HAs and MDs, at EUs with a low, compared to a medium or high, patient volume.

The *stability* of staff resources is another important variable considered in the study. Some of the data in this case were obtained from the supervising nurses (SRNs) at the various EUs, in response to the following questions: "Considering both their quantity *and* quality (or adequacy), how *stable* over time would you say are the resources available to the emergency unit?" The question was asked about the physicians and about the nurses working in each unit. On the average, SRNs see the nursing staff of their respective units as "very stable," but depending upon the particular unit the situation ranges from "extremely stable" to only "fairly stable." Stability is even more variable for the medical staff. In this case, the range is from "extremely stable" to "not so stable," although on the average the SRNs see the medical staff as more stable in EUs with a high patient volume and EUs located in SMSA/urban areas. On the stability of either the medical or nursing staff, the data show no differences between institutions with and without medical teaching affiliations, or institutions with and without emergency personnel training programs.

Certain additional data about staff stability were provided by HAs, who were asked to indicate how easy or difficult it is for their respective institutions to "recruit and maintain professional nursing staff for the emergency unit." Overall, the HAs indicated only some difficulty in this connection, reporting midway between "it is fairly easy" and "not as easy as it should be" (but not very difficult). On the average, hospitals apparently do not experience great difficulty in this area. As with other measures, however, here too there are substantial interunit differences, and some institutions experience considerable difficulty while others do not. At the same time, the data show no appreciable differences in this respect among the several groupings of EUs.

Length of service is another indicator of staff stability. In this regard, of all MDs working at the thirty EUs at the time of data collection, 44.3 percent reported having been associated with their respective units four years or more, and 73.6 percent reported having been associated with their units for at least one year. The corresponding figures for RNs, which cover both full- and part-time employees, are 41.8 percent and 73.5 percent, respectively. These results also indicate considerable staff stability and are consistent with the above findings based on the data from SRNs and HAs. (See also related data on staff size and average hours worked below.)

Clinical Staff Size and Hours Worked

Data on medical staff size and physician hours worked in the EUs studied were obtained from hospital records (RECs) and from the physicians (MDs) themselves. These data concern (1) the average number of MDs working in the various EUs, whether full or part time, (2) the total number of hours worked by these MDs, and (3) the average number of hours worked per MD. (Similar data were also obtained about RNs.) It should be noted that the data from RECs refer to the "most recent week" prior to fieldwork for which the information was available at each institution (five hospitals were unable to supply the information). The parallel data provided by MDs, on the other hand, were obtained from those particular doctors who were working in each EU during fieldwork, and with reference to an "ordinary work week."

For the twenty-five EUs for which data from RECs were available, the average number of physicians working in the various units "during the most recent week" was 7.8 per unit (the number ranging across EUs from a low of 1 to a high of 22). During that same week, these physicians worked a combined total of 151 hours (across EUs the number ranges from 25 to 252 hours). And the average number of hours worked per physician was 24.5, ranging across EUs from a low of 3.9 to a high of 48.0 hours. Other things being equal, the higher this number, the more likely it is that a unit has a relatively stable medical staff.

The corresponding numbers and ranges based on the self-reported data by the MDs are 6.8 physicians per EU (range: 3-13 MDs), 124 total hours worked by all these physicians combined (range: 25–231 hours), and an average of 21.1 hours worked by each physician (range: 3.6–28.0 hours), respectively.

As the above ranges suggest, there are large differences among individual EUs in the number of MDs who work there, the total hours worked by them, and the average number of hours worked per MD. According to both sets of data, the number of hours worked per MD is highest, on the average, for EUs with a high patient volume and lowest for EUs with a low patient volume (the medium-volume units occupy an intermediate position). Similarly, it is higher for the EUs of hospitals that are not church-operated compared to those that are, and also for the EUs of hospitals with medical teaching affiliations compared to institutions without such affiliations.

Nonmedical Staffing Pattern and RN Hours Worked. The average number of full-time equivalent (FTE) positions budgeted in the various EUs for registered nurses (including supervising nurses), licensed practical nurses (LPNs), technicians, and other nonmedical personnel turns out to be 13.3 FTE positions. Across institutions, however, this number varies widely, from a low of only 1.0 positions to a high of 31.0 positions. Almost half of these budgeted positions, or an average of 6.6 per EU, are for RNs. An additional 2.8 positions are for LPNs. And, of the remaining FTE budgeted positions, 1.1 are for technicians and 2.8 are for other nonmedical personnel (clerks, secretaries, and the like) working in the EU. All of these figures, which were computed by the research staff, are based on data obtained from hospital records.

For each of the nonmedical groups involved, and all of them combined, the average number of budgeted positions per unit is larger for EUs having a high patient volume (these average a total of 21.6 nonmedical positions each) than for EUs with a medium patient volume (which average 12.4 positions) or a low patient volume (which average only 6.0 positions). The EUs of hospitals in SMSA/urban areas also average a larger number of FTE budgeted positions for nonmedical staff than their counterparts in non-SMSA areas (15.1 versus 9.2). The same pattern holds true for EUs in hospitals with teaching affiliations, and also

emergency personnel training programs, than for their counterparts in hospitals that do not have these characteristics.

Even more important, perhaps, is the fact that all of these
patterns hold true also when one considers RN staffing separately.
As pointed out above, the thirty EUs in the study average a total of
6.6 FTE budgeted positions for RNs, almost exactly half of all the
budgeted positions for nonmedical personnel. Across EUs,
however, this number ranges from a low of 2.5 to a high of 14.3,
indicating great variability in highly skilled nurse staff resources.

Other data from RECs show that the average number of
RNs actually working in the EUs studied during the "most recent
week" was 8.9 per unit, ranging across units from a low of 4 to a
high of 16. These same nurses worked a combined total of 239
hours during that week, the number ranging across EUs from 104
to 568 hours. And the average number of hours worked per RN
was 26.7, ranging across individual units from a low of 10.6 to a
high of 36.0 hours. The corresponding numbers and ranges based
on the self-reported data by the registered nurses working in the
thirty EUs during fieldwork are very similar: 8.8 RNs (range: 4–
17), 242 hours (range: 102–512), and 27.1 hours (range: 17.1–37.3),
respectively.

Both the average number of RNs and the total hours worked
per RN are greater for EUs having a high, compared to medium or
low, patient volume. They are also greater for EUs operated by
hospitals with medical teaching affiliations than hospitals without
them and, to a lesser extent, also for institutions located in SMSA
compared to non-SMSA areas. On the whole, these patterns are
similar to the corresponding medical staff patterns discussed
above, suggesting that some EUs have richer or more stable
clinical staff resources—both medical and nursing.

Clinical Staff Hours in Relation to Patient Volume

Further analysis shows that, for the thirty EUs in the
sample, the ratio of patient visits to RN hours worked (during the
most recent week) averages about 1.50 visits per RN hour worked,
ranging across institutions from a low of 0.57 to a high of 5.25
when using hours from hospital records in the denominator, and

from 0.52 to 4.06 when using self-reported hours by RNs. Other things being equal, a high ratio is likely to indicate that staff resources are being efficiently used, and a low ratio the opposite. It is also possible (but less probable) that a high ratio indicates a heavy workload or insufficient staffing in some cases, while a low ratio indicates exceptionally demanding patient visits. Based on the available evidence from the study, it is not possible to explain the great variability in the obtained ratios on the basis of observed interinstitutional differences in workload or patient composition. More probably, the EUs studied differ very substantially in the work efficiency of their RNs, and this accounts for most of the variability in the obtained ratios. (See also related discussion of the economic efficiency of EUs in Chapter Seven.)

The corresponding ratio of patient visits to physician hours worked averages 2.48 for the thirty EUs when physician hours are taken from hospital records, and 3.26 when self-reported hours by the MDs are used in computing the ratio. (Most of the discrepancy between the two figures is undoubtedly due to the fact that the time base for hours worked is the "most recent week" in the case of the data from RECs compared to "an ordinary work week" in the case of the data from MDs.) The former figure ranges from 0.59 to 4.57 across individual EUs, and the latter ranges from 0.53 to 12.17 visits per physician hour worked. In relation to patient volume, therefore, interinstitutional differences are even greater for physician hours worked than for registered nurse hours worked.

Finally, the ratio of patient visits to physician hours worked is greater for EUs with a high, compared to a low or medium, patient volume; for EUs in church-operated hospitals compared to other hospitals; for EUs in hospitals that have emergency personnel training programs compared to those that do not; and for EUs in SMSA compared to non-SMSA areas. The corresponding patterns for the ratio of patient visits to RN hours worked are very similar, except that in this case the ratio is also higher for EUs in hospitals with medical teaching affiliations compared to hospitals without such affiliations.

Staff Adaptability to Changing Levels of Patient Volume

In recent years, patient volume in EUs has been increasing at a significant rate, and this trend is likely to continue, at least for the foreseeable future. Regardless of this general trend, patient volume at a particular EU may also change from time to time, usually upwards but sometimes downwards as well. One potentially important issue in this connection concerns the relative ability of EUs to handle a considerable increase in patient visits with current staffing levels—without adverse effects on the quality of care. A related issue concerns the likely effect on the quality of care that a comparable decrease in patient visits might have, again assuming current staffing levels.

To explore these issues, certain data were obtained from the MDs and RNs working in the various EUs, and also from the hospital administrators (HAs) of the various institutions. The question asked of these respondents on the first issue was "If, in the next two months, patient visits were to *increase by 10-15 percent* but the quality of patient care were to remain at its current level, how well could the present staff of this emergency unit handle the increased patient volume?" This was followed by a second question: "Considering the number of patients that the staff now sees on an average day, what effect would a *10-15 percent decrease* in patient visits have on the quality of care provided by this emergency unit?"

On the average, MDs believe that their respective units could handle a 10-15 percent increase in patient volume with only "some minor difficulties" (the grand mean for the thirty EUs is 2.07, on a six-point scale in which 1.00 corresponds to "without any difficulties"). At the same time, the capabilities of individual EUs vary considerably (EU mean scores range from 1.20 to 3.50 on the scale used). The RNs are less optimistic than the MDs but, on the average, they too believe that their respective units could handle the increased volume with only "minor" to "moderate" difficulty. The corresponding estimates by HAs indicate an intermediate level of optimism. Overall, then, even though there is considerable variability across EUs, the data indicate that, with present staffing levels, the EUs in the study apparently would be able to respond well to a 10–15 percent increase in patient visits.

The data from the second question indicate that the effect of a 10–15 percent decrease in patient visits on the quality of patient care would be very small. Still, there are considerable interinstitutional differences in this respect. In some of the units, for example, respondents estimate that the quality of care would improve "moderately" to "considerably" (depending upon the group of respondents involved) while in other units it would improve "very little," if at all.

Apparently, on the average, with their current staff, hospital EUs would be able to handle a rather substantial increase in patient volume without any adverse effects on the quality of care, and with only minor to moderate difficulty. The quality of care in the same EUs, on the other hand, would be unlikely to improve significantly following a 10–15 percent reduction in patient volume. These findings suggest that, overall, the staffing levels of EUs at the time of data collection were probably reasonably adequate and sufficient to provide quality care considering the workload (specifically, the quantity of work as represented by the number of patient visits).

Perceived Institutional Strengths and Weaknesses

The final section of this chapter considers the problems and strengths of EUs, as perceived by several key groups. Most of these data were obtained by means of open-ended questions in the personal interviews completed by respondents. Accordingly, they are likely to reflect what these individuals themselves considered salient or significant.

Included at the beginning of each interview were two questions concerning the "most important strengths" and "major problems" of EUs. The problems and strengths actually mentioned in response to these questions were, after preliminary examination, grouped by the research staff into the following categories: organization and supervision; staff resources; nonstaff resources (funds, equipment, and the like); work relations within the EU; staff involvement and satisfaction; costs, charges, and economic efficiency; tension and strain within the EU or between it and other hospital units; staff performance and quality of care; relations with the parent hospital; and relations with the community.

Most Important Strengths of EUs

The question asked about strengths was "What are the *two* or *three* most important areas, or respects, in which you consider this emergency unit to be *particularly strong or especially outstanding?*" It was asked of emergency unit physicians (MDs) and registered nurses (RNs), and of the selected hospital physicians (HMDs) and hospital administrators (HAs).

First, according to the MDs from all thirty EUs combined, their respective units are strongest in staff performance (quality of care) and staff resources, these two areas accounting for about two-thirds of all the strengths mentioned by MDs. These same areas are also the two most frequently mentioned by RNs. Further, staff performance/quality of care is the strength most frequently mentioned by both MDs and RNs not only for the total sample but also when the various groupings of EUs are considered separately. The same pattern, moreover, also is found concerning staff resources.

Three other areas in which the MDs and RNs consider their units as being particularly strong, though less so than in the above two areas, include relations with the parent hospital, relations with the community, and nonstaff resources. Together, the five areas account for 96 percent of all the strengths mentioned by MDs and 90 percent of those mentioned by RNs, when the data from all the thirty EUs are considered. Strengths in all other areas (including those of work relations within the EUs, tension and strain, economic efficiency and costs, staff satisfaction and involvement, and organization and supervision) were mentioned infrequently, not only by MDs and RNs but also by the remaining groups of respondents.

Thus, for example, nearly two-thirds of all the strengths mentioned by HMDs and HAs again are in the areas of staff performance/quality of care and staff resources. These groups, however, mentioned staff resources more frequently than did the MDs and RNs. Other areas in which the HMDs and HAs consider the EUs to be particularly strong include relations with the community, nonstaff resources, and relations with the parent hospital. These three areas were mentioned with about equal frequency by the HMDs, while the HAs mentioned relations with the community more than twice as often as the other two areas. Taken together, the five areas specified account for 93 percent of all the strengths mentioned by HAs and 95 percent of all the strengths mentioned by HMDs. Finally, the top three areas of strength mentioned by the community respondents (CRs) are staff performance or quality of care, relations with the community, and staff resources—in that order.

Obviously, the different groups of respondents show remarkable agreement in their views concerning the major strengths of the EUs in the sample (as they did earlier concerning the goal priorities of EUs). The strengths of a particular EU, of course, may or may not conform to the above patterns, regardless of the specific source(s) of data. Moreover, a complete picture of the strengths and weaknesses of hospital EUs can be developed only after reviewing all of the findings of the study. Nevertheless, the views of the several groups of respondents about the overall strengths of their institutions are very similar.

Patient Perceptions of Strengths

The patients (PATs) who participated in the study as respondents also seem to agree with the other respondent groups concerning the strengths of EUs. Specifically, in response to the question "Thinking back to your visit, what aspects of your experience in the emergency room did you find the most satisfactory?" the patients (from the twenty-eight EUs involved combined) mentioned the following aspects: waiting time or length of visit (19 percent of all responses), the staff's attitudes or actions (18 percent), the quality of care received (14 percent), the EU's staff resources or staff at large (10 percent), the doctors who treated them (8 percent), and the nurses (7 percent) in the emergency unit.

Clearly, staff resources and the quality of care were favorably evaluated by the patients.

Perceived Major Problems or Weaknesses

The specific question asked of respondents about institutional problems was "At the present time, what sorts of problems does the emergency unit of this hospital face? What would you say are the *major* problems or key issues?"

Although some of the greatest strengths of these organizations are in the areas of staff resources and relations with the community, some of their most important problems are also in these areas. According to both MDs and RNs, for example, most of the major problems faced by EUs are concentrated in the area of resources. Specifically, for the thirty EUs in the sample combined, staff resources and nonstaff resources together account for 58 percent of all the problems mentioned by MDs, and 63 percent of those mentioned by RNs. However, staff resources are more problematic than other resources according to the RNs, while the reverse is the case according to the MDs. In some institutions, staff resources were mentioned by some respondents both as a strength (for example, "good medical staff") *and* as a problem (for example, "not enough nurses").

Other areas in which both the MDs and RNs perceived major problems, but on a much smaller scale, include relations with the community (mentioned by 17 percent of the MDs and 9 percent of the RNs), relations with the parent hospital (8 percent of MDs, 9 percent of RNs), and staff performance or quality of care (8 percent of MDs, 6 percent of RNs). Additionally, a few of the problems cited by RNs concern the EU's organization or supervision (8 percent of RNs). In general, however, problems in these latter areas were mentioned much less frequently, by both MDs and RNs, than were problems in the resource areas.

The HMDs and HAs also provided information about the current major problems faced by EUs. Briefly, both of these outside groups of respondents, like the doctors and nurses working in the EUs, mentioned staff resources and nonstaff resources as the top two problem areas. The third most frequently mentioned problem area by both HAs and HMDs is that of relations with the community (the same area that placed third according to MDs). These three areas together account for two-thirds of all the problems mentioned by either HAs or HMDs. Thus, the several groups of respondents show a high degree of agreement about both the problems and strengths of hospital EUs.

In summary, staff performance/quality of care ranks first or second among the most important strengths of EUs mentioned by each of the several groups of respondents. This is consistent with the earlier finding about the emphasis placed by EUs on the quality of patient care as a high goal priority. The area of staff resources is also generally considered as a top strength, occupying first or second place among the strengths most frequently mentioned by respondents (when staff performance places first, staff resources places second, and vice versa). This same area, however, also occupies a prominent place among the current major problems of EUs mentioned by the respondents. Other frequently mentioned strengths include relations with the parent hospital and relations with the community—areas that are also frequently seen as problematic.

Concerning problems, the nonstaff resources of EUs are mentioned first or second most often by all the responding groups (these resources are also seen as one of the top three strengths of EUs by one group, the RNs). The same is true about staff resources. Other problems among the three most frequently mentioned by at least one of the several groups of respondents include relations with the community and relations with the parent hospital. These same areas, however, are also seen as strengths by at least one group of respondents.

Reputation of EUs

Finally, on the assumption that reputation may be a good, though indirect, indicator of institutional strengths/weaknesses, most groups of respondents—including the MDs, RNs, HMDs, and CRs—were asked the following question about their respective EUs: "At the present time, *what kind of reputation* does this emergency unit have in the community outside?" The response alternatives were (1) an excellent reputation, (2) a very good reputation, (3) a good reputation, (4) a fair reputation, and (5) a rather poor reputation.

As might be expected, the reputation attributed to individual EUs by the several groups of respondents varies a great deal—from exactly midway between "excellent" and "very good" on the above scale down to only a "fair reputation" (depending on the particular group of respondents considered). On the average, however, the reputation of the thirty EUs in the sample is evaluated as "good" to "very good" by all four groups of respondents. More specifically, the CRs and MDs evaluate it as almost "very good," and the HMDs and RNs evaluate it as midway between "good" and "very good." The grand means of the mean evaluations given to the thirty EUs by the four groups on the five-point scale used are 2.26, 2.27, 2.49, and 2.55, respectively; and the corresponding ranges of EU mean scores on reputation based on the data from CRs, MDs, HMDs, and RNs are 1.60-3.20, 1.50-3.29, 1.89-3.80, and 1.50-3.71. These results are consistent with the findings about the perceived top strengths of EUs, which include "relations with the community."

According to all four groups of respondents, on the average, the EUs of large hospitals have a better reputation in the community than their counterparts in medium-sized hospitals, which in turn have a better reputation than their counterparts in small hospitals. The reputation attributed to EUs, in other words, appears to correlate positively with the size of the parent hospitals. Even the small hospital EUs, however, are evaluated by all groups as having a slightly better than just "good" reputation on the average.

Similarly, according to all four groups of respondents, the EUs of hospitals with medical teaching affiliations, on the average, have a better reputation in their communities than do their counterparts in hospitals without medical teaching affiliations. Exactly the same pattern holds true, moreover, for the EUs of hospitals that have and do not have emergency personnel training programs. All groups agree, in effect, that the former have a better reputation in the community (considerably better, according to the MDs and RNs) than do the latter. Finally, on the average, the reputation of EUs located in SMSA areas does not differ from the reputation of EUs located in non-SMSA areas, according to the evaluations provided by most of the respondent groups involved. (The relationship of EU reputation to EU effectiveness is discussed in Chapter Seven; for additional details, see Georgopoulos, Cooke, and Associates, 1980.)

In conclusion, it should be noted that not all EUs conform to the above general patterns. Interinstitutional differences concerning the reputation and specific patterns of problems and strengths that characterize particular EUs exist and should be expected. Additionally, certain differences among the views of the several groups of respondents in this connection likewise exist. On the whole, however, these differences are minor; intergroup agreement, as reflected in the patterns of findings just discussed, is high. Regardless of the level of intergroup agreement in any particular area, however, the data generally show considerable interinstitutional differences on most measures and for most areas studied, including the areas of organizational structure, problem solving, and effectiveness.

Summary

This chapter provides a descriptive overview of the distinguishing organizational characteristics of hospital EUs. The selected characteristics form a fairly comprehensive picture of the organizational situation of these health service systems at the time the data were collected. Some changes may have taken place since then on some of the characteristics discussed, but there is no reason to suspect that the basic picture has not remained very similar. Major organizational characteristics in the hospital field such as those considered in this chapter usually change slowly. In any event, since the relationships investigated in this research are all based on measures using data from the same time period, whatever changes may have occurred since the time of fieldwork would not affect the relationships found between the organization and effectiveness of hospital EUs.

Chapter Four

Evaluating Institutional Effectiveness

According to the research model employed, adequate assessment of the effectiveness of hospital EUs at the institutional level requires both multiple criteria and cross-hospital comparisons using properly aggregated data. In addition, of course, it requires valid and reliable measures. In the present study, EU effectiveness was evaluated with data from several independent sources, so as to take into account a number of legitimate perspectives, using not only multiple criteria but also multiple methods of measurement. The primary criteria employed, respectively representing clinical and economic performance, were the quality of patient care, or clinical efficiency, and the cost of service, or economic efficiency. These criteria were assessed at the institutional level, and quality was measured separately for the care provided by the medical and nursing staff at the EUs studied.

Each primary criterion was assessed using several specific measures, which, after careful analysis of their methodological properties (including discriminability, reliability, and validity), were combined into a single index. The resulting index in each case was in turn examined for methodological adequacy and statistically validated against measures that were not incorporated into it but that were expected—on substantive, theoretical, or methodological grounds—to correlate with the criterion being measured by the index.

Although focusing on clinical and economic efficiency as the principal criteria of EU effectiveness, the study also measured five secondary criteria and examined both their interrelationships and relationships to the primary criteria. The secondary criteria were: promptness of medical attention to incoming patients (the inverse of "patient waiting time"); staff satisfaction with the EU, or "social efficiency"; patient satisfaction; emergency unit responsiveness to meeting the community's changing needs and expectations regarding emergency medical services; and institutional reputation in the community for both the EU and its parent hospital. Before we discuss the approach and indices used to measure clinical and economic efficiency, certain issues concerning the concept and assessment of institutional effectiveness should be examined.

The Concept of Effectiveness

Perhaps the most fundamental question in the health services field today is that of institutional effectiveness. Regarding hospital emergency services, organizational researchers do not have established measures or even agreed upon methods for assessing institutional effectiveness. This is also true for hospitals and other complex organizations. Researchers agree, however, that the concept of institutional or system effectiveness is complex and multifaceted rather than unidimensional.

In the present study, the overall effectiveness of a hospital EU is viewed as the joint outcome of economic, clinical, and social performance—an outcome that reflects the relative success with which an EU is able to solve a number of major problems, including adaptation to the environment and system maintenance problems, resource acquisition and allocation problems, coordination and integration problems, and problems of internal strain. In essence, what effectiveness entails is the ability of an EU as a system to achieve and maintain high levels of output, in terms of quality, cost, acceptance, and related aspects, and do so without incapacitating its resources and without undue strain for its members (for a more formal definition of organizational effectiveness, see Georgopoulos, 1975, p. 186).

In complex organizations and institutions having multiple functions and goals, the various aspects of effectiveness may or may not be positively interrelated, and inconsistencies in intercriterion relationships are common (see Seashore, Indik, and Georgopoulos, 1960). Great care is therefore necessary in selecting particular criteria to the exclusion of others. In the present study, the different criteria of EU effectiveness were not expected to correlate highly, or even significantly, with one another, and one interesting task was to ascertain the pattern of relationships among the various criterion measures. Only some of the reasons for this apparent anomaly are found in the complex nature of effectiveness *per se;* others concern the nature of organizational rationality that is characteristic of hospitals and hospital EUs.

Organizational Rationality and System Effectiveness

The level of rationality in a system such as a hospital EU depends upon the quantity and quality of all the knowledge that is used in defining goals and specifying outcomes, in identifying appropriate means or resources for achieving these outcomes, and in evaluating performance. Because knowledge is always imperfect and incomplete and the ability of people to assimilate and process information is finite, the level of rationality that is possible for the system is similarly limited and imperfect. Within these limits, the level of organizational rationality that is feasible depends largely on the degree to which system objectives are agreed upon, understood, and accepted by all the participants—doctors, nurses, administrators—so that all are motivated to work and cooperate toward their accomplishment.

When system goals and priorities are unclear, inconsistent, or incompatible with one another, when means are uncertain, and when the criteria for performance evaluation are ambiguous, multiple, or unstandardized, a high level of organizational rationality is difficult to achieve and maintain. Health service institutions are especially prone to experiencing difficulties of these kinds. Even more generally, however, for organizations having multiple functions and goals, high levels of rationality are not easy to attain. But hospitals and hospital EUs face additional complications in this connection. These stem from the fact that organizational rationality at these institutions encompasses not only economic but also clinical and social components.

Clinical rationality reflects the patient care decisions made in the EU. These are mainly under the control of the doctors, although nurses and others may also contribute. The principal concern is to generate and implement decisions that are expected to meet the clinical needs of patients, as defined by the doctors, or facilitate professional performance. Quality of performance, as defined by current standards of professional practice, is the major if not sole underlying criterion. Financial costs incurred in formulating and implementing clinical decisions generally are of only secondary importance to those who make such decisions. The main objective of clinical rationality, in short, is professional-clinical efficiency. Clinical rationality, however, may promote the quality of patient care but interfere with cost efficiency, which depends upon the economic rationality of the system.

Economic rationality is mainly, if not exclusively, concerned with economic efficiency. It reflects decisions and controls, in both clinical and nonclinical areas, that are likely to maximize the output(s) of the system (for example, the number of emergency patient visits processed), while minimizing the costs of output (which are associated with the system's investment in staff resources, work facilities, and the like). To the extent, however, that these costs are determined by the medical decisions made in the system—decisions that are intended to promote clinical efficiency often without regard for financial considerations or cost consequences—the economic rationality of the system might be jeopardized. The reverse could also occur, of course; an overriding concern for economic rationality could jeopardize clinical efficiency.

Finally, social rationality depends on the extent to which decisions in the system, whether clinical or nonclinical, are based on means-ends considerations which show concern for the participants as individual human beings regardless of their roles or status in the system. From the point of view of the participants—doctors, nurses, administrators, technicians, secretaries—social efficiency means job satisfaction and personal goal attainment in return for their work contributions. From the point of view of the organization, it means maximizing the levels of member motivation, loyalty, and involvement so as to promote cooperation toward the attainment of system objectives. In short, social rationality is intended to promote the social, or social-psychological, efficiency of the system.

The three kinds of rationality are not independent of each other; they are interrelated, but not in a simple manner. Generally, they are not positively correlated or mutually reinforcing (that is, a high level of one kind of rationality does not necessarily imply a high level of another), nor can they substitute or compensate for one another to any significant extent. Some minimal level of each appears to be essential to achieving an overall rationality that can assure or maximize effective organizational functioning. In the present study, the institutional effectiveness of a hospital EU is viewed as the joint outcome of the clinical, economic, and social efficiency levels achieved by the system as a whole—the three kinds of efficiency which correspond to the three components of rationality just discussed.

To the extent that decisions, actions, and problem-solving efforts, in both clinical and nonclinical areas, take all three components of rationality into account, the overall effectiveness of the system should be enhanced. It is extremely difficult, however, for a hospital or hospital EU to maximize all three kinds of rationality and corresponding kinds of efficiency simultaneously. A hospital cannot keep raising the level of patient care quality, for example, while also reducing costs, or even holding costs constant, on a continuing basis. Beyond some upper limit, clinical efficiency cannot be increased without jeopardizing economic efficiency, and vice versa. Until that limit is reached, however, for most hospital EUs there is probably substantial room for improving both economic and clinical efficiency.

Institutional effectiveness requires that no single component of rationality be maximized at the expense of the others, nor be insufficiently taken into account. Ideally, major decisions and actions in the system should take into account all three kinds of rationality at all times. Only then will the overall organizational rationality and institutional effectiveness of the system be optimized.

In practice, of course, a particular institution might intentionally emphasize one type of efficiency (and rationality) at the expense of another. From a theoretical and methodological point of view, however, any assessment of the overall effectiveness of hospital EUs that does not take into consideration all three kinds of efficiency would be seriously incomplete and inadequate. This is not to say that the three should be given equal attention or weight. Clinical efficiency, as reflected in the quality of care provided at the various EUs (and also in the goal priorities of EUs, discussed in Chapter Three), is undoubtedly the most critical component of institutional effectiveness and the single most important criterion to consider. It is the *sine qua non* of effectiveness, however significant the other two criteria might be. From an institutional point of view, economic efficiency is usually more important than social efficiency. In this research, therefore, economic efficiency and clinical efficiency were used as the primary criteria of EU effectiveness, and social efficiency was included among several secondary criteria, recognizing, of course, that a certain level of social efficiency might well be a requisite to achieving high economic and clinical efficiency.

Approaches and Methods for Evaluating the Quality of Care

Although a considerable amount of health services research has been devoted to measuring the quality of patient care in hospital settings, nearly all of this work has been concerned with inpatient care or care in outpatient clinics, and not with the care provided at hospital emergency units. Typically, such research has been concerned with the quality of care at the individual patient (and individual physician) level or for patients in particular diagnosis-related groupings on a case-by-case basis. This also holds true for research on the quality of emergency care (for some interesting research of this kind, see Frazier and Brand, 1979; Greenfield and others, 1981; Pascarelli, 1982). Much less work has been done to measure the quality of care provided to the aggregate of patients at a hospital, an entire inpatient service or outpatient clinic, or a hospital emergency unit as such. Nevertheless, the available research literature concerning the assessment of patient care quality is instructive and will be briefly reviewed at this point, with special emphasis on its relevance to evaluating the quality of care provided at hospital EUs.

Basic Approaches to Assessment

Most approaches to assessing the quality of care or clinical efficiency have focused on either structures, processes, or outcomes (a distinction first made by Donabedian, 1966). Those focusing on structure tend to be concerned with patient care plans and treatment protocols; those focusing on process tend to be concerned with the activities of providers/performers; and those focusing on outcomes tend to be concerned with the impact of structures or processes, being particularly dependent (in a relatively direct way) on the appropriateness of clinical activities and on how well such activities are performed. Some approaches, of course, have relied on combinations of structure, process, and outcome measures (see, for example, Flood, Scott, Ewy, and Forrest, 1982; Forrest, Scott, and Brown, 1976; Scott, Forrest, and Brown, 1976).

Structure-Based Measures. Most measures of the quality of care considered to be structure-based overlap the domain of other problem areas as conceptualized in the present study. For example, Donabedian's (1966) list of structural measures includes such variables as the adequacy of facilities and equipment, the qualifications of medical staff, and the organization of medical staff. Other structure-based measures include staff/patient ratios, timeliness of supportive services, indicators of staff skill, and the like. Generally, however, these measures are not direct indicators of patient care quality; rather, they are concerned with how the organization is set up to perform the patient care task.

Some structure-based measures have focused on patient care plans or treatment protocols. Gibson, Bugbee, and Anderson (1970), for example, analyzed the operation of hospital emergency services in terms of written policies, both clinical and administrative, and the recency with which these policies had been revised. The policies and protocols examined were considered relevant to such things as professional responsibility, permissible treatment, conditions under which definitive treatment cannot be provided, use of observation beds, treatment permits, wound closure, and transfer to other hospitals.

Process Measures. Measures of process typically focus on the activities of performers, primarily doctors or nurses. For example, Brook and Appel (1973) attempted to assess the therapeutic process by questioning physicians as to whether the process was adequate or inadequate. Brook and Stevenson (1970) estimated the adequacy of diagnostic and therapeutic processes, using criteria developed for the diagnosis and minimum treatment of various diseases. Williamson (1971) similarly studied diagnostic processes— procedures carried out in order to furnish the doctor with facts on which to base his diagnosis—and therapeutic processes (planning, implementing, evaluating). Payne and others (1976) developed a "physician performance index" (also used by Rhee, 1976) based on disease-specific criteria and the following aspects: history, physical examination, lab and radiology tests, special procedures, and therapy. Lewis and others (1969), using a "critical incident technique," related critical incidents to outcomes such as disability, discomfort, and satisfaction. In the field of emergency care, Kresky (1982) recommends using process measures.

The common denominator for all of these process-based measures is their focus on the work activities of performers. Though free from some of the difficulties associated with structure-based measures, process-linked measures do present problems. First, their precise relationship to patient outcome is unclear. Second, some of the activities performed by physicians may not be directly related to, or even contribute to, changes in the condition of the patient. Third, process measures are often based on records (typically on retrospective reviews of records), which are seldom complete or unproblematic; the nonuniformity and variable quality of medical records make it difficult to assess the activities of performers accurately or in sufficient detail. Fourth, the cost of collecting data on clinical activities from records or through observation often outweighs the benefits. Reliable data on the quality of staff activities are probably easier and less costly to obtain from the performers (that is, the doctors and nurses involved) and their co-workers and peers. Further, such data can be as accurate, reliable, and valid as data from records in assessing clinical efficiency.

Outcome Measures. Compared to measures of process, measures that focus on outcomes may provide a more direct indication of change in patient condition but a less direct indication of clinical staff performance. Further, outcome measures do not necessarily reflect only those changes resulting from clinical services to a patient during the EU visit but may also reflect changes due to patient behavior and to follow-up care, including self-care at home. Outcome measures may be confounded by the characteristics of patients, the severity of condition, and the extent to which the problems of patients had progressed ("staging") by the time of entry into the EU.

Ideally, of course, outcome measures should closely reflect the effects of clinical practices and services. Donabedian (1966) refers to such measures as "situation-specific proximate" outcomes—measures that are somewhat between process measures and measures of patients' end-states after the patients have left the care-delivery unit. Most outcome measures, however, have not been situation-specific proximate measures, although they have focused on end-states. Some researchers, for example, have used a continuum of states or stages that ranges from complete recovery to death (see, for example, Shapiro, 1967; Lewis and others, 1969; Brook and Stevenson, 1970; Williamson, 1971; Forrest, Scott, and Brown, 1976). The present study makes use of a similar kind of continuum—the patient management continuum (see Chapter Six).

One frequently used outcome measure is death rate. This may be a more economical, but less sensitive, measure than other measures based on the continua described above, particularly for assessing quality of care in hospital EUs. Roemer, Moustafa, and Hopkins (1968) used death rate adjusted for case severity for measuring the quality of care provided to hospital patients. Severity-adjusted death rates also have been used by Neuhauser (1971) and by Goss and Reed (1974), who questioned the validity of the death rate measure because they did not find it to be related to variables such as the technical adequacy, control status, and teaching status of the hospital. They advocate using case fatality rates instead, that is, the deaths attributed to a given diagnosis expressed as a percentage of deaths for all diagnoses treated. Neuhauser suggests using measures of disability, infection rate, and adverse drug reactions. Others (for example, Shortell, Becker, and Neuhauser, 1976) suggest using medical-surgical death rates and postoperative complication rates. None of these approaches, however, is appropriate for measuring, at the institutional level, the quality of patient care provided at hospital EUs, where patient stay is shorter than one day.

Generally, outcome measures such as death rates are determined only in part by staff performance. They are also determined by the patient's condition (medical, demographic, social, economic) and behavior and by other factors (for example, facilities), as well as by the interaction of these variables. In addition, some outcome measures require following up and assessing the patient's condition after discharge and so are expensive and relatively inappropriate for measuring the quality of hospital emergency services.

Other Approaches. Other measures of quality focus on "overall" care rather than on specific structures, processes, or outcomes. Georgopoulos and Mann (1962), for example, developed a measure of overall care based on ratings of the quality of medical and nursing care by the medical and nursing staff in general hospitals, which they validated using a panel of experts and other data. Similar measures have been used by Denton and others (1967), Neuhauser (1971), Shortell, Becker, and Neuhauser (1976), and Payne and others (1976). The major advantages of such measures are that (1) they can be used to assess quality for large aggregates of patients or at the institutional level (rather than just at the individual patient level or for a given diagnosis) and (2) they are relatively inexpensive and reliable indicators at least of perceived quality. They are therefore not only useful but probably also indispensable for assessing quality at the institutional level. For the reasons specified above, some of the measures developed in the present study used ratings by doctors and registered nurses of the quality of medical and nursing care provided to patients in their respective EUs.

In the present research, several major aspects of EU effectiveness were considered, and, correspondingly, multiple criteria were used to assess effectiveness at the institutional level. Moreover, EU effectiveness was examined from several points of view, using data not only from the medical and nursing staff but also from other key groups in the hospital, from patients, and even from selected individuals in the community, in addition to data from records. The principal criteria of institutional effectiveness, of course, were clinical efficiency and economic efficiency, the former as reflected in the quality of patient care provided to EU patients. Because clinical efficiency is considerably more complex and more difficult to evaluate than economic efficiency, the study relied on both previously used approaches and on new methods, as discussed in Chapters Five and Six. A summary of previously used methods and techniques to measure patient care quality is presented next.

Data Collection Methods and Measurement Techniques

Researchers have used many data collection techniques in their efforts to measure the quality of patient care in hospital settings. Generally, however, three major methods have been employed: (1) review of existing documents, such as the patient's medical record (for example, Morehead, 1967; Roemer, Moustafa, and Hopkins, 1968; Sanazaro and Williamson, 1970); (2) observation of ongoing activities in the patient care setting with information recorded at prescribed intervals over time (for example, Haussman, Hegyvary, and Newman, 1976); and (3) surveys relying on questionnaires or interview data from clinical staff and others (for example, Georgopoulos and Mann, 1962; Neuhauser, 1971; Payne and Lyons, 1972; Payne and others, 1976; Shortell, Becker, and Neuhauser, 1976).

Medical records have been a frequent source of data for assessing quality. Peer reviews and audits of various kinds have relied heavily on such records (for example, see Morehead, 1967; Sanazaro and Williamson, 1970; Williamson, 1971; Avery and others, 1976). The main problem with medical record reviews, as Peterson (1963) pointed out long ago, is finding relevant and accurate data in records that are sufficiently specific and comparable across situations. Other problems include incompleteness and the fact that the medical record may not truly reflect what was actually done or not done by the performers. Richardson (1972) has delineated several obstacles that need to be overcome in using records, even when judgments are made by qualified experts. These obstacles include personal clinical bias, careless record review in which information is overlooked, misinterpretations of recorded events, geographical differences in stringency of judgments, and reluctance by some judges to criticize their peers.

Observation is a relatively infrequently used, and also costly and cumbersome, method of data collection for assessing clinical efficiency. In one of the few studies using this method, Lewis and others (1969) relied on observations based on a "critical incident technique." Observing their own work, nurses recorded information on the date and time that a decision-making problem arose and on the critical question as seen by the nurse; additional data about the management of the patient were also recorded. In another study (Johnson and Rosenfeld, 1969), trained observers recorded average time spent by clinical staff in the examining room. More recently, in a study attempting to assess the quality of nursing care (Haussman, Hegyvary, and Newman, 1976), nurse observers filled out work sheets on a 10 percent sample of patients. The work sheets contained subsets of criteria from a master list.

In reviewing studies based on observation, Peterson (1963) pointed out that the major problems are cost, observer bias, and reproducibility. The latter two problems can be reduced by increasing the observation period (a minimum of two or three days might be necessary for adequate agreement among observers); an increase in the observation period, however, exacerbates the problem of cost. Moreover, for comparative studies such as the present one, covering relatively large numbers of patients or institutions, observation would be so cumbersome and inefficient as to be unsuitable. For measuring quality at the system or institutional level, in short, observation could not be the method of choice.

Finally, survey methods employing interviews and questionnaires have been used in a variety of ways to measure the quality of care, in most cases relying on physicians and nurses as primary data sources (for example, Georgopoulos and Mann, 1962;

Denton, 1967; Neuhauser, 1971; Payne and Lyons, 1972; Payne and others, 1976; for a critique and evaluation of the usefulness of such measures, see Price, 1972). The clinical judgment approach employed by Georgopoulos and Mann (1962) in a comparative organizational survey of general hospitals, for example, relied on structured interviews and questionnaires for obtaining evaluations of the quality of medical care and nursing care from physicians and professional nurses. These measures were then validated with expert ratings and other data. Klein, Malone, Bennis, and Berkowitz (1961) used interviews with administrators to obtain ratings of difficulty of illness, medical management, and the quality of care provided in outpatient clinics. Berkowitz and others (1962) used a similar interview method with experts, clinicians, and patients. In another study, Neuhauser (1971) administered questionnaires to expert evaluators to obtain quality of medical care ratings on a five-point scale. More recently, among other methods, Scott, Forrest, and Brown (1976) administered questionnaires to patients to assess their recovery.

One major advantage of the survey method is the feasibility and economy of gathering evaluative data from a variety of relevant respondents, large samples of individuals and institutions, and different care-delivery settings. Still another advantage is that, properly used, this method yields measures of both good reliability and apparent validity. As with all other methods, however, the question of validity has not been definitely settled. Nevertheless, in combination with the "quasitracer patient conditions" approach employed by the present study, the questionnaire and interview method seemed especially suitable.

Evaluation Perspectives, Controls, and Adjustments

Just as there are different methods for measuring the quality of care or clinical efficiency, so there are different legitimate (or at least useful) perspectives: the perspective of the performers (doctors and nurses), their professional peers, the patients, outside experts, and others. Accordingly, researchers have to guard not only against method variance but also against "bias," or variance associated with the perspectives of evaluators. For example, doctors may give greater weight to diagnostic performance and less weight to socioemotional care compared to nurses. On the other hand, doctors and nurses may weigh medical treatment considerations about equally.

Further, patients' evaluations of quality of care and their own satisfaction may or may not correlate with physician or nurse evaluations of the same variables. Patients may give a great deal of weight to such things as discomfort experienced, waiting time, and personal attention received but be unable to judge the clinical performance of their doctors and nurses. Similarly, outside experts may rely disproportionately on ideal or normative standards, paying little attention to situation-specific constraints, compared to peer reviewers from within the same institution as the performers.

How much and how systematically the perspectives turn out to differ in particular studies of particular settings such as the EU are empirical questions. It is not likely, however, that measures of quality associated with these different perspectives would be totally unrelated or mutually exclusive. For one thing, with the exception of patients' evaluations, all other perspectives involve professional clinical judgment and a technical knowledge base that is shared by the evaluators to one extent or another.

Still, apart from the problem of method variance, the issues of bias, unreliability, and the like must be carefully considered. Good methodological studies concerned with these issues in a major or systematic way are rare in the patient care literature, and those that are available generally involve peer review measures (for example, see Neuhauser, 1971; Williamson, 1971; Richardson, 1972; Brook and Appel, 1973; Payne and others, 1976). Nevertheless, the importance of relying on multiple perspectives is obvious. Thus, in their study of institutional differences in the quality of surgical care, Scott, Forrest, and Brown (1976) included the patient's own assessment of ability to return to normal functioning, in addition to various outcome and process measures not based on patient responses. Similarly, the clinical judgment approach used by Georgopoulos and Mann (1962) relied on evaluations by physicians, professional nurses, and others, while also pooling the data provided by the different groups of performers.

Often, regardless of approach, method, or perspective employed, the measures used to assess quality of care or clinical efficiency are confounded by extraneous factors or suffer from lack of comparability, the latter being an especially troublesome problem in comparative analyses. Accordingly, some studies have made an effort to control or adjust for "case-mix" in order to improve the comparability of measures. For example, Gibson (1976) concluded that it is important to control for patient characteristics and the severity of the patient's illness in developing outcome measures in EU settings. Avery and others (1976) reviewed two techniques of controlling for factors that may influence outcomes but are beyond the control of the care-delivery unit. One is the so-called "staging" technique in which patients are allocated into subgroups on the basis of relative risk of adverse outcomes associated with the patient's condition at the time of arrival (see also Scott, Forrest, and Brown, 1976). The second is a multivariate technique that adjusts separately for each factor (for example, patient age, sex, socioeconomic status) that may affect the outcome in spite of the quality of care given.

In their study of interinstitutional differences in the quality of surgical care, the Stanford Center for Health Care Research staff used as "controls" patient characteristics such as age, sex, physical status, and extent of the disease to predict the probability of a poor outcome. Scott, Forrest, and Brown (1976), of the Stanford group, also used a sample of physicians as expert raters to determine the difficulty and uncertainty of various types of operating procedures (see also Flood, Scott, Ewy, and Forrest, 1982; Forrest, Scott, and Brown, 1976). Controls for severity have been used by a number of other researchers: Shortell, Becker, and Neuhauser (1976) asked a panel of eleven physicians to rate the probability of death for certain conditions on a four-point scale; a study by Semmlow and Cone (1976) included an injury severity score based on the area of body burned; and Feller and Crane (1970) conducted an empirical study to estimate survival for burn patients based on the patient's age and size/depth of burn (see also Feller, Flora, and Bawol, 1976).

According to Krischer (1976), most severity indices sum severity subscores based on attributes that describe the patient's illness or injury (for example, location) and the characteristics of the patient (for example, age, sex, medical history). In the Cumulative Index Rating Scale developed by Linn, Linn, and Gurel (1968), impairment scores for each of twenty-three organ areas were summed to form the index. Krischer points out that such indices are based on two major assumptions: "ordinality" (the severity index for one profile of subscores is greater than or equal to the same severity index for a second profile of subscores if and only if the severity of the first profile is greater than or equal to the severity of the second profile); and "additivity" (the different subscores make independent contributions to the composite severity index). He further points out that while the majority of severity indices violate these assumptions, they still are useful. For example, although the Injury Severity Score (ISS) developed by Baker and others (1968) does not conform to the assumptions of additive value functions, Semmlow and Cone (1976) report data from a sample of 8,850 patients, collected from the Illinois Trauma Registry, showing that the ISS bears a strong linear relationship to mortality rates, length of stay, and percentage of patients requiring major surgical procedures.

Finally, one way of controlling for patient case-mix is to use high-homogeneity conditions as "tracers." Kessner, Kalk, and Singer (1973) used this method to evaluate neighborhood health centers in terms of how well they reached at-risk populations (for example, to assess how well hypertensive adult males in the community were being treated). These researchers also specified a number of criteria for selecting tracers: (1) tracers should be relatively well defined and easy to diagnose; (2) prevalence of the condition used as tracer should be high enough to permit adequate study; (3) the condition under study should be sensitive to the quality or quantity of care received; and (4) the techniques for the professional management of the condition should be well defined.

The present study of hospital emergency services developed and made use of a similar, or analogous, approach—the "quasi-tracer patient conditions approach"—on which it relied heavily for assessing the quality of care (see Chapter Five). Although the measures of quality obtained through this approach have a built-in adjustment for patient case-mix and severity, two additional measures of severity were also considered. One of these concerns the proportion of emergency patients who, after arriving at the EU, were admitted to one of the hospital's intensive care units or were sent to the operating room. The other involves the proportion of patients who arrived at the EU by ambulance. Both measures are probably indicative of the severity as well as the complexity of patient inputs and therefore seemed important to explore.

Economic Efficiency

Although conceptually economic efficiency is a much simpler phenomenon than clinical efficiency, operationally it also presents a variety of difficulties. Some of these are associated with the unavailability of required data at many health care institutions. Others concern the accuracy or comparability of available data, and still others concern the merit of different measurement options.

The term *efficiency,* of course, always implies a ratio (generally a ratio of input to output or investment to return), but the question of how to measure the terms of this ratio, especially the numerator, presents unresolved problems and unsettled issues, particularly in the health services field. Health care economists are not in agreement in this regard, and their orientations and preferences vary considerably. More important, when the present study was undertaken, past research was of little direct relevance to the measurement of the overall economic efficiency of hospital EUs. The project's consulting economists (Sylvester I. Berki and Paul J. Feldstein) agreed with each other and others in the field that, all things considered, the number of patient visits to the EU probably would be the best and most appropriate measure of output (that is, the denominator of the ratio), and their recommendation was followed.

With this issue resolved at the outset, the study considered several measurement options regarding economic efficiency, including the use of one or more of the following: (1) gross staff productivity or staff hours worked in relation to output during a particular time period; (2) payroll costs in relation to output; (3) charges for patient care (hospital charges, physician fees) per patient visit; (4) some adaptation of Feldstein's (1967) "costliness index"; and (5) some measure of "cost per case," such as that used by Shuman, Wolfe, and Hardwick (1972) or by Lave, Lave, and Silverman (1972). The first three options would yield measures of economic efficiency that do not control for patient case-mix; the last two would yield measures that do. Given the economic and financial data actually available at the institutions studied, however, the last two options did not prove feasible, whatever their merits.

In the end, after careful consideration of several alternatives and associated problems, especially problems relating to the quality and availability of relevant data, the index developed in the present study to assess the economic efficiency of hospital EUs incorporates a total of four specific measures, as follows: (1) physician time per patient visit to the EU (an indicator of physician productivity); (2) registered nurse time per patient visit to the EU; (3) total EU payroll expenditures, for all personnel except physicians, per patient visit; and (4) "current total costs to the hospital of an average patient visit to the EU," as estimated/calculated by each institution. The first three measures were computed by the research staff using relevant data from institutional records in each case. (Complete data were available for twenty-six of the thirty EUs in the sample.) The index and measures used for economic efficiency are discussed in detail in Chapter Seven.

Social Efficiency and Other Critiera

Finally, in addition to the primary criteria of clinical and economic efficiency, the present research measured and examined five secondary criteria each of which was considered, on both pragmatic and scientific grounds, to be a potentially important indicator of institutional effectiveness. These include staff satisfaction with the EU (for both doctors and nurses), an important indicator of the social efficiency of hospital EUs; patient satisfaction with the care received; promptness of medical attention to incoming patients; EU responsiveness in meeting the community's changing needs and expectations regarding emergency medical services (a measure of organizational adaptation); and the reputation of EUs in their respective communities according to the selected community respondents (CRs) and the patients (PATs) who participated in the study.

Each of these secondary criteria was considered interesting and important in its own right to include. Some of them (for example, patient satisfaction) are of significant interest to many in the emergency medical services field. Equally important, given the current state of knowledge in this area, it was deemed methodologically desirable to use several criteria such as these for the purpose of complementing, and to some extent also validating, the primary criteria. In addition, the secondary criteria specified represent legitimate perspectives that ought to be explicitly acknowledged and, if possible, taken into account when evaluating the overall effectiveness of hospital EUs. Finally, most of these criteria are relatively easy to measure. The nine specific measures used in the study to represent the five secondary criteria of EU effectiveness are described in Chapter Eight, following the discussion of the primary criteria and their measurement in Chapters Five, Six, and Seven.

Summary

Discussed in this chapter were the concept of institutional effectiveness, as it pertains to hospital emergency services, and some of the underlying rationality issues that it entails; the problem of assessing EU effectiveness by focusing on such major criteria as economic, clinical, and social efficiency; and certain approaches and methods for evaluating the quality of patient care at the institutional level.

Chapter Five

Clinical Efficiency:
The Quality of Patient Care

Evaluation of the quality of patient care provided at the various EUs turned out to be a complex and difficult task, in part because it required measurement at the institutional level rather than just at the individual patient/individual physician level. Since no standard or generally acceptable methodologies were available for assessing the quality of either medical or nursing care, apart from the widely held view that at least partial reliance on medical "peer judgment" at some point in the process is indispensable, the study found it necessary to devise its own methods, including the "quasitracer patient conditions" approach discussed below. The measurement procedures developed also had to take into account the possibility of major case-mix differences among EUs, and especially the possibility that the level of severity of patient problems treated might differ significantly from one EU to another. Finally, the specific measures used had to be statistically valid and reliable as well as substantively meaningful and appropriate to all EUs.

In view of these considerations and the discussion in Chapter Four, the index developed to assess the quality of medical care at the institutional, or EU, level incorporates three measures: (1) an evaluation of the quality of medical care by significant peers from the parent hospital (namely, the HMDs group of selected hospital physicians, described in Chapter Two), that is, peers of the physicians (MDs) who were actually providing this care at each EU; (2) a rating of the quality of medical care by the registered nurses (RNs) working at each EU, that is, by significant co-workers of the MDs who were the principal performers; and (3) the quasitracer patient conditions measure. This last measure is based on data provided by EU MDs and RNs concerning each of ten carefully selected diagnosis-related groupings of EU patients, referred to in this study as quasitracer patient conditions or "quasitracers." Briefly described, this is a composite measure of the quality of medical care provided at each EU to the aggregate of patients in the ten quasitracer conditions combined. It is also a measure of quality that is adjusted for patient volume and that takes into account, in a meaningful way, the relative severity of the patients' medical problems, thus assuring high comparability of measurement across EUs.

The quality of nursing care at the EU level was assessed using similar procedures. The final index in this case also incorporates three measures: (1) an evaluation by emergency unit MDs and RNs of the quality of nursing care provided to patients in the above ten quasitracer conditions; (2) a rating of the quality of nursing care at each EU compared to the EUs of other institutions, based on data from RNs; and (3) a measure that combines an evaluation by physicians of RN performance and a noncomparative rating by MDs and RNs of the nursing care that patients generally receive at each unit.

Finally, for methodological reasons, the medical care index and the nursing care index were also combined into a single overall index of the quality of patient care provided at the various EUs. The measures and index of the quality of medical care will be discussed first.

The Quality of Medical Care

In developing and validating measures that would make it possible to compare hospital EUs on the quality of their patient care, the research relied on several different sources of data and analysis techniques and on several legitimate perspectives.

Institutional and patient records constitute useful but inadequate sources of relevant information for assessing the "medical management of patients" or medical care quality.

Seldom are they sufficiently complete, fully auditable, or satisfactorily standardized to provide the necessary data for generating measures of acceptable validity, reliability, and comparability. Further, however accurate and comprehensive, records are best suited to "retrospective review" or the evaluation of past work and do not necessarily reflect the quality of current clinical performance. Even when excellent records are available, medical judgment must still be relied upon when selecting evaluation standards or specifying variables that would best depict the quality of patient care. Finally, assessing the quality of care at the institutional level through the analysis of patient records is not only a debatable but also a very costly procedure when doing comparative studies of more than a few institutions.

In view of these considerations, the decision in this research was that records should be used, but not as the sole or even main source of data. Interviews and questionnaires completed by the physicians working in the thirty EUs, that is, the principal performers in each case, served as another important source of information. It was also recognized, however, that to some degree the performers might be biased or, worse yet, differentially biased across EUs. Accordingly, evaluations of the quality of medical care were also obtained from the performers' professional peers, namely, selected key physicians (HMDs) from each EU's parent hospital who had contact with, or personal knowledge about, the EU but were not associated with it. (The selected HMDs were described in Chapter Two.) In addition, similar evaluations were obtained from the principal co-workers of the performers, namely, from the registered nurses (RNs) working at each EU (both full time and part time, including those in supervising positions). The selected physicians and registered nurses provided data as knowledgeable "observers" of medical performance and its outcomes at their respective hospital EUs. Finally, information from certain other sources, including various records and the recent EU patients (PATs) who participated in the study, was also used, but only for validation purposes.

Ultimately, four measures of the quality of medical care were developed. Two of these are relatively simple measures, respectively based on ratings by the HMDs and RNs. The third measure is based on data from EU physicians (MDs) and registered nurses (RNs) about ten categories of patients that were used in this study as quasitracer patient conditions. The fourth measure is a composite one, incorporating the other three. It constitutes an index of the quality of medical care at the EU level and is used in this research as the main measure of patient care quality.

Evaluation of Medical Care by Significant Peers: Measure 1

In the personal interviews that they completed for the study, the selected physicians (HMDs) from the parent hospital of each EU were asked, among other things, to rate the quality of medical care provided at the EU. The specific question was "On the basis of your experience and information, how would you rate the *quality of medical care* that patients generally receive in this emergency unit? Would you rate it excellent, very good, good, fair, or rather poor?" These physicians had no difficulty responding. The data provided by the HMDs were subsequently quantified by assigning corresponding scale values to the five response alternatives, 1 for "excellent" through 5 for "rather poor."

Based on these data, a mean rating score was computed separately for each of the thirty hospital EUs. As expected, these mean scores were found to vary considerably across EUs, from 1.22 (belonging to the best-scoring EU) to 3.14. On this measure, the grand mean for the thirty EUs (the average of the thirty scores) turned out to be 2.08, with a standard deviation of .45. Further analysis shows that the between-EU variance in the obtained ratings is significantly greater than the within-EU variance (F = 2.81, df = 29, 178, $p < .01$) and η^2 = .31. In addition to discriminating well among institutions, therefore, Measure 1 is an appropriate one at the EU level and has acceptable reliability. If the validity of the medical peer judgment perspective that this measure reflects is also adequate, the mean ratings in question can be regarded as one acceptable measure of medical care quality at the EU level.

Evaluation of Medical Care by Knowledgeable
Co-Workers: Measure 2

A second measure was derived from the responses of RNs working in each EU—the principal co-workers of EU physicians—

to the following question: "On the basis of your experience and information, how would you rate the quality of *medical care* that patients generally receive in this emergency unit?" Response alternatives were (1) outstanding, (2) excellent, (3) very good, (4) good, (5) fair, (6) rather poor, and (7) poor. This item was included in the self-administered questionnaire that RNs were asked to complete immediately following their personal interview for the study.

Based on these data, mean scores were again computed for each of the thirty EUs. These range across institutions from 1.75 to 3.57 and average 2.71, with a standard deviation of .43. Accordingly, this measure also discriminates well among EUs. Further, the between-EU variance on the obtained ratings is significantly greater than the within-EU variance (F = 2.24, df = 29, 242, $p <$ .01), and η^2 = .21. These results, which are statistically similar to those concerning Measure 1, suggest that Measure 2 is also satisfactory for representing the quality of medical care at the EU level.

In summary, the above measures are appropriate at the institutional level and discriminate well among the EUs studied, each showing considerable interhospital differences in the quality of medical care provided by EUs. The significant response agreement (η^2) found within EUs in each case, moreover, indicates that they are reliable measures. Additionally, these two criterion measures correlate positively and significantly with each other (r = .49, $p <$ .01, N = 30 EUs), as they should on methodological grounds: EUs scoring high (low) on one measure are likely also to score high (low) on the other. Given the independent sources of data involved, this correlation obviously constitutes an important finding; it shows convergent validity for the two measures. Finally, as will be shown below, the same two measures also correlate significantly (r = .42 and $p <$ .05, and r = .59 and $p <$ .01, respectively) with the third measure of medical care.

Quality of Medical Care in Ten Quasitracer
Patient Conditions: Measure 3

The third measure included in the index of the quality of medical care required more complex procedures. It is a measure of quality adjusted for patient volume that was obtained by means of a new approach to assessing the quality of patient care at the institutional level—the "quasitracer patient conditions approach."

Conceivably, the quality of care at different institutions might vary to some extent simply because the level of difficulty of the patient problems varies. Although Measures 1 and 2 may be satisfactory on most counts, they only implicitly take into account possible major differences in patient case-mix, that is, in the heterogeneity and severity of patient conditions. Presumably, the HMDs and RNs did take these factors into consideration when rating the quality of medical care, but it is not certain that they did so satisfactorily from a methodological standpoint. Therefore, it was important to develop another measure of quality—one that could deal with this problem explicitly and systematically and make it possible to ensure rigorous equivalence with respect to comparability across EUs.

The quasitracer patient conditions approach was designed to yield results of high comparability across hospitals while taking into account both patient volume and patient case-mix in a meaningful way. Briefly, the approach called for (1) judicious selection of a manageable number of diagnostic categories or patient conditions with differing medical care requirements across conditions but similar requirements within conditions; (2) collection of certain data about the number of patients treated in each condition; and (3) appropriate evaluations of the quality of care given to these patients, condition by condition, at each of the thirty EUs in the sample. In other words, this measure of medical care quality at the EU level would "control for" the severity of patient problems treated.

Because severity may vary greatly from one diagnostic category to another, it was important that the measure reflect the quality of care given to patients in each of a number of such categories—a number sufficient to "represent" much of the range of problems typically treated at an EU. Ideally, selected categories should differ in terms of accompanying care requirements but still encompass patients whose conditions would be fairly similar in severity within categories. Moreover, each category should be specific or homogeneous enough to have the same medical meaning across institutions. Furthermore, it would be important to select both patient conditions for which clear and precise medical treatment protocols are generally in use (for example, myocardial infarction) and conditions for which treatment protocols are much less standardized across institutions (for example, psychiatric illnesses). Finally, conditions likely to be well managed from a medical standpoint as well as conditions that might not be well managed should both be represented.

On the basis of these considerations, a review of the emergency care literature, advice from two medical consultants to the study (Beverly C. Payne, M.D., and Paul Y. Ertel, M.D.), and suitable pretesting, a total of ten patient categories/diagnostic groupings, hereafter referred to as "quasitracer patient conditions," were finally selected and used. Included among them are both trauma and nontrauma conditions, conditions of high and low incidence of emergency patient visits, conditions requiring highly specialized or complex treatment procedures as well as conditions requiring more routine medical attention, conditions for which explicit medical standards are widely accepted and others for which standards are less well defined, and conditions involving not only internal medicine and surgery but also pediatrics, gynecology, and other services.

As a set, the selected quasitracer conditions were expected not only to account for a significant proportion of the total patient input of each EU in the sample but also to reflect reasonably well the quality of medical care provided to all patients at the EUs studied. The particular quasitracer conditions chosen are shown below in their exact wording, format, and order of presentation to respondents (Exhibit 5-1).

Three of the selected quasitracers may appear unusual to some readers: Drug abuse cases were selected because of the deep social concern about them and because there was reason to believe that hospital EUs are not well prepared to deal adequately with such problems. Rape cases were chosen because they entail both medical and psychological care requirements. Further, according to some previous research (Geis, Chappel, and Cohen, 1975), most rape cases are treated in the emergency room at most hospitals, and treated rather poorly according to another study (Welch, 1975).

Exhibit 5-1. Quasitracer Condition Question on Medical Management.

Please consider the patients in the categories specified who visited this emergency unit over the *past four-six weeks*. On the average, *how well were these patients managed from a medical standpoint*? (Check one for each category.)

The Medical Management of Emergency Patients in This Category Was:

Category (Condition):	Excellent (1)	Very good (2)	Good (3)	Fair (4)	Rather poor (5)	There were no such patients (0)
Acute myocardial infarction, cardiac arrest, and ventricular fibrillation cases	☐	☐	☐	☐	☐	—
Lacerations of the face or neck involving *more than skin*	☐	☐	☐	☐	☐	—
Acute psychiatric illnesses—suicide (depression), acute psychoses	☐☐	☐☐	☐☐	☐☐	☐☐	—
Fractures or dislocations	☐☐	☐☐	☐☐	☐☐	☐☐	—
Acute upper respiratory infections with stridor, epiglottitis, and asthmatic bronchitis cases	☐☐	☐☐	☐☐	☐☐	☐☐	—
Rape cases	☐☐	☐☐	☐☐	☐☐	☐☐	—
Infants *with* blood disorders, dehydration, congenital anomalies, or respiratory distress syndrome	☐	☐	☐	☐	☐	—
Spinal injuries or closed head injuries *with* subdural hematomas or neurologic deficit	☐☐	☐☐	☐☐	☐☐	☐☐	—
Drug abuse cases	☐☐	☐☐	☐☐	☐☐	☐☐	—
Burns of the face, ears, hands, feet, or perineum, *and* burns involving 10% or more of total body surface area with 2%	☐	☐	☐	☐	☐	

Finally, respiratory infections were selected because they are often said to "clutter" hospital emergency rooms and because of the trend toward increased use of emergency care facilities for nonemergency care.

The question in Exhibit 5-1, designed to elicit evaluations of the quality of "medical management of patients" (that is, the quality of medical care) in each quasitracer condition, was asked of the MDs and RNs working in each of the thirty EUs. It was included in the questionnaire forms that respondents from these two groups filled out (individually and privately) immediately after their personal interviews. This question was preceded by a companion question designed to elicit data about the number of patients in each of the same ten quasitracer conditions. That question was as follows:

Considering all patient visits to this emergency unit over the *past four–six weeks,* approximately how many patients do you estimate there were in each of the categories specified? (Check one for each category.)

The Number of Emergency Patients Was:

Category (Condition)	Consid- erable (1)	Moder- ate (2)	Small (3)	Very small (4)	Zero (There were no such patients) (5)
Acute myocardial infarctions	☐	☐	☐	☐	☐

[categories continue as in Exhibit 5-1].

Measure 3 of the quality of medical care focuses exclusively on the ten quasitracer conditions specified, and represents the average quality of medical care at each EU for the aggregate of patients in this set of conditions during the most recent four–six-week period, as assessed by MDs and by RNs. The measure was derived from the data obtained with the two quasitracer questions in a way that adjusts for patient volume—that is, for the number of patients in the different conditions—while taking into account the severity of patient problems by assessing quality separately for each of the ten conditions. The construction of Measure 3 required three steps: (1) analyzing the data on patient volume, (2) analyzing the data on medical management (quality), and (3) combining these two sets of data in order to obtain the desired measure.

Analysis of Patient Volume. The data from MDs about patient volume were first aggregated at the EU level. Specifically, using the five-point response scale provided, means were computed separately for each quasitracer condition and EU involved. Thus, for each of the thirty EUs, ten means were computed—one for every quasitracer. These ten means were then averaged to estimate average patient volume at each EU for all ten conditions as a set. Similarly, the means obtained for the thirty EUs for each particular condition were averaged to estimate patient volume in the thirty EUs for each of the ten quasitracers. Next, the same series of operations was repeated exactly with the data on patient volume provided by RNs, and the corresponding statistics were computed.

The top segment of Table 5-1 presents the results of the computations just described and the relationships between MDs' and RNs' assessments. The table shows mean patient volume in the thirty EUs by quasitracer condition, listing the average volume for each condition, according to MDs (column 1) and RNs (column 2). The corresponding standard deviations are also shown (columns 3 and 4). As assessed by both MDs and RNs, mean patient volume in the thirty EUs is highest for fractures and dislocations and lowest for rape cases. The four most populous conditions, according to both assessments, are fractures or dislocations, upper respiratory infections, facial lacerations, and myocardial infarctions, in that order. The four least populous conditions, again according to both MDs and RNs, are rape cases, followed by spinal injuries, infant disorders, and burns. The intermediate-volume conditions are drug abuse and psychiatric illnesses. This pattern, however, may not reflect the volume in a particular EU because, as the standard deviations in columns 3 and 4 indicate, mean patient volume for specific quasitracers varies a great deal from one EU to another.

The results in Table 5-1 show that average patient volume for the ten quasitracer conditions, as assessed by MDs, ranges across individual EUs from 2.59 (on the five-point scale used) to 3.93, the mean being 3.23 and the standard deviation .35. The corresponding figures for patient volume as assessed by RNs are

2.58 to 3.73, 3.11, and .31, respectively. Thus, both measures indicate substantial interinstitutional range. The Cronbach coefficient alpha for the former measure is .89 and for the latter .86, indicating high reliability for both. Moreover, the two measures correlate highly and significantly (r = .74, p < .01), indicating good convergent validity. And, if they are combined (not shown in Table 5-1), the resulting index correlates .94 with the measure based on the data from MDs and .92 with the measure based on the data from RNs, and its Cronbach alpha is .91.

Table 5-1 also shows the correlation between patient volume as assessed by MDs and patient volume as assessed by RNs separately for each of the ten quasitracers (column 5). These condition-specific correlations range from r = .14 (for respiratory infections) to r = .73 (for psychiatric illnesses). All are positive, and all except the smallest two of the ten involved are statistically significant (p < .05).*

Finally, if the means on patient volume for the ten quasitracers were rank-ordered, the resulting rankings for the MDs (column 1) and RNs (column 2) data would be identical. The rank-order correlation between these two sets of ranks approaches unity (ρ = .98, p < .01, N = 10 quasitracers).

From these findings, it is clear that the assessments of patient volume at the EU level, provided independently by the two professional groups (MDs and RNs) most directly responsible for treating the patients, are in close agreement and have satisfactory reliability as well as convergent validity. Before they could be accepted as appropriate measures at the institutional/EU level, however, they were also subjected to an analysis of variance. Specifically, the assessments of patient volume by MDs were analyzed separately for each quasitracer (1) to determine whether the between-EU variance on those assessments is larger than the within-EU variance and (2) to ascertain the level of respondent agreement (or "interrater agreement") within EUs by computing

*If these condition-specific assessments by MDs and RNs are combined, condition by condition, the alphas for the resulting indices corresponding to the ten quasitracers (in the order that they are listed in Table 5-1) are .56, .40, .84, .49, .24, .78, .76, .78, .72, and .73.

Table 5-1. Patient Volume and the Quality of Medical Management of Patients in Selected
Quasitracer Conditions at the Emergency Units (EUs) Studied, as Assessed by
Emergency Unit Physicians (MDs) and Registered Nurses (RNs).

Quasitracer Condition	Mean of EU Means (N = 30 EUs), Data from		Standard Deviation (N = 30 EUs), Data from		Correlation Between MD Means and RN Means (N = 30 EUs)[a]	df[b]		Between- Versus Within-EU Variance (One-Way Analysis of Variance)					
								F		$p \leq$		η^2	
	MDs (1)	RNs (2)	MDs (3)	RNs (4)	$r =$ (5)	MDs (6)	RNs (7)	MDs (8)	RNs (9)	MDs (10)	RNs (11)	MDs (12)	RNs (13)
Myocardial infarctions	2.85	2.54	.57	.55	.38	29, 157	29, 231	3.41	4.11	.01	.01	.39	.34
Facial lacerations	2.63	2.52	.47	.41	.26	29, 158	29, 231	1.42	1.53	.09	.05	.21	.16
Psychiatric illnesses	3.41	3.36	.53	.45	.73	29, 158	29, 231	2.40	2.82	.01	.01	.31	.26
Fractures or dislocations	2.05	1.80	.43	.30	.35	29, 157	29, 231	3.49	2.00	.01	.01	.39	.20
Upper respir. infections	2.06	1.97	.57	.41	.14	29, 160	29, 231	2.05	1.67	.01	.02	.27	.17
Rape cases	4.37	4.38	.42	.49	.64	29, 154	29, 229	3.21	7.63	.01	.01	.38	.49
Infant disorders	3.89	3.71	.42	.48	.62	29, 157	29, 231	1.55	2.12	.05	.01	.22	.21
Spinal injuries	3.97	3.89	.42	.46	.65	29, 157	29, 229	1.85	3.03	.01	.01	.26	.28
Drug abuse cases	3.26	3.05	.57	.61	.56	29, 160	29, 231	2.91	4.41	.01	.01	.35	.36
Burns of face, ears, etc.	3.77	3.88	.47	.39	.59	29, 159	29, 231	2.98	1.88	.01	.01	.35	.19
Average Volume for All Conditions	3.23	3.11	.35	.31	.74								

Assessments of the Quality of Medical Management of Patients by Quasitracer Condition

	MDs	RNs	MDs	RNs	r =	MDs	RNs	MDs	RNs	MDs	RNs	MDs	RNs
Myocardial infarctions	1.82	1.79	.39	.34	.38	29, 153	29, 231	1.89	1.87	.01	.01	.26	.19
Facial lacerations	1.92	1.99	.30	.36	.09	29, 147	29, 218	1.00	2.12	.48	.01	.16	.22
Psychiatric illnesses	2.70	3.11	.52	.47	.58	29, 130	29, 201	1.58	2.55	.04	.01	.26	.27
Fractures or dislocations	1.91	1.98	.44	.41	.42	29, 160	29, 234	2.57	3.65	.01	.01	.32	.31
Upper respir. infections	1.91	2.12	.34	.41	.38	29, 157	29, 225	1.44	2.43	.08	.01	.21	.24
Rape cases	2.64	2.93	.65	.62	.59	25, 62	23, 109	1.80	2.20	.03	.01	.42	.32
Infant disorders	2.28	2.25	.41	.50	.62	27, 93	29, 167	1.64	2.45	.04	.01	.32	.30
Spinal injuries	2.45	2.30	.49	.44	-.03	28, 94	29, 164	1.38	1.67	.13	.02	.29	.23
Drug abuse cases	2.45	2.77	.42	.44	.35	29, 187	29, 221	1.31	1.79	.15	.01	.22	.19
Burns of face, ears, etc.	2.11	2.34	.46	.39	.44	29, 113	29, 155	1.75	1.22	.02	.22	.31	.19
Average Quality for All Conditions	2.21	2.34	.29	.33	.48								

[a] $N = 30$ EUs except for the assessments of quality for rape cases ($N = 23$), infant disorders ($N = 28$), and spinal injuries ($N = 29$). The product-moment correlations in column 5 are all statistically significant ($p \leq .05$) except those concerning patient volume for facial lacerations and respiratory infections and those concerning quality for facial lacerations and spinal injuries.

[b] If all eligible respondents from all 30 EUs had found it possible to assess patient volume/quality for any given quasitracer, the maximum possible degrees of freedom would be 29, 181 in the case of MDs and 29, 241 in the case of RNs. The greatly reduced degrees of freedom associated with some assessments of quality, especially by MDs, are mainly a consequence of the very small or zero patient volume (too small to evaluate quality) in one or more of the four least populous conditions (rapes, spinal injuries, infant disorders, burns) in various EUs.

the η^2 statistic. The same procedure was repeated with the data provided by RNs.

The results from this last series of analyses are also summarized in Table 5-1 (top segment, columns 6–13). Briefly, the obtained F ratios are all larger than 1.00—significantly larger for all ten quasitracers in the case of the data from RNs and for all but one of them, facial lacerations, in the case of the data from MDs. The corresponding η^2 values (columns 12 and 13) range between .21 (for facial lacerations) and .39 (for myocardial infarctions) for the data from MDs, and between .16 (for facial lacerations) and .49 (for rape cases) for the data from RNs. These results indicate significant homogeneity of responses within EUs.

Overall, then, the assessments of patient volume in the various quasitracer conditions by MDs and RNs yield measures that are appropriate at the EU level of aggregation and are also reliable and valid. Because the two independent assessments correlate highly, it was finally decided to combine them into a single (and more stable) measure by averaging, separately for each EU, the two means computed for each particular quasitracer based on the data from MDs and RNs. The resulting index (which is used later in conjunction with the quality of care in the ten quasitracers) correlates highly and significantly with both of these component measures, as might be expected. The component-to-index correlations for the various quasitracer conditions range between .82 and .94 for the MDs' component measure, and from .66 to .92 for the RNs' component measure, depending upon the particular quasitracer involved. (These product-moment correlations are all statistically significant; $p < .01$ and $N = 30$ EUs in each case.)

Data on Quality. The second series of analyses focused on the MD and RN evaluations of medical care quality for the same quasitracers. The overall procedure was to repeat the data aggregation steps and computations performed above for patient volume. The results of these analyses, involving the data about the quality of the "medical management of patients," are summarized in the bottom segment of Table 5-1.

On the average, according to both MDs (column 1) and RNs (column 2), the quality of medical care in the EUs studied is best for myocardial infarctions and second best for fractures and dislocations; it is poorest for psychiatric illnesses, second poorest for rape cases, and third poorest for drug abuse cases. The other quasitracer conditions occupy intermediate positions with respect to medical care quality. If the ten quasitracers are rank-ordered and compared to one another in terms of their respective mean scores on quality (columns 1 and 2), the rank-order correlation of quality based on the data from MDs and from RNs turns out to be .93 ($p < .01$, $N = 10$ quasitracers). The two sets of ranks are extremely similar.

For the ten quasitracers aggregated as a set, moreover, the quality of medical care as assessed by MDs correlates positively and significantly ($r = .48$, $p < .01$, $N = 30$ EUs) with the quality of medical care as assessed by RNs (Table 5-1, bottom segment, column 5). Based on the MDs measure, the average quality of medical care for all ten conditions combined ranges across individual EUs from 1.72 (on the five-point scale used) to 2.79, the mean being 2.21 and the standard deviation .29; and the corresponding figures based on the RNs' measure are 1.75 to 3.34, 2.34, and .33. Both measures indicate considerable interinstitutional differences in medical care quality. Equally important, both appear to be highly reliable measures—the Cronbach alpha for the former being .85 and for the latter .92. And when the two measures are combined, the resulting index correlates .82 with the MDs' measure and .89 with the RNs' measure, and its alpha equals .91.

The correlations for the ten quasitracers between quality as evaluated by MDs and quality as evaluated by RNs (column 5) across the thirty EUs range from –.03 (for spinal injuries) to .62 (for infant disorders). All except one of these ten product-moment correlations are positive (the single negative correlation is not significant), and all but two of them are statistically significant ($p < .05$). If the assessments of quality by the two groups are combined condition by condition (by averaging, separately for each EU, the obtained means based on the data from MDs and from RNs) into a single index, the component-to-index correlations for the ten quasitracers turn out to range between .69 and .90 for the MDs' component measure, and between .66 and .91 for the RNs' component measure, depending upon the particular condition considered. All of these product-moment correlations, of course, are statistically significant ($p < .01$, $N = 30$ EUs in all cases), and the Cronbach alpha for the resulting index that encompasses all ten of the quasitracers is .91, indicating excellent reliability for this index.

Finally, Table 5-1 presents the results of the analyses of variance performed on the assessments by MDs and RNs of medical care quality for each quasitracer condition (columns 6–11), along with the corresponding η^2 findings (columns 12–13). Very briefly, the F ratios are ≥ 1.00 for all the quasitracers and data from both groups of respondents. Moreover, the majority of the F ratios in the case of the data from MDs, and all but one of the ratios in the case of the data from RNs, indicate that the between-EU variance on medical care quality is significantly greater ($p <$ .05) than the within-EU variance. Similarly, the η^2 values range from a low of only .16 (for facial lacerations) to .42 (for rape cases) in the data from MDs, and from .19 (for three of the ten conditions) to .32 (for rape cases) in the data from RNs, indicating "interrater" agreement within EUs. The F ratios are somewhat stronger for the evaluations by RNs (show more inter-EU variability) compared to those by MDs, while the η^2 findings are somewhat stronger in the data from MDs (show more intra-EU agreement among individual respondents) compared to those from RNs. Overall, the results from both groups uphold the appropriateness of aggregating the assessments provided by MDs and RNs to derive measures of medical care quality at the institutional/EU level. They also show satisfactory agreement among respondents within EUs regarding the quality of medical care to patients in each quasitracer condition.

In summary, the quasitracer measures of quality based on the data from MDs and RNs properly aggregated and combined at the EU level are clearly reliable and appropriate for institutional-level analysis, have good apparent and convergent validity, and discriminate well among hospital EUs. If they also discriminate among the quasitracer conditions, as they should, they can be used with confidence to construct a composite measure of medical care quality that takes into account patient case-mix and patient volume. Table 5-2 presents the empirical evidence on this issue,

Table 5-2. Intercorrelations of the Quality of Medical Care Provided to Emergency Unit (EU) Patients in Ten Quasitracer Conditions, Based on Assessments of Quality by EU Physicians (MDs) and Registered Nurses (RNs).

	1	2	3	4	5	6	7	8	9	10
1. Myocardial infarctions	.38	.78	.11ns	.51	.60	.49	.31	.46	.29ns	.46
2. Facial lacerations	.71	.09ns	-.08ns	.50	.57	.49	.11ns	.29ns	.20ns	.38
3. Psychiatric illnesses	.56	.31	.58	.22ns	.07ns	.19ns	.31	.15ns	.52	.56
4. Fractures or dislocations	.70	.88	.51	.42	.66	.38	.56	.28ns	.49	.45
5. Upper respir. infections	.75	.76	.46	.74	.38	.57	.65	.18ns	.34	.35
6. Rape cases	.47	.53	.39	.38	.58	.59	.57	.16ns	.30ns	.62
7. Infant disorders	.57	.58	.30ns	.66	.68	.35	.62	.23ns	.39	.54
8. Spinal injuries	.48	.64	.45	.57	.50	.71	.39	-.03ns	.23ns	.25ns
9. Drug abuse cases	.75	.52	.70	.63	.55	.51	.41	.40	.35	.60
10. Burns of face, ears, etc.	.56	.60	.27ns	.54	.58	.64	.43	.43	.55	.44

Quasitracer Condition (rows and columns 1–10)

Upper triangle: Intercorrelations Based on Data from MDs

Lower triangle: Intercorrelations Based on Data from RNs

Diagonal: Correlation (Agreement) Between MDs' and RNs' Assessment for Each Condition

Note: These are all product-moment correlations of quality across conditions, computed on the assessments by MDs and RNs, aggregated at the EU level. $N = 30$ EUs except for some correlations involving missing data, all of which are associated with the conditions of rape, infant disorders, and spinal injuries (for which the N ranges between 24 and 29). All correlations except those accompanied by the designation "_ns_" are statistically significant ($p \leq .05$).

showing the intercorrelations for the quality of medical care provided by the EUs studied to patients in the various quasitracer conditions. Two sets of intercorrelations are shown: one for quality as assessed by MDs (upper-right triangle) and one for quality as assessed by RNs (lower-left triangle).

The results in Table 5-2 show that the quality of medical care as assessed by MDs varies considerably from one quasitracer condition to another. The relevant correlations range widely, between -.08 (quality for psychiatric illnesses versus burns), the only negative coefficient among the forty-five involved, and .78 (quality for myocardial infarctions versus facial lacerations). In most cases, however, the quality of medical care for a particular condition correlates positively and significantly with the quality of care for the others. Thus, the level of quality does not vary randomly across quasitracers in the EUs studied. At the same time, the intercorrelations generally are of moderate size, averaging only .43 (and two of the quasitracers—psychiatric illness and spinal injuries—do not correlate significantly with the rest). Therefore, in their assessments of quality, the MDs clearly discriminate among the quasitracers. The RNs also discriminate, though less sharply than do the MDs. In the case of the RNs, the corresponding correlations range between .27 and .88, the average intercorrelation being .57. It must be noted that all but two of the forty-five correlations are statistically significant, indicating a certain consistency in the quality of care among the quasitracer conditions studied.

Finally, if the assessments of the quality of medical care by MDs and RNs are combined and averaged at the EU level (separately for each of the ten quasitracers), the corresponding forty-five intercorrelations based on these combined assessments (not included in Table 5-2) range from a low of .09 to a high of .88, and the average intercorrelation is .55. These results also suggest that some hospital EUs consistently tend to provide better medical care than others regardless of the particular patient condition considered.

Quality Adjusted for Patient Volume. The ultimate objective of the preceding analyses concerning Measure 3 was to make it possible to construct a measure of quality for the ten quasitracer conditions as a set that would also take into account interinstitutional differences in the number of patients associated with these conditions at the various EUs. The process of constructing the desired measure involved several steps. First, based upon the number of patients in each quasitracer at each particular EU, quasitracers were classified, separated for each EU, as either *high* (above median) or *low* (below median) on patient volume (for that specific EU). Second, separately for each quasitracer, the distribution of the thirty EUs on quality of care (based on the assessments by MDs and RNs combined) was dichotomized at the median, and each EU was classified either as a high-quality or a low-quality EU (with respect to that particular quasitracer). Thus, the quality of care was considered high or low by comparison to quality for the same quasitracer in the other EUs, while patient volume was considered high or low by comparison to volume in the other quasitracers within the same EU.

Next, for any given quasitracer, those EUs that placed high on *both* quality of care and patient volume were given a score of 1 (best possible); those that placed high on quality but low on volume were given a score of 2; those that placed low on *both* quality and volume were given a score of 3; and those that placed low on quality of care but high on patient volume (most "damaging" circumstance) were assigned a score of 4. Finally, the scores assigned to each particular EU on the ten quasitracers were averaged to obtain a single overall score of the quality of medical care that the aggregate of patients in this set of quasitracer conditions receive at each particular EU—an overall score of quality adjusted for patient volume. This overall score constitutes Measure 3 of the quality of medical care.

The theoretically maximum possible range of EU scores on this measure would be from 1.50 (if all of the five high-volume quasitracers in a particular EU also scored high on care quality *and* the five low-volume quasitracers likewise scored high on quality) to 3.50 (if all of the five high-volume quasitracers scored low on quality *and* the five low-volume quasitracers also scored low on quality). Within this range, the smaller the score, the better the quality of care would be at an EU. The actual scores received by the thirty EUs on medical care quality as assessed by the quasitracer patient conditions approach just described range from

1.50 (for the best-scoring EU) to 3.50 (for the poorest-scoring EU) and average 2.46, with a standard deviation of .71. Because the observed range coincides exactly with the theoretically maximum possible range that this measure could yield, the interinstitutional differences in medical care quality revealed by this measure are very substantial.

Other findings show that Measure 3 (which takes into account patient volume and incorporates the combined evaluations of quality by MDs and RNs) correlates highly with the corresponding measure based on the assessment of quality only by MDs ($r = .80$, $p < .01$, $N = 30$ EUs) or only by RNs ($r = .82$, $p < .01$, $N = 30$ EUs). The latter two measures, which in effect are components of Measure 3, also correlate significantly ($r = .54$, $p < .01$, $N = 30$ EUs).

The initial plan was to construct Measure 3 solely on the basis of the data obtained from MDs, that is, the performers themselves. This would have maximized the independence of data sources used to construct the three measures of medical care: Measure 1, it will be recalled, is based on data from HMDs (the professional peers of the performers) and Measure 2 on data from RNs (the principal professional co-workers of the performers). In view of the preceding findings (which, among other things, demonstrate the reliability of the RN assessments and their agreement with the MD assessments), however, that plan was modified so that a more stable measure could be developed by combining the evaluations provided by RNs with those provided by MDs.

Further analysis shows that Measure 3, which adjusts for patient volume, also correlates highly with its unadjusted counterpart—that is, with the combined MD and RN assessments of quality that are similarly aggregated at the EU level but *not* adjusted for patient volume ($r = .90$, $p < .01$, $N = 30$ EUs). Thus, Measure 3 yields almost the same outcome as its nonadjusted counterpart would in terms of the levels of quality of medical care found to characterize the thirty EUs in the study.

Even more important, the stability of Measure 3 remains virtually unaffected when the four least populous of the ten quasitracer conditions (see Table 5-1) are omitted entirely from consideration. More specifically, the correlation between Measure 3, which is based on data for all ten quasitracers, and its modified counterpart, which would involve only the data for the six most populous quasitracers, approaches unity ($r = .98$, $p < .01$, $N = 30$ EUs). Retention of the relatively more unstable data on quality pertaining to the four least populous quasitracers (compared to the other six quasitracers), therefore, has not affected the integrity of the obtained measure. In view of these results, incidentally, it appears that the total number of quasitracers that might be required to develop a reasonably satisfactory measure of medical care quality at the EU level could be as low as six (instead of the ten used in the present study)—provided, of course, that conditions of extremely low patient volume are not included.

It is also important from a methodological standpoint that, even though Measure 3 was confined to a very specific subpopulation of EU patients (the aggregate of patients belonging to the set of the ten quasitracer conditions), it still correlates positively and significantly with the two measures of medical care quality that are not restricted to patients in any particular conditions. More specifically, it correlates .42 with Measure 1 ($p < .05$, $N = 30$ EUs) and .59 with Measure 2 ($p < .01$, $N = 30$ EUs). Thus, hospital EUs scoring high on the quality of medical care for their patients in the ten quasitracer conditions (Measure 3) are also likely to score high on quality for all of their patients (Measure 1 and/or Measure 2), and vice versa. In effect, Measure 3 is a good indicator of medical care quality not only for the patients in the ten quasitracers but also for the total group of patients visiting each EU. Evidently, those EUs that provide high/low quality of medical care to patients in the selected set of conditions also tend to provide high/low quality of care to the rest of their patients.

In the final analysis, Measure 3 is a purer and probably better measure than either of the other two measures of medical care quality because it explicitly and systematically takes patient volume and patient condition into account. The other two measures, however, share the advantage of taking into account all of the patients, not just those belonging to the selected quasitracer conditions, besides being simpler and more economical measures to develop and use.

Final Index of Quality of Medical Care: Measure 4

The three measures of medical care quality discussed in the preceding pages eventually were combined, separately for each EU, to construct a composite measure of medical care quality at the institutional level: Measure 4. This is the *final index of the quality of medical care* developed and used in this research. To construct this index, the scores registered by each EU on the three component measures were summed, without introducing any weights,* to yield an overall score of quality at the EU level. The resulting index scores range from 4.67, for the best-scoring EU, to 10.21, for the poorest-scoring EU (the maximum possible range of scores on this index being 3.50–15.50). The grand mean of the thirty EUs on this index is 7.25, and the corresponding standard deviation is 1.31. Clearly, the developed index (Measure 4) discriminates well among EUs. Moreover, it correlates highly with all three of its components, as follows: .73 with Measure 1, .82 with Measure 2, and .88 with Measure 3 of medical care. Finally, the statistical reliability of the index is relatively good (R = .75). Reliability for this and other similarly constructed indices was computed using the following formula:

$$R = \frac{k \cdot r_{x_i x_j}}{[1 + (k - 1) \cdot r_{x_i x_j}]},$$

where k = the number of component measures and $r_{x_i x_j}$ = the average intercorrelation among the component measures. The validation of all quality of patient care measures developed in this research is discussed in detail in Chapter Six.

Consideration of Possible Adjustment to the Medical Care Index. The relationship of the medical care quality index to a

---

*Although the evaluation of medical care by nurses might appear to be more heavily weighted than the evaluation by physicians, this is not the case. The evaluations by RNs are incorporated in only two of the three specific measures of medical care, and the same holds true of the evaluations of medical care by physicians (MDs and HMDs). Moreover, the actual/observed range of EU scores on the three component measures of the medical care index is quite similar.

number of variables that might reflect the severity of condition of the patients treated at the various EUs was also examined. The main purpose of this examination was to determine whether an adjusted medical care index might be also desirable to construct and use in subsequent analyses. The results proved negative. Very briefly, the quality of medical care in the EUs studied, as represented by Measure 4, turns out not to correlate significantly with any of the likely adjustors considered. Specifically, it correlates (1) only .29 with the proportion of EU patients during the most recent quarter who, according to data from records, were sent by the EU to one of the intensive care units or operating rooms of the parent hospital; (2) only .26 with the percentage of EU patients during the most recent four weeks who, according to data from records, arrived by ambulance; and (3) only .16 with the percentage of EU patients "over the past four weeks" who, in the judgment of the physicians working in each EU, arrived in "life-threatening condition" and, conversely, only -.09 with the percentage of patients who "had a problem that could have been handled in a doctor's office instead of the emergency unit." For all correlations in the present series, $p > .05$. (Descriptive statistics on the variables in this series may be found in Chapter Three.)

In view of these findings, it was concluded that adjustment of the medical care index would be neither appropriate nor feasible. An additional possibility of refining the medical care index by controlling for hospital size was also considered, but, based on the obtained results concerning the magnitude of the relationship between parent hospital size and the quality of patient care in hospital EUs (see Chapter Nine), this was also deemed unnecessary. Therefore, all subsequent analyses involving the quality of medical care will rely on the index discussed above (Measure 4).

The Quality of Nursing Care

As with medical care, three different measures were developed and combined to yield an index of the quality of nursing care at the EU level. The first measure, which takes into account patient case-mix, was constructed using data from RNs (the performers) and MDs (the performers' principal professional co-workers) about the quality of nursing care in the ten quasitracer conditions discussed above (see Table 5-3). A similar question to the one used for assessing the medical management of patients in the quasitracer conditions (see Exhibit 5-1) was used for assessing the quality of nursing care in the same conditions. This measure of nursing care quality was computed in exactly the same manner as was Measure 3 of medical care, and will be described here only briefly, simply by summarizing the results of the lengthy series of analyses that replicated those reported above concerning the medical care measure.

Quality of Nursing Care in Ten Quasitracer
Conditions: Measure 1

For the aggregate of patients belonging to the selected quasitracer conditions, the quality of nursing care as assessed by RNs correlates positively and significantly ($r = .47$, $p < .01$, $N = 30$ EUs) with the quality of nursing care as assessed by MDs (before these assessments are adjusted for patient volume). The Cronbach alpha is .83 for the former measure and .89 for the latter. If the two assessments are combined into a single index, the MDs' component correlates .86, and the RNs' component correlates .85, with the resulting index. The Cronbach alpha for this index is .90. Apparently, both groups provided reliable evaluations of the quality of nursing care given to patients in the quasitracer conditions at their respective EUs, and their evaluations show sufficient agreement for the purpose of combining them into a single measure.

Moreover, the F ratio and η^2 findings (Table 5-3) are similar to those presented earlier about medical care (Table 5-2), except that the overall pattern of results for nursing care is weaker than the pattern for medical care. Other results show that, according to the combined MD and RN assessments measure, the quality of nursing care in the EUs studied does not vary randomly from one quasitracer condition to another. On the other hand, the average intercorrelation among the ten quasitracers on this measure is not high ($r = .54$, $p < .01$), and the range of the forty-five correlation

Table 5-3. Quality of Nursing Care in Selected Quasitracer Conditions in the Emergency Units (EUs) Studied, as Assessed by EU Physicians (MDs) and Registered Nurses (RNs).

	The Quality of Nursing Care by Quasitracer Condition														
	Mean of EU Means (N = 30 EUs), Data from		Standard Deviation (N = 30 EUs), Data from		Correlation Between MD Means and RN Means (N = 30 EUs)[a]	Between- Versus Within-EU Variance (One-Way Analysis of Variance)									
						df[b]		F		$p \leq$		η^2	
Quasitracer Condition	MDs	RNs	MDs	RNs	$r =$	MDs	RNs	MDs	RNs	MDs	RNs	MDs	RNs
Myocardial infarctions	1.91	1.57	.39	.22	.46	29, 154	29, 229	1.59	.98	.04	.50	.23	.11
Facial lacerations	1.95	1.88	.37	.26	.27	29, 148	29, 216	1.28	1.42	.18	.08	.20	.16
Psychiatric illnesses	2.44	2.93	.47	.34	.56	29, 130	29, 206	1.67	1.26	.03	.18	.27	.15
Fractures or dislocations	2.01	1.86	.34	.31	.44	29, 160	29, 233	1.58	2.39	.04	.01	.22	.23
Upper respir. infections	2.00	2.01	.35	.27	.11	29, 155	29, 227	1.36	1.24	.12	.20	.20	.14
Rape cases	2.53	2.65	.57	.58	.29	25, 66	24, 112	1.69	1.64	.05	.04	.39	.26
Infant disorders	2.29	2.14	.38	.44	.25	27, 92	29, 163	1.17	1.14	.28	.08	.26	.20
Spinal injuries	2.26	2.14	.42	.35	.09	28, 96	29, 164	1.08	1.29	.38	.16	.24	.19
Drug abuse cases	2.42	2.60	.42	.36	.45	29, 136	29, 220	1.32	1.43	.14	.08	.22	.16
Burns of face, ears, etc.	2.13	2.20	.41	.49	.42	29, 114	29, 154	1.13	1.98	.32	.01	.22	.27

Note: N = 30 EUs except for the assessments of quality for rape cases (*N* = 22), infant disorders (*N* = 28), and spinal injuries (*N* = 29).

[a] The five largest correlations in the set are statistically significant (*p* < .05). The corresponding correlation for all quasitracer conditions combined is .47 (*p* < .01).

coefficents involved is very considerable, .12 to .80. As with medical care, therefore, the present measure also discriminates well among quasitracers.

When the MD and RN assessments are combined (condition by condition, and separately for each EU involved), adjusted for patient volume, and averaged for the ten quasitracers, Measure 1 of the quality of nursing care is obtained (in exactly the same manner as Measure 3 of the quality of medical care). This measure correlates .75 with the quality of nursing care as assessed only by RNs and adjusted for patient volume, and .82 with the quality of nursing care as assessed only by MDs and adjusted for patient volume. (The latter two measures correlate less strongly with each other but still significantly: $r = .43$, $p < .01$, $N = 30$ EUs.) The same measure, which is adjusted for patient volume, also correlates highly ($r = .90$, $p < .01$) with its counterpart that is not adjusted for patient volume. Finally, Measure 1 of the quality of nursing care, which makes use of the data for all ten quasitracers, correlates very highly ($r = .94$, $p < .01$) with the corresponding measure that omits from consideration the data obtained for the four least populous of the ten quasitracer conditions.

Hospital EU scores on Measure 1 of the quality of nursing care range from 1.50 to 3.50, the observed range coinciding with the theoretically maximum possible range. The mean for the thirty EUs on this measure is 2.46, and the standard deviation is .74. Overall, the present measure is somewhat weaker in comparison to the quasitracers measure of medical care quality but still meets the usual criteria of apparent validity, discriminability, and reliability satisfactorily. It is therefore, an acceptable and reasonably adequate measure of the quality of nursing care at the EU level.

Comparative Evaluation of the Quality of
Nursing Care: Measure 2

The second measure of the quality of nursing care was obtained by aggregating to the EU level the responses of RNs to the following questionnaire item:

Considering the emergency units of all other hospitals with which you are familiar, how would you estimate the *quality of nursing care* provided in this particular emergency unit? (Check one.)

_____ (1)   The quality of nursing care in this emergency unit is outstanding *compared to* most other units

_____ (2)   It is much better than in most other emergency units

_____ (3)   It is generally better

_____ (4)   It is about the same as in most other units

_____ (5)   It is somewhat poorer

_____ (6)   It is generally poorer

_____ (7)   The quality of nursing care in this emergency unit is much poorer *compared to* most other units

_____ (8)   I can't judge

Eighty percent of all eligible respondents were able to use the above scale and evaluate the quality of nursing care comparatively; nearly all of the remaining respondents selected the "I can't judge" alternative. The EU means on the resulting measure range from 1.50, for the best-scoring unit, to 3.43 at the other extreme; the grand mean for the thirty EUs is 2.58; and the standard deviation is .46. These results indicate that the measure discriminates well among institutions. The between-EU variance on this measure is not significantly greater than the within-EU variance (F = 1.35, df = 29, 183, p = 12). However, the F ratio is larger than 1.00 and approaches significance at the .05 level. Moreover, the corresponding η^2 = .17, which indicates significant interrater agreement within EUs. Accordingly, aggregation of the data to the EU level is appropriate.

Finally, Measure 2 of nursing care, which is not restricted to any particular subgroup of patients, correlates positively and significantly (r = .41, p < .05, N = 30 EUs) with Measure 1, which is. Such a relationship between different measures of essentially the same criterion variable was, of course, expected. The obtained correlation is only modest, however, even though Measure 1 is partially based on data provided by the RNs. This suggests that the two measures are not confounded by their partial reliance on a common source of data.

Composite Measure of Quality of Nursing Care: Measure 3

The third measure of nursing care incorporates two different but related components, one involving an evaluation of nursing *performance* and the other an evaluation of nursing *care*. The first component consists of the mean of the responses of physicians (MDs) from each EU to the following questionnaire item about the performance of professional nurses at their respective insitutions:

For the purpose of answering this question, please assume that, even in the very best emergency units and under the most favorable circumstances, *not every member of the PROFESSIONAL NURSING STAFF is doing outstanding or excellent work consistently.* With this assumption in mind, please indicate about how many of the professional nurses in this emergency unit are doing outstanding or excellent work consistently. (Check one.)

_____ (1) *More than 3 out of every 4* nurses are doing outstanding or excellent work consistently
_____ (2) About 3 out of every 4 nurses
_____ (3) About 2 out of every 3 nurses
_____ (4) About 1 out of every 2 nurses
_____ (5) About 1 out of every 3 nurses
_____ (6) About 1 out of every 4 nurses
_____ (7) *Fewer than 1 out of every 4* nurses are doing outstanding to excellent work consistently.

The second component combines, at the EU level, the ratings by MDs and RNs of the quality of nursing care in their respective institutions based on a seven-point scale. The specific questionnaire item in this case, for both groups, was:

On the basis of your experience and information, how would you rate the *quality of nursing care* that patients generally receive in this emergency unit? (Check one.)

_____ (1)   Nursing care in this emergency unit is *outstanding*
_____ (2)   Excellent
_____ (3)   Very good
_____ (4)   Good
_____ (5)   Fair
_____ (6)   Rather poor
_____ (7)   Nursing care in this emergency unit is poor.

Measure 3 of nursing care was derived by summing and averaging, without any weights, the mean scores of the thirty EUs on the above two components, which were found to correlate positively and significantly ($r = .50$, $p < .01$, $N = 30$ EUs). The resulting scores of individual EUs on this measure range from 2.01 (best-scoring unit) to 2.92 (poorest-scoring unit), the grand mean for the thirty EUs is 2.47, and the standard deviation is .27. (In the present case, the obtained range was mathematically reduced due to the successive averaging of EU scores on the several scales involved.) Measure 3 correlates highly with both of its components: .87 with the nursing performance component and .86 with the nursing care component ($p < .01$ and $N = 30$ EUs in both cases), and has acceptable reliability ($R = .67$).

Final Index of the Quality of Nursing Care: Measure 4

As in the case of medical care, the three measures of the quality of nursing care discussed above were combined to yield a single index. The procedure involved a simple summation of the scores that each EU received on the three measures. The resulting index scores range across EUs from 5.38 (for the best-scoring EU) to 9.76 (for the poorest-scoring EU), with a mean of 7.52 and a standard deviation of 1.20. The obtained scores indicate considerable interinstitutional differences in the quality of nursing care provided at the various EUs, though less wide-ranging differences than those found for the quality of medical care.

This final index of the quality of nursing care, Measure 4, correlates highly with its three components, as follows: .88 with Measure 1 (the quasitracers measure of nursing care), .76 with Measure 2, and .73 with Measure 3 (in all cases $p < .01$ and $N = 30$ EUs). Its statistical reliability also is relatively high, $R = .73$. In subsequent analyses, therefore, this index will be used as the main measure of the quality of nursing care provided at the EUs studied.

Index of the Overall Quality of Patient Care

It was possible also to construct an all-inclusive index of the *overall quality* of patient care by combining the nursing care index with the medical care index. The procedure required only a simple summation of the scores achieved by each of the thirty EUs on these two indices (the resulting product in each case being equal also to the sum of scores on the six more specific measures subsumed by the two indices). EU scores on this overall index of patient care quality range from 10.05 (best score) to 18.61 (poorest score), the grand mean for the thirty EUs is 14.77, and the standard deviation is 2.25. As might be expected, the obtained index correlates very highly with both the nursing care index ($r = .89$) and the medical care index ($r = .91$), and its statistical reliability also is high ($R = .93$).

Because this is a global index, which does not differentiate between the level of medical care quality and the level of nursing care quality at a hospital EU (that is, between the two principal components of "clinical efficiency"), and which "masks" differences between these two components and assigns equal importance to them, it is a problematic index. It is a less pure and less meaningful measure analytically than are the separate indices of medical and nursing care quality on which it is based. The lower the correlation between medical and nursing care quality, moreover, the lower the usefulness of such a global index would be. Because the results from the present study (see Table 5-4) show that these two criterion variables correlate significantly but not very highly, use of the overall index must be cautious and limited to special-purpose analyses. In nearly all subsequent analyses, no use will be made of this all-inclusive index. Instead, the research will routinely rely on the two purer indices of patient care quality—the separate indices of the quality of medical and nursing care.

Interrelationships Among the Quality of Care Measures

The product-moment correlations among all of the measures of medical, nursing, and overall patient care discussed in the preceding pages are presented in Table 5-4. These suggest several important conclusions. First, the global index of the overall quality of patient care correlates very highly, and at about the same level, with the indices of medical and nursing care: .91 and .89, respectively. In fact, it also correlates highly with most of the components of these less inclusive indices (components that, indirectly, it also subsumes), the specific coefficients ranging between .53 and .87.

Second, the indices of medical and nursing care quality correlate .61. Therefore, only about 37 percent of the variance in nursing care quality across hospital EUs could be accounted for by knowledge of interinstitutional differences in the quality of medical care, and vice versa. (In other words, EUs scoring high on the quality of medical care may or may not score high also on the quality of nursing care, and vice versa.) Therefore, it is necessary to treat these two indices—which constitute the principal measures of clinical efficiency in the study—separately in subsequent analyses. In other words, it is important to retain both indices in analyzing interinstitutional differences in the quality of patient care, in examining the relationship of such differences to differences in organizational structure and problem solving, and in determining the sources and correlates of such differences more generally.

The results in Table 5-4 also show that the three specific measures of the quality of medical care intercorrelate positively and significantly; $r = .50$ on the average. In addition, they correlate highly, .81 on the average, with the index of the quality of medical care. Of the three, the quasitracers measure correlates best with the index. The corresponding findings about nursing care show a

Table 5-4. Interrelationships Among the Criterion Measures of Patient Care Quality.

	Quality of Medical Care				Quality of Nursing Care				Overall Index
	Measure 1	Measure 2	3	Index (4)	1	Measure 2	3	Index (4)	
Quality of Medical Care									
Measure 1: Evaluation of Quality by Medical Peers (Non-EU Physicians)	--	.49	.42	.73	.36	.17ns	.24ns	.34	.61
Measure 2: Rating of Quality by Co-workers (EU Registered Nurses)		--	.59	.82	.49	.38	.17ns	.49	.74
Measure 3: Quality for Ten Quasitracer Patient Conditions (Adjusted for Patient Volume)			--	.88	.73	.28ns	.21ns	.61	.84
Index of Quality of Medical Care (Measure 4)				--	.68	.34	.25ns	.61	.91
Quality of Nursing Care									
Measure 1: Quality for Ten Quasitracer Patient Conditions (Adjusted for Patient Volume)					--	.41	.49	.88	.87
Measure 2: Quality by Comparison to Other Institutions						--	.53	.76	.60
Measure 3: Composite Measure of Nursing Performance and Nursing Care							--	.73	.59
Measure 4: Index of Quality of Nursing Care								--	.89
Overall Quality of Patient Care									
Overall Index of Quality of Patient Care									--

Note: The correlations shown are product-moment correlations based on institutional-level measures ($N = 30$ EUs in all cases). All of the correlations except those accompanied by the designation "*ns*" are statistically significant ($p < .05$), and most are significant at the .01 level.

similar though slightly weaker pattern; the average correlation among the three specific measures in this case is .47, and their correlation with the nursing index averages .79. Here, too, the quasitracers measure correlates best with the index.

More important, the three specific measures of medical care on the average correlate only .38 with the three specific measures of nursing care. Five of the nine correlations involved in this set, in fact, are not statistically significant. The only high correlation among the nine is that between the two quasitracers measures (r = .73), and this in part is a result of the common procedures used to develop these two measures, both of which are adjusted for patient volume. Further, while the three specific measures of medical care on the average correlate .81 with the medical care index, they correlate only .46 with the nursing care index. And, conversely, the three specific measures of nursing care correlate .79, on the average, with the nursing care index but only .49 with the medical care index. The two indices themselves correlate only .61. Clearly, then, the results in Table 5-4 show excellent discriminant validity for these two indices of the quality of patient care. The two indices indeed measure different though related aspects of clinical efficiency.

Summary

This chapter was concerned with the assessment of one major aspect of institutional effectiveness—the quality of patient care, or the clinical efficiency, of hospital EUs. The data used to construct the desired measures were analyzed and discussed in detail, along with the methodology and procedures used to assess quality at the EU level. Several specific and substantively meaningful measures of the quality of medical care were developed, including one based on a new approach to assessing quality—the quasitracer patient conditions approach. These were then combined into a single index. The same was done regarding the quality of nursing care. The available evidence shows that the obtained indices of the quality of medical and nursing care provided at the EUs studied are internally consistent, have acceptable statistical reliability, and discriminate well among EUs.

They also have good apparent validity. Further, the results to be presented in Chapter Six concerning their validation confirm the adequacy of these indices even more convincingly. In short, the study was able to develop measures of medical and nursing care that are both methodologically satisfactory and substantively acceptable. Chapter Six provides additional evidence for this conclusion, extending and supplementing the findings that were discussed in Chapter Five.

Additional Measures of Clinical Performance

The analyses presented in Chapter Five have produced a great deal of evidence showing that the separate indices of the quality of medical and nursing care developed in this research (1) are statistically reliable and capable of differentiating satisfactorily among hospital EUs, (2) have both apparent face validity and good discriminant validity when compared to each other, and (3) incorporate specific measures of quality which rely on data from several independent sources and show good convergent validity. Still, the validity of these major indices of clinical efficiency must be further assessed. Accordingly, a series of additional analyses of available data were performed to investigate the validity of the two indices more thoroughly; the results of these analyses are presented in this chapter, with special emphasis on the medical care index.

These special analyses involved the determination of relationships between the indices of the quality of medical and nursing care and validating measures derived from data concerning:

1. The promptness of medical attention to incoming patients as reflected in patient waiting time (a frequent problem for hospital EUs).
2. Patient satisfaction (one possible criterion of clinical efficiency).
3. Patient death rates.

4. Certain aspects of care culled from the emergency visit records of recent patients by means of a physician review or "medical audit" of records from a subsample of the EUs studied.
5. Evaluations of the overall quality of patient care by non-EU physicians and by community respondents associated with the various EUs.
6. The appropriateness of clinical procedures and the performance of patient care activities at the various EUs, using data based on the concept of a "patient management continuum" and a "patient visit staging" approach to assessing the quality of care.*

Promptness of Medical Attention to Incoming Patients (Patient Waiting Time)

Patients visiting a hospital EU often have to wait for considerable lengths of time before they are seen by a physician. Although waiting time may not correlate highly, or even directly, in all cases with the quality of medical care received or the clinical efficiency of the institution, it is not unreasonable to expect some relationship. Most, if not all, hospital EUs are concerned about the problem and make some effort to minimize waiting time for their patients. Some are unsuccessful, however, and lengthy delays are not infrequent. At any rate, short waiting times are indicative of greater promptness of medical response to the patients' problems, and promptness of medical attention was expected to correlate positively with the quality of medical care given to EU patients.

Data from the present study show that the percentage of patients visiting the various EUs who were "seen by a doctor within the first fifteen minutes after arriving" ranges across institutions from a low of 28 percent to a high of 95 percent, the average for the thirty EUs being 56 percent with a standard

---

*In addition, in Chapter Eight the primary criteria of EU effectiveness, which include the economic efficiency index (discussed in Chapter Seven) and the indices of the quality of medical and nursing care, are compared to several secondary criteria of effectiveness involving EU staff satisfaction, or "social efficiency," EU responsiveness to community needs and expectations, and institutional reputation.

deviation of 18 percent. These figures are for patients visiting each EU "in the past four weeks," according to combined estimates provided by the physicians (MDs) and registered nurses (RNs) working in the various EUs.* The estimate by MDs correlates positively and significantly with the estimate by RNs ($r = .59$, $p <$ .01), and the two estimates correlate highly (.91 and .87, respectively) with the combined estimate, which has good reliability ($R = .74$). This measure of promptness, therefore, is methodologically sound.

According to related estimates by the patients who participated in the study as respondents, incidentally, average waiting time before the patient was seen "by either a nurse or a doctor" amounted to fourteen minutes for the twenty-eight EUs involved. EU means differed greatly on this measure as well, however, ranging from one minute to forty-one minutes. Obviously, patient waiting is a major problem for at least some of the institutions.

The index developed in Chapter Five to assess the quality of medical care provided to patients at the EUs in the sample correlates positively and significantly ($r = .43$, $p < .01$, $N = 30$ EUs) with the percentage of patients seen by a doctor within fifteen minutes of their arrival at the unit, that is, with the above measure of promptness of medical attention. The better the score of an EU on medical care quality, the higher the percentage of its patients likely to have been seen by a doctor within fifteen minutes after their arrival (or the shorter the patient waiting time), and vice versa. The same index correlates even more highly with the percentage of patients seen by a doctor within fifteen minutes as estimated by RNs only ($r = .53$, $p < .01$).

In contrast, the quality of nursing care index does not correlate significantly with the percentage of patients seen by a doctor within fifteen minutes of arrival, as estimated by either MDs

---

*As estimated by MDs only, the percentage of patients seen by a doctor within fifteen minutes ranges across EUs from 10 percent to 97 percent and averages 53 percent, with a standard deviation of 23 percent. The corresponding figures based on the estimates by RNs only are 30 percent to 96 percent, 60 percent, and 19 percent, respectively. For the former measure, $F = 3.76$ and $p < .01$, and $\eta^2 = .38$; for the latter, $F = 6.61$ and $p < .01$, and $\eta^2 = .45$.

only (r = .09, p > .05) or by MDs and RNs combined (r = .25, p > .05). Finally, the global index of the quality of overall patient care discussed in Chapter Five occupies an intermediate position: it correlates significantly (r = .39, p < .05) with the percentage of patients seen by a doctor within fifteen minutes as estimated by MDs and RNs combined, but the correlation is not as strong as with the medical care index.

These results involving promptness of medical attention as represented by patient waiting time provide further support for the validity of the medical care index. The data show that the quality of medical care as assessed by this index is significantly higher in EUs having a higher percentage of their incoming patients seen by a doctor within fifteen minutes of their arrival (or a lower patient waiting time).

Patient Satisfaction

Logically, patient satisfaction, unlike promptness of medical attention, should correlate positively with the quality of *both* medical and nursing care. The extent to which EU patients are actually capable of evaluating the quality of their care accurately and validly, however, is not known. Obviously, patients must be considered less capable of making sound technical judgments about care quality than their physicians and nurses, yet, they alone are best qualified to indicate whether and to what extent they are satisfied with the care that they received. In any case, their perspective is important to consider in its own right, as one legitimate criterion variable.

On the aggregate, the patients visiting an EU during the same time period should be able to provide a reasonably accurate (though probably incomplete) evaluation of the care that they received, or at least of some aspects of the staff's performance and behavior. To the extent that they can, a positive though probably not high correlation between patients' evaluation of their care and the indices of medical and nursing care quality should be expected. Accordingly, the patients who participated in the study (PATs) were asked several questions about their care and the EU staff. The data that these questions yielded were aggregated to the EU level in the usual manner, and the resulting measures were examined in relation to the indices of the quality of medical and nursing care.

First, PATs were asked: "All things considered, how satisfied are you with *the care that was given to you in the emergency room* during this visit? (Check one)." The response alternatives, forming a five-point scale, ranged from "(1) I am completely satisfied" to "(5) I am not satisfied at all." Based on this question, mean patient satisfaction scores range widely across EUs, from 1.14 to 3.00 on the five-point scale used; the grand mean for the twenty-eight EUs for which data are available is 1.98, and the standard deviation is .44.

As represented by this *general* measure of satisfaction, patient satisfaction turns out to correlate positively and significantly, and at about the same level, both with the index of the quality of medical care ($r = .40$, $p < .05$) and the index of the quality of nursing care ($r = .41$, $p < .05$). Hospital EUs with better scores on either of these two indices (neither of which involves data from patients) also score better on mean patient satisfaction with the care received.

Since the patient satisfaction measure represents satisfaction with the overall care received, it is not surprising that it yields a very similar relationship to the indices of medical and nursing care. Nor is it surprising to find that the same measure correlates best with the global index of overall patient care quality ($r = .45$, $p < .01$), which subsumes the medical and nursing care indices combined (see Chapter Five). Perhaps more important for present purposes is the fact that these results provide additional and independent validating evidence for the indices of the quality of medical and nursing care.

The PATs were also asked two *specific* questions about the care that they received separately from the medical and nursing staff. One question was "Overall, how *well* would you say the doctor (or doctors) who treated you in the emergency unit *took care of you?*" The question was then repeated with reference to the nurses. In both cases, the response alternatives ranged from "extremely well" to "not well at all," forming a five-point scale. Corresponding measures of the care received, as assessed by the patients, were obtained by aggregating the data from each of these two questions to the EU level.

The results show that, as might be expected, the general measure of patient satisfaction correlates positively and significantly with the more specific measures of patient satisfaction with the care received from EU doctors ($r = .81$, $p < .01$) and EU nurses ($r = .46$, $p < .01$). Note that the correlation is much stronger with medical than with nursing care. This difference is worth noting because the more specific measures concerning the care received from nurses and physicians also correlate significantly with each other ($r = .42$, $p < .05$). The correlations obtained between these two measures and the indices of the quality of medical and nursing care also are positive but not statistically significant at the .05 level, ranging between .21 and .28. Apparently, EU patients have a better sense of the quality of their *overall* care, which they associate more closely with the care that they received from the physicians than from the nurses, than they do about medical or nursing care considered separately.

Finally, the patients were asked a series of questions about "the staff who took care of you in the emergency room," which included the following five items: (1) "To what extent did the staff who took care of you make an effort to *really understand* your problem?" (2) "On the whole, how satisfied were you with the way the emergency room staff *explained* to you how your problem should be handled?" (3) "How *considerate* were (they) of you *as a person?*" (4) "To what extent did the staff who took care of you *really know* what they were doing?" (5) "Compared to what you might have expected before you got there, *how good a job* did the emergency room staff do for you?"

Each of these items could be answered by selecting one of five responses, ranging from most to least favorable. The data from each item were first aggregated, and means were computed at the EU level. Then, based on these means, the interrelationships among the items were examined. As expected, the five items were found to correlate positively, and in most cases significantly, with each other, the average interitem correlation for the series being .45 ($p < .01$, $N = 28$ EUs). The five items were then combined into a single and more stable index of *EU staff performance as assessed by patients,* for which the Cronbach coefficient alpha is .77.

This index of staff performance as assessed by the patients (or "patient satisfaction with the EU staff") correlates significantly and at about the same level with the aforementioned measures of the care received from the doctors and from the nurses as evaluated by the patients ($r = .51$ and $r = .49$, respectively, and $p < .01$ in both cases). Additionally, it correlates even more highly with the general measure of patient satisfaction with the care received ($r = .73$, $p < .01$) discussed above. The same five-item index of EU staff performance correlates .54 ($p < .01$) with the quality of nursing care index, .46 ($p < .01$) with the global index of the overall quality of patient care, and .31 ($p = .06$) with the index of the quality of medical care, adding to the previous evidence for the validity of these indices. The fact that the patients' assessment of staff performance correlates better with nursing than medical care suggests that patients responded to the above five items concerning staff performance mostly with reference to the nonmedical staff, quite probably having the nursing staff principally in their minds. On the whole, the results in this section consistently show a positive relationship between the quality of patient care and patient satisfaction at the EUs studied, thus serving to validate the quality of care measures.

EU Patient Death Rates

Patient death rates and certain measures obtained through a special review of patient records by two knowledgeable physicians also were examined in relation to the indices of medical and nursing care quality.

Of the thirty EUs in the sample, twenty-three were able to provide information from records about the number of deaths "during the most recent quarter" and also distinguish between patients classified as "dead on arrival" and those who "died while in the emergency unit" (for more descriptive details, see Georgopoulos, Cooke, and Associates, 1980). Based on these data, death rates per thousand patient visits were computed separately for the two categories as well as for both of them combined. The data show that, across institutions, the rate for "dead on arrival" does not correlate with the rate of deaths "while in the emergency unit" (r = .07, p > .05, N = 23 EUs). Both rates, however, correlate significantly with overall death rate, or total death rate, although the former correlates with it much more strongly (r = .93, p < .01, N = 21 EUs) than does the latter (r = .42, p < .05, N = 21 EUs).

These two rates, however, fail to correlate significantly with either the medical or the nursing care index, the specific coefficients being near zero. The overall death rate comes marginally closer than either of the two more specific rates to showing a very slight relationship with the two indices of the quality of care, which is in the right direction but not statistically significant. Specifically, the overall death rate correlates -.10 with the index of the quality of nursing care and -.23 with the index of the quality of medical care (p > .05 and N = 21 EUs in both cases). Interestingly, however, the overall death rate correlates significantly with one of the three specific measures of medical care quality included in the index—namely, the quasitracers measure (r = -.44, p < .05, N = 21 EUs). In this case, the higher the quality of medical care, the lower the patient death rate at the EU level.

The somewhat stronger tendency of the overall patient death rate to be associated with the quality of medical (compared to nursing) care is not surprising, and the obtained results are not inconsistent with respect to the validity for the medical care index. The results, however, are too weak to be consequential or conclusive. Perhaps more stable data on death rates (for example, data covering longer periods of time than one quarter and more cases) from more hospital EUs would (if accurate) have yielded a statistically significant, though probably still small, relationship with the quality of medical care at the EU level.

Measures from Medical Review of Patient Records

The next series of findings involves certain measures obtained from a review of patient records (RECs). Among the various data collected were copies of the emergency visit records of those patients who were included in the study as respondents (PATs). Among the twenty-eight EUs allowing inclusion of their patients in the study were ten having fifteen or more patients take part in the research. The emergency visit records of these patients (a total of 239 records) were subjected to a special audit by two research-oriented physicians who agreed to perform this task for the present study.

After discussion of the task and a brief practice period with patient records from an EU not belonging to this subsample, the two physicians independently examined each patient record and scored it, on a five-point scale, for legibility of physicians' entries, legibility of nurses' entries, comprehensiveness of the record (completeness in terms of medical and nursing entries), sufficiency of detail for understanding the patient's problem, severity of the patient's problem, appropriateness of diagnosis, appropriateness of treatment, and the "overall quality of the record."

The scores given to the 239 patient records by the two physicians correlate fairly highly for all of these variables except severity, about which the two physicians showed the least agreement. The specific product-moment correlations (each based on N = 239 records), all of which are statistically significant, range from .59 and .61 for the two legibility measures, respectively, to a low of .27 for the severity variable. In other words, those patient records that were rated "high" (or "low") on a particular variable by one of the two physicians also were likely to be rated "high" (or "low") by the other. Moreover, across the ten EUs represented, the mean rating given by one physician to the patient records from each particular EU on each variable involved correlates significantly with the corresponding mean rating given to the same records by the second physician. This holds true for all the variables measured except severity and appropriateness of diagnosis. The relevant rank-order correlations (in all cases N = 10 EUs) range from a low of .02 for appropriateness of diagnosis and .09 for severity of medical problem, at the low side, to a high of .79 for the comprehensiveness variable and .87 for the overall quality of the record.*

---

*Incidentally, one of the two physicians reported that he had inadvertently scored the records for the "overall quality of patient care as reflected in the patient record" rather than for the "overall quality of the

In short, with the exceptions noted, the two physicians agreed well in their ratings, both at the individual patient record level and at the institutional, or EU, level. Accordingly, for each of the variables involved, excluding the severity variable that was set aside, their ratings were combined and averaged for further analysis.

Results based on these combined ratings show a number of interesting patterns. First, across institutions, the legibility of physician entries into the patient record shows no relationship whatsoever to the legibility of nurses' entries ($\rho = .14$, $p > .05$, $N = 10$ EUs). On the other hand, the comprehensiveness of patient records, which correlates very highly with sufficiency of detail ($\rho = .92$, $p < .01$, $N = 10$ EUs), as might be expected, also correlates highly with the overall quality of the records ($\rho = .92$, $p < .01$, $N = 10$ EUs). In turn, both the overall quality and comprehensiveness of patient records correlate very highly with appropriateness of diagnosis ($\rho = .82$ and $.94$, respectively), and also with appropriateness of treatment ($\rho = .92$ and $.85$, respectively). Moreover, the appropriateness of treatment and the appropriateness of diagnosis also correlate highly ($\rho = .88$, $p < .01$, $N = 10$ EUs).

None of the above variables correlates significantly with the index of the quality of nursing care. The relevant rank-order correlations, all of which are based on $N = 10$ EUs, range between .04 and .24 depending upon the variable examined in relation to the index. The pattern of relationships between the same variables and the index of the quality of medical care is stronger, each variable showing a somewhat higher correlation with the medical

---

patient record itself." Thus, the results also include the serendipitous finding of a significant positive relationship between the quality of patient records and the quality of patient care as reflected in the records. It must be kept in mind, however, that the corresponding measures are each based on information from only one rater. The same physician reported a "clear impression" that the quality of patient records seemed to vary systematically across EUs. The other physician also reported a general impression based upon his review of the same patient records— namely, that most EUs appeared to manage those patients who presented serious problems very well but did not appear to be doing an equally good job with the rest of their patients.

than with the nursing care index. Specifically, the index of medical care quality correlates .41 with the appropriateness of treatment measure, .33 with the appropriateness of diagnosis measure, .27 with the overall quality of patient records, .26 with the sufficiency of detail in these records, and .20 with the comprehensiveness of the records.

If the global index of the quality of overall patient care (discussed in Chapter Five) is used in the analysis, the corresponding correlations are all slightly higher, and in the right direction, as follows: .48, .50, .39, .44, and .42, respectively. Only the first two of these, however, approach significance at the .05 level (which would require a $\rho = .56$). Perhaps emergency visit records reflect the quality of overall patient care, or the quality of medical and nursing performance combined, better than they reflect the quality of either nursing or medical care. At any rate, the results from the present series of analyses provide only marginal support for the validity of the overall care index and possibly also the medical care index. The obtained relationships are directionally right in all cases but obviously weak. A more extensive review of a larger number of patient records, using more reviewers and institutions, might have yielded more definite conclusions, about both the validity of the indices and the usefulness of emergency visit records for developing measures of patient care quality more generally. Such a review had been planned and discussed in the research proposal, but the sponsoring agency decided specifically that this part of the study would not be funded by the research grant awarded for the project.

Evaluations of the Quality of Overall Patient Care by Non-EU Physicians and by Community Respondents

The selected hospital physicians (HMDs) who provided the data for Measure 1 of the quality of medical care also evaluated the quality of overall patient care comparatively, by answering the following question during their interview: "Considering the emergency units of all other hospitals with which you are familiar, how would you evaluate the *overall quality of patient care* provided in this emergency unit? *Overall*, is the *quality of patient care* here much better, generally better, about the same, somewhat poorer, or generally poorer compared to these other facilities?"

The response alternatives were assigned scores from 1, for "much better," to 5, for "generally poorer," and the data were aggregated to obtain means at the EU level. The between-EU variance on these scores is significantly greater than the within-EU variance ($F = 2.43$, $p < .01$) and $\eta^2 = .30$. EU means on the measure range from 1.50 (for the best-scoring EU) to 3.40 (for the poorest-scoring EU), yielding a grand mean of 2.31 and a standard deviation of .55. Therefore, this measure too is statistically satisfactory. More important, it correlates positively and significantly with all three indices of the quality of care developed in this study, as follows: .59 with the index of overall patient care quality, .56 with the index of the quality of medical care, and .49 with the index of the quality of nursing care. All of these product-moment correlations are statistically significant ($p < .01$, $N = 30$ EUs). Clearly, these results strongly support the validity of all three indices of the quality of care at the EU level.

The individuals from each community who were interviewed for this research, both because of their special contacts with the EUs and because they represent one additional perspective of interest, were also asked about the overall quality of patient care in the particular EUs with which they were familiar. Specifically, these community respondents (CRs) were asked to evaluate overall quality both comparatively, by answering the same question as the HMDs, and noncomparatively, by answering the following question: "On the basis of your experience and information, how would you rate the overall quality of patient care that patients generally receive in this emergency unit? Would you rate it excellent, very good, good, fair, or rather poor?" In the usual manner, the response alternatives were assigned values ranging from 1, for "excellent," to 5, for "rather poor," and the data were aggregated to the EU level.

Nearly 20 percent of the CRs were unable to evaluate the quality of care comparatively. Accordingly, the data from that question were excluded from any further consideration (even though the distribution of EU scores based on them correlates highly, $r = .71$, with the distribution of EU scores based on the data obtained from the noncomparative rating provided by the same respondents). On the other hand, CRs had no difficulty rating the quality of patient care by answering the second (the noncomparative) question. EU mean scores based on this rating vary from 1.00 (for the best-scoring EU) to 3.00, yielding a grand mean of 1.93 and a standard deviation of .45. The interinstitutional range is obviously considerable, and the distribution of EU means approximates a normal distribution. At the same time, however, the F ratio is only marginal, and the η^2 value clearly fails to meet the established methodological standards of the study (F = 1.47 with p = .22, and η^2 = .07). Accordingly, results involving this measure must be viewed with caution.

With respect to the validity issue, analysis shows that the CRs' noncomparative rating of the overall quality of patient care correlates positively, though not highly, with the three care indices, as follows: .35 ($p < .05$) with the overall index of the quality of patient care, .28 ($p > .05$) with the index of the quality of medical care, and .35 ($p < .05$) with the index of the quality of nursing care. Interestingly, moreover, the CRs' noncomparative evaluation of the quality of care correlates positively and significantly with the HMDs' comparative evaluation (r = .40, $p < .05$). On the whole, the relationships between these two measures of care and the indices of the quality of care developed in this study support the validity of the indices.

Finally, it may be methodologically important as well as substantively interesting to note that, across hospital EUs, the quality of patient care as rated by CRs also correlates positively and significantly with overall patient satisfaction (r = .51, $p < .01$, N = 28 EUs) and with EU staff performance as assessed by the patients (r = .45, $p < .01$, N = 28 EUs). Both of the latter measures, it may be recalled, were found to correlate significantly with the quality of care as assessed by the indices developed for this purpose, which incorporate no data from the patients.

Appropriateness of Procedures and the Performance of Care Activities: The Patient Visit Staging Approach

An alternative approach to that adopted for assessing the quality of patient care at the institutional level was also used in this research, but mainly for exploratory and validation purposes. This supplementary approach, which focuses on evaluating patient care processes instead of outcomes, involves the concept of *patient visit staging*. This concept is analogous to that of "disease staging," as discussed by Gonnella and Goran (1975) and used by Forrest, Scott, and Brown (1976) to assess the quality of inpatient surgical care in hospitals. Briefly, the staging approach involves assessing the sequence of distinct phases or stages that EU patients typically go through. Each emergency visit, in other words, can be examined in terms of a *patient management continuum* that encompasses a number of different stages, which together define it.

From the standpoint of the EU as an organization, the patient management continuum represents the work inputs, transformation processes, and outputs of the system and reflects the system's work cycle. The stages on the continuum are not totally fixed or entirely exclusive, and some of them occasionally may be "short-circuited" during the patient care process. Nonetheless, they are fairly well differentiated, at least with respect to most patients most of the time, and readily recognizable as such by the clinical staff.

More specifically, with regard to either a single patient visit or an aggregate of such visits, the patient management continuum may be meaningfully divided into the following stages:

1. Receiving and registering the patients who arrive for care at the EU (patient entry).
2. Initial screening of patients by the staff (triage), usually by a nurse.
3. Examination and testing of patients (patient workup).
4. Diagnosis.
5. Treatment.
6. Preparation of the patients for discharge (including "patient teaching" and instructions for "follow-up care").
7. Patient visit disposition and discharge (patient exit).

Each stage generally involves a characteristic set of work activities and clinical procedures. These activities and procedures (and the outcomes associated with each stage) are outlined in Table 6-1.

Table 6.1. A Professional Management Continuum (Stages/Phases) of a Patient Visit to a Hospital EU.

		System Inputs		Transformation Phases				Outputs
Stage → Focus ↓		Patient Entry into EU (1)	Initial Screening (Triage) (2)	Assessment of Patient (Examination, Testing) (3)	Diagnosis (4)	Treatment (5)	Preparation for Discharge and Post-Care (6)	Disposition (Patient Exit from EU) (7)
Structures:	Performance programs (patient care plans, treatment protocols)	Procedures for facilitating patient entry into the EU, admission rules	Criteria and specifications for initial screening and triage	Patient assessment plans, objectives, procedures (history, physical, lab work, X-ray)	Diagnostic protocols and decision requirements	Treatment arrangements, types of treatment specified for various conditions	Provisions for patient teaching, care continuity, and post-care	Disposition rules/routines, arrangements for patient to leave the EU
		Who is to assist patient entry, admit, and receive patient?	Who is to do screening and sorting, on what basis (e.g., severity)?	Who sees patient, who may examine/test, consultants and data used?	Who makes, records, confirms, revises diagnosis?	Who carries out what treatments, under whose supervision?	Who is to instruct the patient, explain post-care requirements?	Who completes what steps for patient exit, who assists in patient exit?
Processes:	Staff activities (clinical)	Appropriateness of activities for patient admission and entry	Were right screening and sorting specifications followed?	Were appropriate data obtained? Were the right tests/exams ordered and completed?	Was diagnosis made following appropriate procedures?	Were right treatments prescribed, ordered, and given?	Were instructions and provisions for post-care appropriate?	Was disposition appropriate? Was exit timely?
		How well did the performers carry out these activities?	How well were they implemented? Was staff prompt, sensitive?	How well did the performers carry out the patient assessment tasks?	How well/carefully was the patient diagnosed?	How well were the treatment/therapy tasks executed?	How well did the performers prepare the patient for discharge?	How well was the patient disposition effected?
Outcomes:	Impact on patient (activity) outcomes	Smooth patient entry, emotional impact on the patient	Correct assignment of patient, allocation to right phase; time elapsed until patient first seen	Thoroughness and accuracy of assessments made	Correctness and promptness of diagnosis of patient's problems and needs	Correctness of treatment decisions, efficacy of therapy, impact on patient's status	Patient teaching efficacy re: care requirements and follow-up	Cumulative impact on patient's medical, physical, psychological condition; total waiting time between entry and exit; patient satisfaction

Within any particular EU, of course, the activities associated with any one stage of the patient management continuum might tend to be better performed than those associated with another, regardless of the level of overall performance. Further, EU staffs could differ substantially with respect to how well they perform the activities associated with one or more stages. Similarly, the appropriateness of clinical procedures from the point of view of maximizing clinical efficiency could also vary significantly, both across stages and from one EU to another. Therefore, the determination of interinstitutional differences along this patient management continuum may be a plausible and useful (though untested) approach to assessing the quality of care at the EU level, much like the quasitracer patient conditions approach (see Chapter Five). For this reason, it was also explored in this research but on a more limited basis than the quasitracers approach.

For this exploration, undertaken primarily for the purpose of validating the principal indices of the quality of care developed by the study, relevant data were obtained from EU physicians (MDs) and registered nurses (RNs) concerning five of the seven stages distinguished on the patient management continuum. Specifically, with reference to each particular stage (see Table 6-1), except diagnosis and treatment, MDs provided data about the *appropriateness* of procedures while RNs provided data about the *performance* of corresponding activities.

In the case of RNs, the following question was asked:

Generally, *how well performed* (or how well carried out) are each of the following activities in this emergency unit? (Check one for each activity.)

On the Whole, These Activities Are:

Activities:	Extremely Well Performed (1)	Very Well Performed (2)	Fairly Well Performed (3)	Not so Well Performed (4)	Not Well Performed (5)
Receiving and registering patients who visit this emergency unit	☐	☐	☐	☐	☐

The initial screening
(triage) of patients ☐ ☐ ☐ ☐ ☐

. . . etc.

In the case of MDs, the question was:

From the standpoint of enabling the medical and nursing staff in this emergency unit to provide patients with emergency care of the *highest quality possible* at reasonable cost, *how appropriate* would you say are each of the following procedures? (Check one for each kind of procedure.)

On the Whole, These Procedures Are:

Procedures (for):	Completely Appro- priate (1)	Very Appro- priate (2)	Fairly Appro- priate (3)	Not so Appro- priate (4)	There are no such procedures in this unit (0)
Receiving and regis- tering patients	☐	☐	☐	☐	☐
The initial screening (triage) of patients	☐	☐	☐	☐	☐

. . . etc.

The RNs from the various hospital EUs had no difficulty evaluating the performance of activities associated with each specified stage: The overall nonresponse rate averaged less than 10 percent for every stage except that of "disposition and discharge," for which it was 12 percent. The MDs, on the other hand, apparently had some difficulty with the question about appropriateness: The overall nonresponse rate in their case averaged 19 percent (exactly the same for all of the stages specified). According to the obtained data, this nonresponse was not primarily due to the absence of procedures at some of the EUs. The greater complexity of the question asked of MDs compared to the one asked of RNs probably was the main reason. The best guess is that, if the "at reasonable cost" qualification had not been included in the stem of the question, the nonresponse rate would have been much smaller. (Incidentally, this qualification may have been disregarded by some of the MDs, since the measure of appropriateness based on these data shows no significant relationship to the economic efficiency of EUs as measured by the index discussed in Chapter Seven.)

Measures of Appropriateness and Performance

The data provided by the MDs who were able to assess appropriateness were aggregated to the EU level, and means were computed separately with reference to the appropriateness of procedures for the five stages of receiving, screening, examining-testing, preparing for discharge, and discharging the patients. The range of EU means is very substantial for all five kinds of procedures, being smallest (but still quite large) in the case of "examination and testing" procedures, for which EU means range from 1.37 to 2.50, with a grand mean of 1.95 and a standard deviation of .27. The interinstitutional range is largest in the case of patient screening procedures. The relevant F ratios for the measures corresponding to the five procedures are all greater than 1.00, ranging from 1.12 to 1.65, but most of them do not reach statistical significance at the .05 level. The corresponding η^2 values, on the other hand, are all acceptable, ranging from .16 to .23.

Further analysis shows that, across EUs, the appropriateness of each kind of procedure, as measured with the above data, correlates positively and significantly with the appropriateness of the others. The specific product-moment correlations among the five kinds of procedures range from .34 to .75 ($p < .05$ and $N = 30$ EUs in all cases), depending upon the particular pair examined, and average .54 (the median intercorrelation is .49). Therefore, there is considerable uniformity regarding the appropriateness of procedures across the five stages of the patient management continuum for which data were collected.

Given these findings, it was decided to combine and average the five appropriateness scores (means) received by each EU in order to develop a single, and more reliable, index of the appropriateness of procedures at the EU level. As might be expected, the five components that it subsumes correlate highly with the resulting index, .79 on the average, the specific correlations ranging from .67 to .86 ($p < .01$ in all cases). The Cronbach alpha for this index also is high—specifically, .84. In other words, the obtained index is statistically reliable and internally consistent. The scores of the thirty EUs on this index, indicating the average appropriateness of procedures at each institution for the five stages specified, show considerable interinstitutional variation. Specifically, based upon the five-point scale used, they range from 1.50 to 2.70 and yield a grand mean of 2.06 with a standard deviation of .27.

The data from RNs concerning the performance of activities corresponding to the same five stages were similarly aggregated and analyzed at the EU level. These data also indicate sizable interinstitutional differences in performance at each particular stage. (Interestingly, the range of obtained EU means is smallest for the examination-testing stage and largest for the patient screening stage—the same pattern found with the appropriateness measure based on data from MDs.) The corresponding five F ratios for the performance measure are all greater than 1.00 and statistically significant ($p < .05$), ranging from 1.65 to 2.77; and the relevant η^2 values are also acceptable, ranging from .18 to .26.

As with appropriateness, there is substantial uniformity from one stage to another with regard to how well performed the various activities are in the EUs studied. Specifically, the average intercorrelation of the performance of activities corresponding to the five stages examined is .60 (the median intercorrelation is .59). The ten specific product-moment correlations in this set range between .40 and .82, depending upon the particular pair of stages considered ($p < .05$ and $N = 30$ EUs in all cases).

When the performance scores of EUs on the five stages are combined, the resulting index of performance correlates highly with each of its five components, the specific product-moment correlation coefficients ranging between .74 and .89 and averaging .82 ($p < .01$, and $N = 30$ EUs in all cases). The Cronbach alpha for this index is .86, indicating high reliability. The scores of individual EUs on this performance index range from 1.60 to 2.57 (on the five-point scale used to evaluate performance) and yield a grand mean of 2.15 with a standard deviation of .25.

On statistical grounds, the performance index is clearly stronger than the appropriateness index. Both, however, are acceptable methodologically. As measured by these two indices, the performance of activities and the appropriateness of procedures at the EUs studied are positively related ($r = .34$, $p < .05$, $N = 30$ EUs), as they should on clinical rationality grounds. However, they probably do not correlate as strongly as might be necessary or desirable from the standpoint of promoting high clinical efficiency in hospital EUs. The interest here is not in this issue, however, but in validating the patient care measures discussed in Chapter Five.

Appropriateness and Performance in Relation to the Quality of Care

When the staging indices are examined in relation to the clinical efficiency indices (discussed in Chapter Five), the results show that the "average" appropriateness of procedures associated with the five stages of the patient management continuum specified is significantly related to the index of medical care quality ($r = .40$, $p < .05$), and also the index of overall patient care ($r = .36$, $p < .05$), but not the index of nursing care quality ($r = .24$, $p < .05$). Apparently, most of the MD respondents must have had medical procedures predominantly in mind when assessing appropriateness. This conclusion is consistent also with the fact that the appropriateness of procedures happens to correlate significantly (and more highly than does the performance of activities) with the proportion of patients in the various EUs who were seen by a doctor within fifteen minutes of their arrival ($r = .44$ and $r = .48$, respectively, when the proportion of patients is estimated by RNs only or by RNs and MDs combined).

The nursing care quality index, nevertheless, does correlate significantly with the activity performance index ($r = .53$, $p < .01$). At the same time, the performance of activities correlates even more strongly with the index of medical care quality ($r = .64$, $p < .01$), and also the index of overall patient care ($r = .66$, $p < .01$), than it does with the nursing care index. On the whole, therefore, the results from the present series of analyses provide strong support for the validity of the medical care quality index, while also adding some evidence in support of the nursing care index.

Appropriateness × Performance Index and Its Relationship to Quality of Care

It is possible, of course, that the care procedures for any particular stage on the patient management continuum are entirely appropriate with respect to enabling an EU to provide high-quality care while the activities required to implement the procedures are not well performed. The reverse could also occur— activities may be well performed by the staff, but the procedures that they implement are not as appropriate as they might be. Correspondingly, differences are possible both within institutions, from one stage of the patient management continuum to another, and across institutions, that is, from one EU to another. Theoretically, the quality of patient care should be best at those EUs where patient care procedures are appropriate and related staff activities are well performed. For these reasons, a joint measure of appropriateness and performance—the Appropriateness × Performance Index—was constructed from the above data.

For each of the five stages of the patient management continuum examined, the mean appropriateness scores of the thirty EUs were multiplied by the corresponding mean performance scores. The resulting cross-product score for a given stage and a given EU constitutes a joint score of appropriateness and performance for that particular stage and EU. These joint scores were found to intercorrelate positively across the five stages involved. The ten correlations associated with the five stages, considered two at a time, range from .29 to .83 (the median $r = .50$), and all except the smallest one are statistically significant ($p <$ .05).

In view of these results, the appropriateness × performance scores concerning the five stages were averaged, separately for each EU, to obtain an Appropriateness × Performance Index. The scores on the five stages that this index incorporates correlate highly with the index, $r = .80$ on the average ($p < .01$), and the Cronbach alpha for the index is .84, indicating high reliability for this joint measure of appropriateness and performance.

Even more important for present purposes, the Appropriateness × Performance Index turns out to correlate positively and significantly with all three indices of clinical efficiency developed in this research. Specifically, it correlates .63 with the index of the quality of medical care, .46 with the nursing care index, and .61 with the index of the overall quality of patient care (these are all product-moment correlations for which $p < .01$ and $N = 30$ EUs). These relationships also support the validity of the quality of care indices, and especially the validity of the quality of medical care index.*

In conclusion, the patient visit staging approach described here appears promising and worthy of further study and refinement. In this study, this approach was used as a supplementary method for assessing clinical efficiency; in future research, it might well be employed as a primary method. Here, at any rate, it was used mainly for the purpose of validating the indices of the quality of care developed by other approaches (described in Chapter Five), with encouraging results.

Summary

The analyses discussed in this chapter yielded a great deal of empirical evidence that supports the validity of the quality of care (clinical efficiency) indices described in Chapter Five. On the whole, this evidence, along with the related evidence presented in Chapter Five, shows that the quality of medical care index meets accepted standards of discriminability, reliability, and validity rather rigorously. Moreover, its components, particularly the

*It is also interesting to note, in this connection, that the Appropriateness × Performance Index also correlates positively and significantly ($p < .05$) with the three specific measures included in the index of the quality of medical care, as follows: .38 with the quality of medical care as rated by the selected hospital physicians (HMDs), .58 with the quality of medical care as rated by the registered nurses (RNs), and .57 with the quasitracer patient conditions measure of the quality of medical care.

quasitracer patient conditions component, are theoretically as well as substantively meaningful; and its correlates include important aspects of clinical efficiency, which were measured with data from several independent sources and which represent several legitimate perspectives. In short, this index is not only satisfactory from a statistical and methodological standpoint but is also promising on theoretical and pragmatic grounds. Accordingly, use in its present form for assessing the quality of medical care provided at hospital EUs, and for research and analysis purposes, appears to be fully warranted by the data and research results that are now available.

The index of nursing care quality is somewhat weaker than the medical care index but still reasonably adequate from a methodological point of view. The index of the overall quality of patient care, which combines these two indices, is a limited-use index. It was developed for special analysis purposes only, mainly to study the statistical characteristics of the other indices, and not as a principal criterion measure of clinical efficiency or EU effectiveness. Finally, it should be noted that, of the three indices under consideration, the one that warrants the most confidence according to the findings is the quality of medical care index—the one that probably represents the most important component of the clinical efficiency of hospital EUs and therefore also the most important criterion of EU effectiveness.

Chapter Seven

Economic Efficiency

As discussed in Chapter Four, institutional effectiveness encompasses several major outcomes of the performance of the system, including the quality of service provided, or clinical efficiency, and the cost of service, or economic efficiency. Moreover, to adequately understand the relationship between the organization and effectiveness of hospital EUs, in principle one should be able to control for the level of economic efficiency when examining differences in clinical efficiency, and vice versa, unless of course there is no relationship between the two criteria.

Economic efficiency, at any rate, is an important criterion not merely on conceptual-theoretical grounds but also for pragmatic reasons. From the perspective of the parent hospital, for example, an EU must utilize its resources in a productive and efficient way. From the perspective of the patients and the community being served, the fees for service must be reasonable and affordable. High costs and economic inefficiency are usually frowned upon and seen as undesirable by all concerned. Generally, moreover, the level of economic efficiency or inefficiency that characterizes an EU is likely to have correspondingly favorable or unfavorable implications for staff performance and satisfaction within the unit, as well as for the unit's relations with the parent hospital and community.

For both theoretical and practical reasons, therefore, it was essential for the study to assess the economic efficiency of hospital EUs. The data used for this purpose were obtained mostly from organizational records (RECs) containing fiscal, budgetary, personnel, and patient census information. To maximize accuracy, a special form was constructed by the research staff for this purpose (see Georgopoulos, Cooke, and Associates, 1980, pp. 474–481) and completed under the direction of the chief executive officer of each hospital. Further, the information obtained was linked directly to specific time periods (for example, the most recent week, most recent quarter) and, where possible and appropriate, to individual staff members (for example, information about number of hours worked in the EU was obtained separately for each RN in the unit), or at least to homogeneous staff subgroups (for example, full-time LPNs).

Additionally, all but two of the EUs in the sample were regarded as separate "cost centers" within their respective parent hospitals, and this made it possible to obtain information that otherwise might not have been available. Still it was necessary to augment these data from records with certain information provided by the physicians (MDs) and by the registered nurses (RNs) working in the various EUs. Even then, sufficient data for all the desired measures were not available for four of the thirty EUs in the sample.

Because the concept of efficiency implies a ratio of input to output, a number of decisions had to be made prior to data collection on how best to represent the two terms of this ratio. After the issues were discussed with the project's consulting health economists (Sylvester E. Berki and Paul J. Feldstein), it was decided that (1) EU "output" should be represented by the number of patient visits during specific time period(s) and (2) EU "inputs," which basically involve the investment of system resources, should be linked to payroll data and/or staff time worked during the same period(s). Possible use of "adjusted" measures of economic efficiency to control for such things as urban-rural differences was also considered and will be examined below in the light of obtained empirical findings.

The decision about what specific data to collect, of course, was also affected by pragmatic concerns relating to the availability of relevant and accurate information at the participating institutions. Eventually, after the limitations of various methodological alternatives were evaluated, certain options were precluded [for example, using some adaptation of Feldstein's (1967) "costliness index" or "cost per case" measures such as those used by Lave, Lave, and Silverman (1972) or Shuman, Wolfe, and Hardwick (1972)] and others were followed. In the end, based on the available data, and considering both feasibility and methodological constraints, it was possible to develop four specific measures and one composite measure, or index, of economic efficiency.

Measures of Economic Efficiency

The specific measures employed to represent the economic efficiency of hospital EUs at the institutional level are as follows:

Measure 1: Physician time per patient visit to the EU (an indicator of gross "MD productivity").

Measure 2: Registered nurse time per patient visit to the EU (an indicator of gross "RN productivity").

Measure 3: Total EU payroll expenditures per patient visit for all personnel except physicians (an indicator of nonmedical staff costs).

Measure 4: Current "total cost to the hospital of an average patient visit to the emergency unit."

Economic efficiency index: A composite measure, incorporating the preceding four measures equally weighted.

The first two measures reflect the clinical staff resources invested at each EU; the third measure represents total nonmedical personnel costs (including payroll costs for all of the nursing staff, technicians, clerks, and so on, but excluding physician costs); the fourth measure represents total costs to the hospital as calculated by each institution. The first three measures were computed by the research staff from raw data. All of the thirty EUs for which data were available, of course, were given a score on each of the measures. In all cases, including the developed index, the smaller the score on the measure, the higher the economic efficiency level that it represents.

To construct Measure 1 of economic efficiency, the total number of physician hours worked in each EU per week as reported by the physicians themselves (see Chapter Three) was divided by the total number of patient visits to the EU during the "most recent week" (which, for the data obtained from organizational records, coincided with the week of interviewing at each institution). This ratio could not be computed for one of the thirty EUs because of insufficient data. Furthermore, reported hours rather than hours from RECs were used in the computations because the latter information was not available for five of the thirty EUs in the sample. Hours were reported individually by the physicians (MDs) working at each EU during fieldwork week, in response to the question "Ordinarily, about how many hours a week do you work in this emergency unit? (Write in number of hours: ____ Hours per week.)"*

Analysis indicates that the obtained measure is a reliable one, though the distribution of EUs on it is somewhat skewed. The sum of self-reported MD hours worked in each of the various EUs correlates highly and significantly ($r = .72$, $p < .01$, $N = 25$ EUs) with the sum of MD hours based on the comparable information available from hospital records. Across EUs, MD time per patient visit based on physician-reported hours (Measure 1) correlates very highly ($r = .86$, $p < .01$, $N = 24$ EUs) with MD time per patient visit based on the corresponding data from RECs.

According to Measure 1, MD time per patient visit in the EUs studied averaged .46 hours (to obtain this mean, the relevant ratio scores were first computed separately for each EU involved and then averaged for the twenty-nine EUs), with a standard deviation of .34 hours. Across institutions, it ranged from .08 hours in the lowest-scoring EU to 1.88 hours in the highest-scoring EU. Based on physician hours from RECs, physician time per patient

---

*Obviously, though greatly overlapping, the MDs responding to this question were not all identical with those for whom work hours had been recorded at every institution; and the specific week that respondents had in mind was not necessarily identical to that for which recorded hours were available or for all of the respondents involved. Based on the data from institutional records, available for twenty-five EUs, an average of 7.8 MDs per EU worked an average of 24.5 hours per MD during the "most recent week." The corresponding figures based on the physician-reported hours, available for all thirty EUs, are 6.8 and 21.2, respectively.

visit ranged across EUs from .22 to 1.70 hours, averaging .52 hours with a standard deviation of .31 hours (N = 24 EUs). Thus, Measure 1 of economic efficiency shows considerable interinstitutional variability.

For Measure 2 of economic efficiency, the total number of hours worked by RNs in each EU was divided by the total number of patient visits to the EU during the "most recent week" (intentionally selected to coincide with the week of interviewing). Data from RECs were used for both hours and visits in computing this ratio, as they were available for all but one of the thirty EUs studied. According to the data from records, an average of 8.9 RNs per EU worked an average of 26.7 hours a week per person, compared to 8.8 RNs and 27.1 hours, correspondingly, based on self-reported hours by the RNs.

The sum of RN hours obtained from RECs for each of the EUs correlates very highly (r = .91, p < .01, N = 29 EUs) with the sum of self-reported hours by the RNs, lending further confidence in the accuracy of both sets of data. Across EUs, RN time per patient visit based on self-reported hours correlates highly and significantly (r = .78, p < .01, N = 29 EUs) with RN time per patient visit based on RECs (Measure 2).

According to Measure 2, RN time per patient visit in the EUs studied averaged .82 hours, ranging across institutions from a low of .19 to a high of 1.77 hours, with a standard deviation of .38 hours. The distribution of EUs on this measure is essentially a normal one. As in the case of Measure 1, the differences among institutions on Measure 2 are substantial. Results also show that Measure 2 correlates positively and significantly, but not very highly, with Measure 1 (r = .38, p < .05, N = 29 EUs).

To construct Measure 3 of economic efficiency, total payroll expenditures for EU personnel (during the "most recent quarter" preceding fieldwork) were divided, separately for each institution, by the total number of patient visits to the EU during the same quarter. All of the data were obtained from RECs and were available for all but two of the thirty EUs. Actual total payroll expenditures for full-time and part-time personnel in the following categories were used: RNs (including those in supervisory positions), LPNs, aides, technicians, and clerks (if any). To maximize accuracy, where possible these data were obtained both in the aggregate (that is, for the several groups combined) and separately for each group and then combined. Minor discrepancies between the corresponding two sum totals for a few EUs were readily resolved prior to constructing the measure.

According to Measure 3, payroll expenditures for nonmedical personnel averaged \$10.16 per patient visit, ranging across institutions (N = 28 EUs) from a low of \$3.20 to a high of \$36.35, with a standard deviation of \$7.05. Obviously, as with the two previous measures, the differences among institutions are considerable. It is also interesting to note that Measure 3 does not correlate significantly with total RN payroll expenditures per patient visit during the same quarter (r = .02, p > .05, N = 22 EUs), nor with Measure 2, which is linked to RN hours worked during the "most recent week" (r = .15, p > .05, N = 27 EUs). On the other hand, it correlates highly and significantly, and about equally, with both of the following validating measures: (1) total EU expenditures (payroll plus other) per patient visit during the specified quarter (r = .75, p < .01, N = 28 EUs) and (2) total EU revenues per patient visit during the same quarter (r = .72, p < .01, N = 28 EUs). As might be expected, the results also show that, based on the same quarterly data, total expenditures per patient visit correlate highly with total revenues per patient visit (r = .77, p < .01, N = 28 EUs).*

Measure 4, unlike Measures 1, 2, and 3, represents a "current cost" estimate calculated and supplied by each institution (along with other financial and patient visit data) in response to the following question: "At the present time, what is the *total cost* to this hospital of an average patient visit to the emergency unit (including *both* direct and indirect costs but *exclusive* of any physician fees)? Average *total cost* to the hospital per emergency visit: \$ _____ ."

This information was supplied by twenty-eight hospitals. In response to an accompanying question, twenty-two of them

*During that particular quarter, incidentally, total revenues per patient visit averaged \$28.09, and the mean ratio of total EU revenues to total EU expenditures was 1.89 for the EUs in the sample. It should be recalled that all dollar figures shown are pre-1980 figures.

indicated that their cost figure was "based on records," five reported that it was a "best estimate," and one stated that it was "both." Furthermore, in response to a follow-up question, twenty-four or more of these institutions (depending on the particular service specified) indicated that their cost figure did not include costs for any of the following services: X-ray, EKG, laboratory, anesthesia, social services, respiratory therapy, ambulance service. Measure 4 shows that, for the twenty-eight EUs involved, the "total cost to the (parent) hospital" at the time of data collection averaged $24.29 per patient visit, ranging from a low of $.50 to a high of $63.00, with a standard deviation of $14.08. Again, the differences across institutions are substantial.

Additional analysis shows that Measure 4 correlates positively and significantly with (1) the "basic fee" charged by the different hospitals per emergency patient visit ($r = .51$, $p < .01$, N = 27 EUs); (2) "additional charges" per patient visit "over and above the basic fee, but excluding physician fees" ($r = .69$, $p < .01$, N = 24 EUs); and (3) average "total fee" (basic fee plus these additional charges) per patient visit ($r = .73$, $p < .01$, N = 23 EUs). It also correlates with "how high charges for patient care are" in the various EUs, as perceived by the MDs working there ($r = .48$, $p < .01$, N = 28 EUs) and by the patients (PATs) and selected community respondents (CRs) who participated in the study combined ($r = .33$, $p < .05$, N = 28 EUs). The same measure, however, does not correlate significantly with "total EU expenditures per patient visit" ($r = .14$, $p > .05$, N = 27 EUs) or "total EU revenues per patient visit" ($r = .21$, $p > .05$, N = 27 EUs) in the EUs studied—a pattern that contrasts to the one found for Measure 3. Apparently, neither EU revenues nor EU expenditures are closely coordinated to, or rationalized in terms of, the cost of emergency patient visits to the parent hospital.

Economic Efficiency Index

The above four measures were combined to construct a composite measure that would represent the level of an EU's overall economic efficiency. The procedure was relatively simple. First, all participating EUs for which scores on all four measures were available (a total of twenty-six EUs) were individually assigned the appropriate score derived from each specific measure. Then these scores (based on the scales described above) were converted into rank-order scores. Specifically, on each particular measure, the twenty-six EUs were rank-ordered from 1, representing the most efficient unit (as indicated by the original score on that measure), to 26, representing the *least* efficient or most costly unit. Then the four scores obtained for each EU from the four rank-orders were summed to yield a composite score. This constitutes the economic efficiency index value obtained for each EU—a value that in effect is the result of combining the scores from the four component measures equally weighted.*

Theoretically, scores on this index could range from 4 (if the same EU had scored *best,* and therefore had been ranked first, on all four specific measures: $1 \times 4 = 4$) to 104 (if the same EU had scored *poorest,* and therefore had been ranked twenty-sixth, on all four measures: $26 \times 4 = 104$). The actual scores range from 9.00 for the particular EU that scored best overall on economic efficiency to 96.00 for the EU that scored poorest overall. Clearly, this is a very great range; its extremes approach the theoretically possible limit of 4.00–104.00. The mean score of the twenty-six EUs on the economic efficiency index is 54.46, the standard deviation is 21.96, and the median of the distribution is 57.50. (The distribution of EU scores on this index is nearly normal.)

In terms of the developed index, therefore, the present study finds great interhospital differences in the economic efficiency of hospital EUs, that is, substantial variability among individual EUs on this primary criterion of institutional effectiveness. In most subsequent analyses, the economic efficiency criterion will be represented by this index.

---

*On all of the component measures, and on the index, EUs were scored in relation to one another and so that the smaller the rank-order score, the *higher* the economic efficiency level it represents. Accordingly, the *higher* the economic efficiency of an EU, as shown by the index, the *lower* the expended physician time, RN time, EU payroll expenditures, and current total cost to the parent hospital per patient visit are likely to be.

Interrelationships Among the Economic Efficiency Measures

Table 7-1 shows the intercorrelations among the component measures of the economic efficiency index and between them and the index (all scores on all measures having been arranged from most to least favorable). The index correlates positively and significantly, as it should, with its four component measures: .66, .72, .57, and .64, respectively ($p < .01$, N = 26 EUs in all cases). These product-moment correlations are sufficiently high to lend confidence in the index, but not so high as to render any one component interchangeable with the index. The correlations among the component measures are also positive but smaller,

Table 7-1. Interrelationships Among the Criterion Measures of Economic Efficiency at the Emergency Unit (EU) Level.

Criterion Measure	1	2	3	4	5
					(Index)
1. Physician Time per Patient Visit to EU	--	.38*	.30	.54**	.66**
2. RN Time per Patient Visit to EU		--	.15	.36*	.72**
3. EU Payroll Expenditures per Patient Visit (for All Nonmedical Staff)			--	.24	.57**
4. Current Total Cost to the Hospital per Patient Visit				--	.64**
5. Composite Measure or Economic Efficiency Index					--

Notes:
*$p < .05$.
**$p < .01$.
Product-moment correlations are shown. All correlations are in the expected direction. The N ranges between 26 and 29.

On all measures, the EUs involved are scored based on their relative rank in relation to one another and so that the smaller the rank-order score, the *higher* the "economic efficiency level" it represents. Accordingly, the *higher* the economic efficiency of an EU, as shown by the index, the *lower* the physician time, RN time, EU payroll expenditures, and current total cost to the parent hospital per patient visit are likely to be.

ranging from .15 to .54. Those involving component Measures 1, 2, and 4 are also statistically significant, while those involving Measure 3 are not (although the correlation between Measure 3 and Measure 1 approaches significance at the .05 level).

Clearly, the index satisfactorily represents each of the four specific measures that it incorporates, while the latter measures are neither substantively nor statistically interchangeable with one another. The statistical reliability of the economic efficiency index also is reasonably adequate, being .68 ($p < .01$, $N = 26$ EUs).

The reliability coefficient was computed using this formula:

$$R = \frac{k \cdot r_{x_i x_j}}{\left[1 + (k - 1) \cdot r_{x_i x_j}\right]} ,$$

where k = the number of component measures and $r_{x_i x_j}$ = the average intercorrelation among the component measures.

In summary, the obtained index of economic efficiency relies on, and incorporates, several meaningful measures of economic performance, with which it correlates highly (.65 on the average). In addition, the specific components of the index (1) correlate significantly with certain additional aspects of economic performance and have good apparent validity, (2) are relatively unambiguous and have high comparability across institutions, and (3) discriminate well among the institutions studied. Finally, the index itself discriminates sharply and reliably among institutions, while its relationships with certain other economic measures add to the evidence for its validity.

More specifically, with regard to validity, a series of analyses shows that the economic efficiency of hospital EUs, as represented by the index, correlates significantly and as expected with the following aspects of economic performance:

1. Total EU expenditures per patient visit ($r = -.42$, $p < .05$, $N = 26$ EUs).
2. RN payroll expenditures per patient visit ($r = -.38$, $p < .05$, $N = 20$ EUs).

3. "Total fees," excluding physician fees, charged by each hospital per visit to its EU ($r = -.45$, $p < .05$, $N = 21$ EUs).
4. "How high" hospital charges for patient care provided by the EU are regarded by the physicians working there ($r = -.38$, $p < .05$, $N = 26$ EUs).
5. Total EU revenues per patient visit ($r = -.35$, $p < .05$, $N = 26$ EUs).
6. Number of patient visits processed by the EU per RN hour worked ($r = .71$, $p < .01$, $N = 26$ EUs).
7. Number of patient visits processed per physician hour worked ($r = .73$, $p < .01$, $N = 26$ EUs).*

Together, these findings provide good empirical support for the validity of the economic efficiency index. (For the relationships between this index and other criteria of EU effectiveness, including the quality of care and medical and nursing staff satisfaction with the EU, see Chapter Eight.)

Consideration of Index Adjustments

To determine the need for refining it, the economic efficiency index was examined in relation to certain potential "adjustors": parent hospital size, urban-rural location, and patient case-mix as shown by certain indicators of the "severity" of patient conditions.

The research plan called for careful examination of potentially "biasing" effects on the economic efficiency measures that might be associated with these particular variables. It was assumed that, to the extent that differences among hospital EUs on these variables were found to correlate significantly and systematically with economic efficiency differences, as assessed by the index, it would probably be desirable to "correct for" the impact of such differences on the index. This could be accomplished by developing a companion *adjusted* index through regression analysis or,

---

*The last two ratios, incidentally, which themselves correlate positively and significantly ($r = .64$, $p < .01$, $N = 29$ EUs), should not be confused with the ratios involved in computing Measures 1 and 2 of economic efficiency (as described earlier in this chapter.)

alternatively, by *controlling* for the influence of biasing variables analytically when studying the relationship between economic efficiency and other variables of interest. Such corrections and adjustments proved unnecessary, however, because none of the potential adjustors turned out to correlate significantly with the original index of economic efficiency.

First, the results show that parent hospital size (as represented by number of beds) does not correlate significantly with the economic efficiency of EUs as represented by the index ($r = .16$, $p > .05$, $N = 26$ EUs). Second, the eighteen EUs located in SMSA (urban) areas do not differ significantly in average level of economic efficiency from the eight EUs that are located in non-SMSA (rural) areas. The mean score of the former group of institutions on the economic efficiency index is 57.89 and that of the latter group is 46.75 (the mean for all of the twenty-six EUs involved, as reported earlier, being 54.46). The difference between these two means is not statistically significant ($t = 1.20$, $p > .05$). Furthermore, the between-group variance (that is, between SMSA and non-SMSA institutions) on EU economic efficiency as assessed by the index is not significantly greater than the within-group variance ($F = 1.12$, $df = 17, 7$, and $p > .05$). In addition, these results remain essentially the same if parent hospital complexity instead of size, or community complexity instead of the SMSA variable, is used in the analysis (see Chapter Nine).

Finally, the economic efficiency of hospital EUs, as assessed by the index constructed for this purpose, fails to correlate significantly with any of the following "severity" indicators that might possibly have served as adjustors:

1. Percentage of EU patients "during the most recent four weeks" who arrived by ambulance ($r = .04$, $p > .05$), based on data from institutional records.*

---

*It is also methodologically interesting to note in this connection that, across EUs, the percentage of EU patients arriving by ambulance computed with data from hospital records correlates positively with the percentage of such patients as estimated by EU MDs ($r = .37$, $p > .05$, $N = 19$ EUs) or

2. Percentage of EU patients "over the past four weeks" who, in the judgment of the MDs working at the various EUs, arrived in "life-threatening condition" ($r = .15$, $p > .05$).

3. Percentage of EU patients who, according to the same physicians, "had a problem that could have been handled in a doctor's office instead of the emergency unit" ($r = .22$, $p > .05$).

4. Proportion of EU patients "during the most recent quarter" who were sent by the EU to one of the intensive care units or operating rooms of the parent hospital ($r = -.27$, $p > .05$), according to data from institutional records.

In view of these results, there was no reason to make any adjustment to the economic efficiency index. In this research, therefore, only the unadjusted index was retained for use in the various analyses concerning the effectiveness of hospital EUs.

The results presented in this chapter concerning the index and measures developed to assess economic efficiency show consistently large differences among hospital EUs on this primary criterion of institutional effectiveness. In the case of some of the measures, part of the observed interinstitutional variability might conceivably be due to nonuniformity in accounting and record-keeping practices among the hospitals involved. However, given the data collection techniques employed (most of the relevant data were provided by each hospital either in "raw" form or in the simplest form possible, following very detailed instructions and a standardized and pretested procedure, using an identical data collection instrument for this purpose—see Georgopoulos, Cooke, and Associates, 1980, pp. 474-481), most of the variation found undoubtedly reflects true differences among the participating EUs. In addition, an array of descriptive findings based on related data

---

RNs ($r = .34$, $p > .05$, $N = 19$ EUs). These correlations, which are based on a greatly reduced sample size due to lack of data for eleven of the thirty EUs studied, just miss statistical significance at the .05 level (which would require a correlation of .39). The estimates provided by these two key groups themselves correlate positively and significantly ($r = .44$, $p < .01$, $N = 29$ EUs), as they should if accurate and valid.

about various aspects of the financial situation of EUs shows similarly great interinstitutional differences (see Georgopoulos, Cooke, and Associates, 1980, chap. 10).

In view of the differences found, incidentally, it is rather surprising that economic aspects and the financial condition of EUs were rarely mentioned as major problems or strengths by the various groups of respondents who participated in the research. Although "maintaining high standards of patient care" was one of the primary goal priorities of EUs, "keeping the costs of service down" was not (see Chapter Three); nor was "providing care at the lowest cost possible" especially emphasized at the various EUs (see Georgopoulos, Cooke, and Associates, 1980). Perhaps the large majority of respondents were not particularly concerned about economic efficiency or costs, or were unaware of financial problems at their respective institutions.

Although some of these findings might suggest that the financial condition of the EUs in the study was not especially problematic, the findings do not necessarily mean that the economic efficiency of these health service systems was on the average high or even acceptable. The great interinstitutional differences shown by the economic efficiency index alone demonstrate rather convincingly that this could not be the case. In fact, to reiterate, most of the available measures of economic efficiency consistently show large differences among EUs. These differences, of course, may be the result of multiple causes, including organizational structure factors, the relative efficacy of problem solving within the system, and even the quality of services rendered. The results in the chapters which follow provide at least a partial answer in this connection.

Summary

Based on the evidence discussed in this chapter, it may be concluded that, although there is still considerable room for improvement, the validity and reliability of the economic efficiency index developed in this research are reasonably satisfactory. In addition, the index discriminates sharply among individual EUs. For the EUs that participated in the study, at least, this particular index constitutes a meaningful measure of overall economic performance at the institutional level, from a methodological as well as from a theoretical and substantive standpoint. The index may well constitute the best measure of this kind available in the field of emergency medical services at the present time, although its methodological adequacy could undoubtedly be enhanced through further research (for example, research involving more institutions and more economic performance measures). In short, the developed index provides, probably for the first time, a useful tool for assessing and comparing the economic efficiency of hospital EUs.

Chapter Eight

Relationships Among
Criteria of Effectiveness

The interrelationships among the different criteria of emergency unit effectiveness measured in the study are presented in this chapter. The effectiveness of hospital EUs, it will be recalled, was assessed at the institutional level, using economic efficiency (see Chapter Seven) and the quality of medical and nursing care, or clinical efficiency (see Chapter Five), as the main criteria. Certain secondary criteria also were measured, however, in part for the purpose of validating the primary criteria, and in part because of their pragmatic importance to the health services field.

Relationships Among Primary Criteria

Table 8-1 shows the relationship between the economic efficiency and the clinical efficiency of hospital EUs. The former criterion is represented by the economic efficiency index described in Chapter Seven, and clinical efficiency is represented by the indices of the quality of medical and nursing care (and also the index of the overall quality of medical and nursing care) discussed in Chapter Five. Table 8-1 shows both the zero-order correlation between economic efficiency and each index of clinical efficiency and the relationship between economic and clinical efficiency partialling out each of the following variables: EU patient volume, breadth or scope of emergency service, parent hospital size, hospital service complexity, and community complexity. These particular variables are among those structural variables that were

Table 8-1. Relationship Between the Economic and Clinical Efficiency of Hospital Emergency Units.

			Economic Efficiency			
			Correlation When Partialling Out			
Clinical Efficiency	Zero-Order Correlation	EU Patient Volume	Breadth/Scope of Emergency Service	Parent Hospital Size	Hospital Service Complexity	Community Complexity
Quality of Medical Care	-.07	-.10	.15	-.15	-.24	-.04
Quality of Nursing Care	.21	-.01	.36*	.15	.06	.22
Quality of Overall Patient Care	.07	-.06	.28	-.02	-.12	.09

*$p < .05$.

included in the study for investigation as likely major correlates of EU effectiveness (see Chapter Nine) and as possible control variables or moderators of the relationship between organizational problem solving and EU effectiveness (see Chapter Ten).

Patient volume, which is an indicator of both work volume and EU size, was measured by the number of patient visits to the EU during the most recent quarter preceding fieldwork. The breadth or scope of emergency service was measured by the ratio of number of patient visits to the EU to the number of inpatient days in the parent hospital during the same period (this ratio reflects the *de facto* definition of "emergency service" prevailing at the various institutions). Parent hospital size is represented by the number of beds reported by each institution. Hospital service complexity, which is also an indicator of institutional resources, is represented by the number of different clinical, ancillary, and other facilities reported annually by each hospital in the American Hospital Association's *Guide to the Health Care Field*. Finally, community complexity is represented by a composite measure, which incorporates the percentage of families with income below poverty level and the percentage of population classified as minority (both based on U.S. Census data) in the city or community in which each institution is located. The measure in question correlates highly with its two components ($r = .77$ and $.97$, respectively, and $p < .01$ in both cases), which themselves also correlate significantly ($r = .61$, $p < .01$).*

The results in Table 8-1 clearly show that the economic and clinical efficiency of hospital EUs are unrelated. None of the zero-order correlations is statistically significant, and only one of the

---

*Concerning the interrelationships among the five structural variables specified, the data show that community complexity correlates significantly only with parent hospital size ($r = .45$, $p < .01$). Hospital size also correlates significantly with hospital service complexity ($r = .68$, $p < .01$), and with EU patient volume ($r = .64$, $p < .01$). The latter two variables correlate significantly but not highly ($r = .41$, $p < .05$). In addition, EU patient volume correlates with the breadth/scope of emergency service ($r = .41$, $p < .05$) and is the only variable in the set that is related to the breadth of emergency service. The remaining intercorrelations among the five variables (taken two at a time) are not statistically significant.

fifteen relevant partial correlations—between economic efficiency and nursing care partialling out the breadth of emergency service—reaches statistical significance at the .05 level. In effect, EUs which score high on economic efficiency may show any level of clinical efficiency (high, moderate, low), regardless of the particular index of clinical efficiency used, and vice versa.

Further analysis of the scores of the twenty-six EUs on the two criteria in question confirms the lack of any significant relationship between them. For example, when a scatter plot is made of the scores on the quality of medical care index and the economic efficiency index received by the various EUs, the obtained plot shows no relationship whatsoever, either linear or curvilinear, between the two indices. This is not to say that some institutions do not score high (or low) on both indices, when "high" and "low" are defined as above and below the median of the distribution on each index. Eight of the EUs do in fact score better than the median on both indices. Apparently, these particular institutions are able to provide medical care of relatively high quality at relatively low cost. However, when the distributions of EU scores on the two indices are considered in their entirety, the results show no relationship between the two criteria.

As a group and on the average, therefore, hospital EUs have not been able to achieve a high level of performance in both the clinical and economic areas simultaneously. Whether this might be feasible through better organization, better staff performance, or better organizational problem solving cannot be determined on the basis of available data from this research or the existing literature on emergency medical services. Partly because of the lack of previous research in this area, the present study hypothesized no specific relationship between these two key criteria. Nevertheless, the expectation of a small positive relationship would have been justified on the grounds that clearly effective institutional performance probably would imply (at least substantively and pragmatically if not methodologically) attainment of both clinical and economic efficiency at relatively high levels, and ineffective performance would imply the opposite.

The actual findings of the study, of course, do not support such a hypothesis, since the two criteria do not correlate. Still, the data show that eight of the twenty-six EUs involved in the analysis were performing at a level better than the median in the area of economic efficiency as well as in the area of medical care, indicating that better than average performance in both areas simultaneously is not a rare phenomenon.

Relationships Among Secondary Criteria

In addition to the primary criteria of economic and clinical efficiency, the study measured five secondary criteria of institutional effectiveness. To the extent that the secondary criteria actually reflect the institutional effectiveness of hospital EUs, they should correlate with one or more of the indices representing the primary criteria, and possibly also with one another as well.

Secondary Criteria of EU Effectiveness

The secondary criteria measured in the present study are: promptness of medical attention to incoming patients; staff satisfaction, or "social efficiency"; patient satisfaction; EU responsiveness to community expectations and needs concerning emergency medical services; and EU and parent hospital reputation in the community.

Two of these criteria—promptness of medical attention and patient satisfaction—and their measurement were discussed in Chapter Six, where they were used along with other measures to validate the indices of the quality of medical and nursing care. Here they will be considered in relation to the other secondary criteria and in relation to economic efficiency.

Promptness of medical attention is represented by one measure, the percentage of patients seen by a doctor within fifteen minutes of their arrival at each EU. Patient satisfaction is represented by two measures: the patients' perception of the quality of care that they received at each EU and a five-item index of satisfaction with various aspects of EU staff performance as assessed by the patients. This index has a Cronbach alpha of .77, indicating good reliability (see Chapter Six for details). The former measure, patient satisfaction with the care received, is based on data from the following question: "All things considered, how satisfied are you with the care that was given to you in the emergency room during this visit?" (See Chapter Six for details.)

This overall satisfaction measure with the care received, it should be pointed out, is strongly related to patient satisfaction with the care received from doctors ($r = .81$, $p < .01$) and also correlates significantly but less strongly ($r = .46$, $p < .01$) with the patients' evaluations of care received from nurses. Patients' assessments of the care received from doctors and of the care received from nurses also correlate significantly ($r = .42$, $p < .05$) though not highly with each other. Finally, patient satisfaction with the overall care received correlates positively and significantly with the extent to which the patients felt that there were no things that the staff could have done (but did not do) to give them better care ($r = .49$, $p < .01$), and the extent to which the EU seemed "to have enough doctors on hand to take care of all the patients within a reasonable time" ($r = .42$, $p < .05$). Neither of these last two variables, incidentally, is a component of the above-mentioned five-item index of patient satisfaction.

Staff satisfaction with the EU, an indicator of the social efficiency of the system, is represented by two measures, having been measured separately for the physicians (MDs) and registered nurses (RNs) working in the various EUs. More specifically, in their personal interviews, MDs and RNs were asked the following five-point-scale question: "On the whole, what do you think of this emergency unit as a place to work? Would you say it is an excellent place, a very good place, a good place, a fair place, or a rather poor place to work?" In the usual manner, the data from each group were aggregated to the EU level to obtain the desired measures, which show the mean satisfaction of MDs and of RNs at each EU.

The average satisfaction of MDs with the EU as a place to work ranges considerably across EUs, from 1.33 (most favorable) to 3.00, which corresponds exactly to "a good place" on the above scale. The mean of the thirty EUs on this measure is 2.18, and the standard deviation is .40. The between-EU variance for this measure is greater than the within-EU variance of responses ($F = 1.70$, $p < .05$), and the corresponding $\eta^2 = .19$. Accordingly, this is a methodologically acceptable measure. The satisfaction of RNs measure shows a similar statistical picture. EU means in this case range from 1.27 to 3.00, the grand mean being 2.04 and the standard deviation .41. The corresponding F = 2.86, $p < .01$, and the $\eta^2 = .25$.

Responsiveness to community expectations and needs concerning emergency medical services is represented by two indices. The first of these has four components, respectively based on data (aggregated to the EU level in each case) from the hospital administrators (HAs), MDs, RNs, and the selected community respondents (CRs) who participated in the study. These data were obtained with the following question: "On the whole, how adequately would you say this emergency unit is meeting *current community expectations* regarding the services it provides?" The response alternatives ranged from "(1) Extremely adequately" to "(5) Not adequately at all."

The between-EU variance for all except one of the component measures (that based on the data from CRs) is significantly greater than the within-EU variance of responses ($F \geqslant 1.78$, $p < .05$), and $\eta^2 \geqslant .18$ for all four components. The mean scores of the thirty EUs on the component measures are as follows: 2.39 (data from HAs), 2.02 (data from MDs), 2.22 (data from RNs), and 2.31 (data from CRs); and the corresponding standard deviations are .60, .34, .26, and .40. The interinstitutional range indicated by the four measures is considerable (1.67–4.50, 1.20–2.75, 1.73–2.71, and 1.56–3.00, respectively). The product-moment intercorrelations among the four measures are all positive but small to moderate, ranging from .11 (data from MDs and CRs) to .47 (data from MDs and RNs) and averaging .28; and three of the six correlations in the series are statistically significant ($p < .05$). The component-to-index correlations for the four measures are all statistically significant ($p < .01$) and fairly high: .75 (HAs' data), .69 (MDs' data, .64 (RNs' data), and .57 (CRs' data). The Cronbach alpha for the obtained index is .53, suggesting only marginal reliability. Finally, the scores of the thirty EUs on this index range from 1.62 to 2.85, with a mean of 2.23 and a standard deviation of .27.

The second index of EU responsiveness incorporates five components, respectively based on data obtained from the same four groups of respondents involved in the first index plus the selected hospital physician respondents (HMDs) from each institution, using the following question: "The emergency health care needs of communities change from time to time. How well has the emergency unit of this hospital been able to *keep up and respond to* such changes?" Five response alternatives, ranging from "(1) Extremely well" to "(5) Not well at all," were provided in addition to an "I can't judge" option.

The data from each group of respondents were properly aggregated to the EU level and their statistical properties examined before constructing the index. The product-moment intercorrelations among the five component measures range from .00 (data from HAs and CRs) to .47 (data from RNs and HMDs), the median intercorrelation is .32, and six of the ten correlations in the series are statistically significant ($p < .05$). The component-to-index correlations range from .29 to .75, averaging .60, and all except the smallest one are statistically significant ($p < .01$). The index constructed with these components has a Cronbach alpha of .62. The scores of the thirty EUs on this index range from 1.67 to 2.77, with a mean of 2.17 and a standard deviation of .27.

Overall, the two indices of EU responsiveness are statistically weak and only barely acceptable. Of all the secondary criteria of effectiveness, responsiveness is probably the least satisfactorily measured. Evidently, the several groups of respondents did not assess EU responsiveness from a very similar perspective. Intergroup agreement is minimal. Since this is only a secondary criterion, however, it was retained with due consideration for its methodological marginality.

Institutional reputation in the community, the last secondary criterion of effectiveness, is represented by two measures: reputation of the EU itself and reputation of its parent hospital. The latter measure was based on three assumptions: (1) that the reputation of a hospital EU may be a reflection of the reputation of its parent hospital, (2) that both the EU and its parent hospital probably enjoy the same or a similar kind of reputation in the community, and (3) that the public's image of the reputation of a hospital EU is partly defined (and possibly even determined) by the parent hospital's reputation. As anticipated, the two measures in question turned out to correlate fairly highly.

Data for the first measure were obtained from the selected community respondents (CRs). The relevant question, asked in the personal interviews completed by the CRs, was "At the present time, *what kind of reputation* does this emergency unit have in the community, generally speaking? *Does it have* an excellent reputation, a very good reputation, a good reputation, a fair reputation, or a rather poor reputation?" Based on this five-point scale, mean scores were computed separately for each of the thirty EUs in the sample. Across EUs, these scores range from 1.60 (most favorable) to 3.20, yielding a grand mean of 2.26 and a standard deviation of .43. The between-EU variance for this measure is only slightly greater than the within-EU variance of responses (F = 1.22, p = .21), while η^2 = .18. In spite of the F-ratio weakness, the measure was retained, partly because its overall statistical profile is not unsatisfactory and partly because of the particular source of data involved—the respondents in this case were not directly affiliated with any of the hospitals or EUs in the study.

In addition, it is important to point out that the validity of this measure is supported with data provided by several other groups of respondents. More specifically, EU reputation as assessed by the CRs correlates significantly with the reputation of EUs as assessed by the MDs (r = .40, $p < .05$), the RNs (r = .56, $p < .01$), the HAs (r = .42, $p < .05$), and the HMDs (r = .53, $p < .01$).

The second measure of institutional reputation in the community, the reputation of the parent hospital, is based on data from the patients (PATs) who completed questionnaires for the study—patients who had recently visited the EUs in the sample for medical treatment. The specific question answered by the PATs was as follows: "Thinking of this particular hospital, what kind of reputation does it have in the community?" The PATs were given five alternatives, ranging from "excellent" to "poor," and an "I don't know" option.

The data from this question, available for twenty-seven of the EUs in the sample, were aggregated to the EU level in order to construct the desired measure of parent hospital reputation. EU scores on this measure range from 1.11 to 3.71 on the above five-point scale, yielding a grand mean of 2.28 with a standard deviation of .72. The between-EU variance on this measure is significantly greater than the within-EU variance of responses (F = 3.86, $p < .01$), and $\eta^2 = .24$. Methodologically, therefore, this is a good measure.

Finally, the assumption that the reputation of hospital EUs is related to the reputation of their parent hospitals is justified by the fact that these two measures of institutional reputation turn out to correlate fairly highly ($r = .61$, $p < .01$) and by the fact that the reputation of hospital EUs, as assessed by the several groups of respondents whose data were not involved in the construction of the two measures in question, correlates positively with the reputation of parent hospitals. Briefly, the results show that EU reputation as assessed by the MDs, RNs, HAs, and HMDs correlates .64 ($p < .01$), .58 ($p < .01$), .26 ($p > .05$), and .46 ($p < .05$), respectively, with the reputation of the parent hospitals as assessed by the PATs.

Interrelationships Among Secondary Criterion Measures

The product-moment correlations among the measures of the secondary criteria of EU effectiveness discussed above are presented in Table 8-2 (lower-right triangle). First, the results show that the two measures of institutional reputation correlate positively and significantly ($r = .61$, $p < .01$). Second, the same is true of the two measures of EU responsiveness to community expectations and needs ($r = .66$, $p < .01$). And, third, the two measures of patient satisfaction correlate even more highly ($r = .73$, $p < .01$). These relationships are all consistent with the original expectations of the study.

The satisfaction of physicians with the EU as a place to work, on the other hand, is not significantly related to the satisfaction of registered nurses ($r = .25$, $p > .05$), even though a positive and statistically significant relationship had been anticipated. Possibly the specific determinants of satisfaction for the two groups differ sufficiently (the RNs are all employees of the parent hospitals while the MDs are not, and medical staffing patterns are considerably more diverse than those of nursing) to account for this finding. At the same time, the obtained correlation is sufficiently close to reaching statistical significance to argue that a weak, marginal relationship between medical and nursing staff satisfaction cannot be ruled out with certainty. Obviously, more research would be useful in this connection. Meanwhile, because they do not correlate significantly and cannot be incorporated into a single index, the two measures of staff satisfaction must be treated as separate and complementary criterion measures.

The measure of promptness of medical attention to patients is represented by the percentage of incoming patients seen by a doctor within fifteen minutes of their arrival at each EU. This measure, which is based on data provided by the RNs working at the various EUs, correlates very well ($r = .59$, $p < .01$) with a second measure, which is based on data provided by the MDs (not shown in Table 8-2). Further, if these two measures are combined, they both correlate very highly with the resulting composite measure (.91 and .87, respectively). However, because the data from MDs might entail some bias concerning the promptness of medical attention given to patients, only the measure based on the data from RNs was retained for further analysis—the measure that correlates most highly with the promptness composite measure. The results concerning the relationships among the secondary criteria of effectiveness further indicate that, of the five such criteria in the series (and also of the nine criterion measures involved), promptness of medical attention is the most unique, because it correlates significantly with only one other secondary criterion measure (physician satisfaction with the EU).

The findings also show that, as expected, the correlations among the nine measures of the secondary criteria of EU effectiveness range widely, from -.11 to .73. Because the criteria and measures employed represent different aspects of institutional effectiveness, as well as different perspectives, their interrelationships were generally expected to be positive but far from perfect. This indeed turned out to be the case. Nevertheless, the overall picture is one of substantial consistency in the interrelationships found. Thus, all but three of the thirty-six relevant correlation coefficients are in the right direction (positive), and eighteen are

Table 8-2. Interrelationships Among Primary Criteria, Among Secondary Criteria, and Between Primary and Secondary Criteria of Emergency Unit (EU) Effectiveness.

	Primary Criteria				Secondary Criteria								
	1	2	3	4	5	6	7	8	9	10	11	12	13
Primary Criteria													
1. Economic Efficiency (Index measure)	--	-.07	.21	.07	-.21	.33*	.35*	-.12	-.10	.21	.39*	.03	-.04
2. Quality of Medical Care (Index measure)		--	.61**	.91**	.53**	.41*	.39*	.40*	.31*	.50**	.44**	.30	.58**
3. Quality of Nursing Care (Index measure)			--	.89**	.33*	.41*	.56**	.41*	.54**	.68**	.42*	.46**	.56**
4. Quality of Overall Patient Care (Measures 2 + 3)				--	.49**	.45**	.52**	.45**	.46**	.65**	.47**	.42*	.64**
Secondary Criteria													
Promptness of Medical Attention to Incoming Patients:													
5. Percentage of patients seen by a doctor within 15 minutes					--	.44**	.18	.17	.23	.13	.22	-.11	.04
Staff Satisfaction with EU													
6. Physicians—MDs (mean)						--	.25	-.02	.09	.23	.35*	-.11	.20
7. Registered Nurses—RNs (mean)							--	.14	.37*	.49**	.60**	.41*	.31*

Patient Satisfaction with

8. Care received at the EU (mean)	--	.73**	.43*	.26	.72**	.47**
9. EU staff (a five-item index for which $\alpha = .77$)		--	.40*	.07	.52**	.49**
EU Responsiveness in Meeting						
10. Community expectations concerning services (an index with data from HAs, MDs, RNs, and CRs; $\alpha = .53$)			--	.66**	.69**	.45**
11. Community's changing needs (an index based on data from HAs, MDs, RNs, HMDs, and CRs; $\alpha = .62$)				--	.24	.13
Institutional Reputation						
12. EU reputation as rated by selected community respondents—CRs (mean)					--	.61**
13. Parent hospital reputation as rated by emergency unit patients—PATs (mean)						--

Notes:
*$p < .05$.
**$p < .01$.
The correlations shown are product-moment correlations at the emergency unit level. For most coefficients, $N = 30$ EUs, and for the remaining ones the N varies between 24 and 28 EUs.

statistically significant ($p < .05$) as well. The three negative correlations are inconsequential, in fact close to zero, and none approaches statistical significance even at the .10 level. The remaining thirty-three correlations in the series average .36, and the median correlation is .35.

In view of these findings and the strong pattern of relationships (discussed below) between the secondary criterion measures and the measures of the primary criteria of EU effectiveness (especially the quality of medical and nursing care), it is reasonable to conclude that to a certain extent the secondary criteria are in fact indicative of the institutional effectiveness of hospital EUs. For this reason, and also because of their intrinsic value and interest to the field of emergency medical services, they deserve more consideration in future studies. For present purposes, however, the importance of these secondary criteria of effectiveness lies mainly in their use for validating the primary criteria.

Relationships Between the Secondary and Primary Criteria

The results in Table 8-2 show that each of the nine measures representing the secondary criteria of effectiveness correlates positively and significantly with at least two of the four indices representing the primary criteria. In fact, three of the nine measures (physician satisfaction with the EU as a place to work, the satisfaction of registered nurses with the EU, and EU responsiveness to the community's changing needs for emergency medical services) correlate significantly with all four indices. Five other measures (5, 8, 9, 10, and 13) correlate significantly with three indices (specifically, the quality of care indices). The remaining measure (the reputation of EUs according to CRs) correlates significantly with two of the care indices. In all, twenty-nine of the thirty-six correlations between the secondary and primary criteria are both positive and statistically significant, confirming the study's initial expectations in this regard. Of the seven nonsignificant correlations in the series, six involve the criterion of economic efficiency.

Of the primary criteria, economic efficiency (which was previously found not to correlate with clinical efficiency) is significantly related to three of the nine secondary criterion measures—MD satisfaction with the EU as a place to work, RN satisfaction, and EU responsiveness to the community's changing needs for emergency medical services. Interestingly, however, each of these particular measures correlates even more highly with the quality of care indices, that is, with clinical efficiency, than it does with economic efficiency. This difference notwithstanding, staff satisfaction with the EU (an indicator of the social efficiency of this system) apparently facilitates both the economic and clinical performance of hospital EUs. The correlations between the remaining secondary criterion measures and economic efficiency range from −.21 to +.21, suggesting that promptness of medical attention to patients, patient satisfaction, and institutional reputation in the community do not appreciably affect the economic efficiency of hospital EUs, and vice versa.

Unlike economic efficiency, the quality of medical care is positively and significantly related to eight of the nine secondary criterion measures. The exception involves the reputation of EUs as perceived by the CRs, but even in this case the correlation just misses statistical significance at the .05 level. The specific product-moment correlations in the present series range from .30 to .58, and the average $r = .41$, the same as the median correlation. It is also interesting to note in Table 8-2 the relatively high correlation ($r = .53$) found between promptness of medical attention to incoming patients and the quality of medical care index. In contrast, promptness of medical attention correlates only modestly ($r = .33$) with the quality of nursing care index.

The quality of nursing care shows a similar, and somewhat stronger, pattern of relationships to the secondary criterion measures. All nine of these measures correlate positively and significantly with the nursing care index, the second major component of clinical efficiency. The specific correlations in this case range from .33 to .68, the average $r = .49$, and the median $r = .46$. Finally, the overall quality of patient care (represented by the special index of clinical efficiency that incorporates the quality of medical and nursing care indices combined) also correlates positively and significantly with all nine measures of the secondary criteria of EU effectiveness. The specific correlations in this case range from .42 to .65 and average .51.

Other interesting conclusions that may be drawn from the results in Table 8-2 concern particular measures of the secondary criteria and their differential relationships to the indices of the quality of medical and nursing care. For example, MD satisfaction with the EU as a place to work is equally well related ($r = .41$) to the quality of medical and of nursing care, whereas RN satisfaction correlates better with the latter than with the former component of clinical efficiency (.56 versus .39).

Patient satisfaction with the care received correlates about equally with the quality of medical and nursing care (.40, .41), whereas patient satisfaction with EU staff performance correlates better with nursing care than with medical care (.54 versus .31), suggesting that patients mainly considered nursing staff in this case. Similarly, EU responsiveness to the community's changing needs for emergency medical services correlates about equally well with the quality of medical and nursing care (.44, .42), while EU responsiveness in meeting community expectations concerning emergency services correlates more strongly with nursing than with medical care (.68 versus .50). Finally, the reputation of EUs, as assessed by the selected community respondents, also correlates somewhat more highly with the quality of nursing than the quality of medical care (.46 versus .30), whereas the reputation of the parent hospitals as assessed by the patients correlates about equally strongly with these two aspects of clinical efficiency (.56 and .58).

On the whole, while not hypothesized in advance, these relationships are both sensible and consistent with the results of the study concerning medical and nursing staffing patterns.

In conclusion, the findings show that each of the five secondary criteria of EU effectiveness examined in this research (four of which are represented by two measures each) is meaningfully and significantly related to at least one, and sometimes both, of the primary criteria of effectiveness (clinical and economic efficiency). Accordingly, the validity of the primary criteria of EU effectiveness is further confirmed and enhanced by these findings—especially the validity of the indices of clinical efficiency.

Summary

Discussed in this chapter were (1) the empirical relationships found among the indices of clinical and economic efficiency, that is, among the primary criteria of EU effectiveness at the institutional level; (2) the relationships between these major criteria and five secondary criteria of EU effectiveness; and (3) the interrelationships among a total of nine specific measures representing the five secondary criteria.

The results show that the economic efficiency of hospital EUs is unrelated to their clinical efficiency (even when controlling for such important variables as EU patient volume, breadth or scope of emergency service, parent hospital size and complexity, and community complexity). The two components of clinical efficiency are positively related, that is, the quality of medical care correlates significantly with the quality of nursing care, and vice versa—though not as highly as might have been expected—and each of them correlates positively and significantly (but in varying degrees) with at least eight of the nine secondary criterion measures investigated. The interrelationships among the secondary criterion measures also were found to be generally positive, as expected, though smaller and more variable than the relationships of the same measures to the primary criteria of EU effectiveness.

The results presented in this chapter add to the substantial evidence presented in Chapters Five, Six, and Seven supporting the validity of the indices developed to assess the clinical and economic efficiency of hospital EUs. In effect, the secondary criteria validate the primary criteria of EU effectiveness, further enhancing one's confidence in the indices used to measure economic and clinical efficiency.

Chapter Nine

Organizational Structure
and Effectiveness

The main purpose of this research, it will be recalled, was to investigate the relationship between the organization and effectiveness of hospital emergency units (EUs) at the institutional level and, in the process, identify some of the major sources and correlates of interinstitutional differences in effectiveness. Emergency unit effectiveness, or performance, is represented by the indices of clinical and economic efficiency discussed in Chapters Five, Six, and Seven, augmented by the secondary criterion measures considered in Chapter Eight. The principal hypothesis of the study was that differences in EU effectiveness can be substantially accounted for by differences in the organization of the system, especially differences in organizational structure and problem solving. Theoretically, the variability in effectiveness among EUs should be determined by all of the following "independent" variables: (1) the technical competence and personal qualifications of individual staff members; (2) the external environment as it bears upon the resources and patient inputs of EUs; (3) the structural linkages and organizational relations between EUs and their parent hospitals, and especially the resources, services, and support provided by hospitals to the EUs; (4) the nature of work relations and problem solving within EUs; and (5) the structure of the system. Controlling for relevant differences in the environment and individual differences among staff members, however, the effectiveness of EUs is expected to be determined mainly by organizational variables.

The present study, therefore, focused on certain aspects of the structure and internal organization of hospital EUs, that is, on the last three of the above sets of variables. In addition, certain aspects of the system's social environment were explored. These are structural characteristics of the communities being served, which in part may define some of the resources and patient inputs of EUs and thus affect the internal functioning of the system. At least indirectly, environmental context could affect organizational functioning. The main research interest, however, was in the relationship of organizational structure and problem solving to effectiveness.

Work relations and problem solving within the EUs in the areas of resource allocation, coordination and control, staff integration, strain and conflict, and adaptation to the environment were considered particularly important as likely determinants of institutional effectiveness. The same applies to certain structural variables, including medical staffing pattern, personnel training programs, medical teaching affiliation, parent hospital size, service complexity, specialization, patient volume (or EU size), and the institution's breadth of emergency service. Of the many aspects of organizational structure that might be interesting to consider, these staff-linked and size-related variables were selected for special attention, both because of their anticipated importance to EU functioning and because of their pragmatic interest to the health services field.

In this study, the term *structure* is mainly used in a generic sense, to refer to the basic anatomy of a system. (For a discussion of various conceptions of structure, see MacKenzie, 1976.) It involves the particular elements, or component parts, encompassed by a system and their relatively stable (that is, more or less permanent) arrangement in time and space. In the case of human organizations, of course, people are the basic elements. In other words, structure is mainly used in a concrete rather than abstract sense, in a manner analogous to Miller's (1965, 1978) distinction between "concrete" and "abstracted" systems, the main interest of the study being in the above-mentioned variables.* In the abstract sense, on the other hand, *structure* represents patterns of relationships (or interactions) among the elements of a system rather than the elements themselves and their spatiotemporal arrangements. The former (anatomical or concrete) aspects might be thought of as the *alpha structures* of organizations, and the latter (abstracted) aspects as their *beta structures*. Here we are primarily concerned with the former.

It should also be noted that certain structural variables, such as those of heterogeneity, complexity, and specialization, may be properly used to characterize both the alpha and beta structures of organizations. Moreover, regardless of how the component elements of organizational structure are conceptualized, it is important to note that, individually and collectively, they carry with them information and possess particular properties or qualifications that have implications for the capabilities of the system (Georgopoulos and Cooke, 1979). Further, the elements in question are ordered and interlinked (that is, are "organized") in various ways; and, together with their linkages, interrelationships, and functions, they constitute what we refer to as "the system."

Beyond the basic anatomical structure of a system, such as the hospital or hospital EU, a variety of more specific, differentiated, and specialized structures—such as the hierarchical or authority structure, the role structure, the communication structure, and the normative structure—may be distinguished, as may different orders of structure (see Georgopoulos and Cooke, 1979). Among recent studies which, using the same basic research model as the present study, have examined aspects of these structures in relation to organizational problem solving and effectiveness (or output) are those by Argote (1982), Cooke and Rousseau (1981), and Sutton and Ford (1982). For some earlier relevant research, see Georgopoulos (1965, 1972, 1975); Georgopoulos and Mann (1962); and Georgopoulos and Matejko (1967).

*Miller himself defines structure as "the static arrangement of a system's parts (subsystems and components) at a moment (of time) in three-dimensional space" (1965, pp. 209, 211).

Although they are conceptually and analytically distinct, the structures and substructures of a system are all juxtaposed and interdependent. But they are not necessarily highly consistent, either internally or with one another. They may or may not be well integrated or mutually reinforcing, but they are never entirely consistent or perfectly integrated. Therefore, not all aspects of organizational structure or structural variables of interest may be expected to intercorrelate highly or even positively. Nevertheless, partly because of their interdependence, they may affect not only one another but also the behavior of individual elements and the functioning of the total system.

Significance of Organizational Structures

The importance of organizational structure to the performance of a system is not difficult to establish theoretically. Briefly, the structures of an organization, or any other social system, essentially constitute the basic problem-solving framework of the system (for example, see Georgopoulos, 1972; Georgopoulos and Cooke, 1979; Cooke and Rousseau, 1981; Sutton and Ford, 1982). They provide a relatively stable base on which staff groups and members can rely in performing their respective tasks, and they facilitate behavior that is both appropriate to the tasks and consistent with the culture (that is, the norms and values) of the system. More specifically, structures affect both problem solving and performance in at least five major ways:

1. By minimizing uncertainty and ambiguity in the system, and thus facilitating the integration and coordination of interdependent functions and enhancing the orderliness and predictability of behavior.
2. By serving as a ready frame of reference or point of departure for the development, refinement, and implementation of work plans and performance programs, and thus ensuring functional continuity.
3. By reducing unwanted deviations from system-sanctioned behavior patterns internally and by ensuring unity of action toward the environment.

4. By providing a basis for selecting among available means of
    problem solving those that are likely to be acceptable to the
    culture of the system as well as technically appropriate.
5. By facilitating decision making and problem solving, as well
    as the regulation and control of behavior, on an organization-
    wide basis.

Under certain conditions, of course, organizational structure
may also affect performance adversely. This is likely in the case of
(1) highly rigid or inflexible structures (which tend to impede
spontaneity, adaptability, and innovative behavior); (2) unneces-
sarily complex structures (for example, overspecialized structures,
structures with too many hierarchical levels to permit meaningful
member participation in decision making or problem solving);
and (3) structures that are so poorly integrated as to make human
adjustment difficult to achieve (for example, when the formal role
structure is grossly incompatible with the informal social structure
of the system). In any event, different structures may have negative
as well as positive consequences for organizational functioning,
and different structural variables may have different effects on
performance, depending upon the nature and level of the particular variables. One important task of organizational research,
therefore, should be to ascertain empirically, as well as to specify
theoretically, the relationships of particular structural variables,
such as those examined here, to system effectiveness.

In summary, the operational continuity of a system, the
level of uncertainty and predictability of behavior within the
system, the ability of the system to regulate work activities and
control performance, and even its ability to respond to the
environment as a unified entity depend, to an important extent,
upon the structure(s) of the system. Thus, structural variables are
expected to have significant effects on organizational problem
solving and performance.

Reported in this chapter are the relationships found
between the major structural variables included in the research and

emergency unit effectiveness.* The findings are grouped according to the following independent variables: (1) community structure variables, or the environmental context of the system; (2) staff-linked aspects of EU organization, such as medical teaching affiliation; and (3) organizational size and related aspects of structure, such as complexity. Results are shown separately for clinical and economic efficiency, and with respect to the former criterion they are shown separately for the quality of medical and nursing care.

Structural Aspects of the Environment and EU Effectiveness

The environmental context of an organization can affect behavior within the system for a variety of reasons. The relevant external environment of hospitals and hospital EUs may be more or less stable, complex, heterogeneous, and so on, with corresponding implications for internal organizational functioning. Structural characteristics of the immediate community, such as the composition of the population being served, may have important implications both for the nature of patient inputs and for the financial and staff resources available to EUs. Population instability and poverty, for example, could hinder the economic (and possibly also clinical) efficiency of hospital EUs, while high levels of education and income in the community might facilitate it.

In order to explore these relationships, the following characteristics of the city or town in which each EU is located were examined in relation to EU effectiveness: (1) formal education level of community residents, measured by the median number of school years completed by persons twenty-five years old or older; (2) economic status, measured by median family income and (secondarily) by the percentage of families with income below the poverty level; (3) community heterogeneity, measured by the percentage of population classified as minority; (4) community complexity—a

*Partial findings concerning the performance of hospital EUs and its relationship to organizational structure have been reported in a previous publication (Georgopoulos, 1985).

composite measure incorporating the percentage of minority population and the percentage of families below the poverty level; and (5) population stability, measured by subtracting from the population base the percentage of growth or decline during the preceding decade. All of these measures are based on data from the most recent U.S. Census reports available preceding the 1980 census. (The intercorrelations among the six measures examined, which are generally high, may be seen in Table 9-1.)

Certain alternative measures for some of these variables were also considered but omitted from further analysis when they were found to correlate highly with the above measures: The percentage of persons twenty-five years old or older who completed high school correlates .99 with the median number of school years completed by the same group; income per capita correlates .82 with median family income; and average public assistance income in the community correlates .68 with the percentage of families below poverty level and .61 with the percentage of minority population. The latter two variables, incidentally, which are the components of the community complexity measure, correlate .61 with each other but .77 and .98, respectively, with community complexity.

The results concerning the relationship between community structure, as represented by the above variables, and the effectiveness of hospital EUs are summarized in Table 9-1. With only one exception, they show no significant relationship. Specifically, only median family income turns out to be significantly associated with any of the three indices of EU effectiveness. Median family income correlates positively and significantly ($r = .43$, $p < .05$) with the quality of nursing care. It does not, however, correlate significantly with the quality of medical care or with the economic efficiency of hospital EUs.

Given the other findings shown in Table 9-1, the modest correlation obtained between median family income and nursing care quality could be a chance occurrence or might be explained in two other ways: Hospital EUs in the more affluent communities may have more competent nursing personnel (but not more competent medical staff, since income does not correlate with the quality of medical care) or a lighter patient load for the nursing

Table 9-1. Relationships between Community Structure Variables and the Effectiveness of Emergency Units.

| | Emergency Unit Effectiveness | | |
| | Economic Efficiency | Clinical Efficiency | |
Community Structure	Economic Efficiency Index (N = 26 EUs)	Quality of Nursing Care Index (N = 30 EUs)	Quality of Medical Care Index (N = 30 EUs)
Formal Education Level			
Median number of school years completed by persons 25 years or older	-.25	.29	.17
Economic Status			
Median family income	-.23	.43*	.28
Percentage of families with income below poverty level	-.12	-.10	.08
Community Heterogeneity			
Percentage of population classified as minority	-.15	.09	.17
Community Complexity			
Percentage of population classified as minority or below poverty level	-.16	.04	.16
Population Stability			
As indicated by the percentage of population growth or decline since the last census	-.08	-.22	-.09

Notes:
*$p < .05$.
All correlations shown are product-moment correlations at the institutional level.

The community structure variables are interrelated as follows: formal education level correlates .85, -.70, -.50, -.60, and .53, respectively, with the variables listed below it; median family income correlates -.72, -.28, -.43, and .66, respectively, with the variables which follow it; percent of families below the poverty level correlates .61, .77, and -.78, respectively, with the variables which follow; percent of population classified as minority correlates .98 and -.51, respectively, with the variables below it; and community complexity correlates -.62 with population stability. These are all product-moment correlations based on an $N = 30$ communities (cities) in each case, and all except the smallest one of them in this set of 15 are statistically significant ($p < .05$).

staff than their counterparts in the less affluent communities. Either interpretation is plausible, but probably no more plausible than the chance occurrence explanation (see also the regression analysis results reported below).

It is also interesting to note that the percentage of families below the poverty level shows no relationship whatsoever to either the economic or the clinical efficiency of hospital EUs. The same is true of the percentage of the population classified as minority, which correlates .61 with the percentage below poverty level, and of community complexity—the composite variable that incorporates both of these aspects of community structure. The relative stability of the population shows a similar lack of relationship to EU effectiveness. Finally, the formal education level of the population yields a pattern of correlations with the effectiveness indices that is similar to that produced by median family income, although none of the correlations is statistically significant at the .05 level.

These results indicate that the effectiveness of hospital EUs does not appear to be significantly affected by the community structure variables explored to this point (formal education level, economic status, community heterogeneity and complexity, and population stability). The correlations between the economic efficiency of EUs and these variables range between -.08 and -.25, none being statistically significant, and the same is true of the correlations between quality of medical care and the same variables, which range from -.09 to .28. Only the quality of nursing care correlates significantly, though modestly, to one of the measures—median family income.

The general lack of significant relationships between community structure variables and EU effectiveness is further confirmed by regression analyses that were performed to ascertain whether several of these community structure variables jointly, or as a set, are significantly related to EU effectiveness. In these multiple regression analyses (standard least squares regressions), the following community structure measures were used as predictors or independent variables: population stability, median family income, formal education level, and community complexity. The results obtained for the three indices of EU effectiveness may be briefly summarized as follows: (1) for economic efficiency, $F = 1.40$, $df = 4, 21$, $p = .27$, and $R^2 = .21$, with none of the partial correlations associated with the four predictors being statistically significant (by t test) at the .05 level; (2) for the quality of nursing care, $F = 2.09$, $df = 4, 25$, $p = .11$, and $R^2 = .25$, with none of the partial correlations being significant; and (3) for the quality of medical care, $F = 1.35$, $df = 4, 25$, $p = .28$, and $R^2 = .18$, again with none of the partial correlations associated with the predictors being statistically significant. In short, these results show no significant relationship between the four community structure measures as a set and each of the three indices of EU effectiveness, confirming the correlational analyses that examined the several measures separately.

Overall, these findings cast some doubt on organizational theories proposing that conditions of environmental turbulence and instability, or stability, can explain organizational functioning. Although the above measures of community structure are based on U.S. Census reports that were less current than the effectiveness measures, the obtained pattern of results is highly suggestive of no direct association between community structure and EU effectiveness.

This lack of association, however, cannot be generalized to aspects of community structure which were not measured in this research or to independent variables reflecting the nature of interaction between EUs and their relevant external environments. As shown in Chapter Eight, for example, the responsiveness of hospital EUs to the changing needs of the community correlates positively with both economic and clinical efficiency of EUs, and institutional reputation in the community also is significantly related to the quality of patient care provided by the various EUs. Even more important, aspects of system-environment relations, such as the extent of collaboration between hospital EUs and other health care organizations in the community, were found to be strongly related to EU effectiveness (see Chapter Ten and Uzun, 1980).

Other Structural Aspects of the Environment

The study examined two additional aspects reflecting the structure of EU environments that were considered potentially important to EU effectiveness: (1) the urban/rural character of the communities in which the various hospital EUs functioned, represented by SMSA and non-SMSA location, and (2) the relative uncertainty of the patient inputs of EUs, represented by a measure of patient volume heterogeneity for ten medical categories of patients (see Argote, 1982).

To determine whether the urban/rural character of the environment affects EU performance, the EUs located in SMSA communities were compared to those located in non-SMSA communities on the economic and clinical efficiency measures. The results show no significant differences between the two groups on any of the criteria. They do not, however, completely rule out some kind of association between SMSA/non-SMSA location and EU performance because they are suggestive of a possible trend in that direction.

Specifically, clinical efficiency tends to be somewhat better, on the average, for EUs in the SMSA communities than EUs in the non-SMSA communities. For the quality of medical care, $\overline{X}$ = 7.01 for the former group of EUs compared to 7.81 for the latter (t = -1.56, df = 28, and p = .13, two-tailed test). The results concerning the quality of nursing care are very similar: $\overline{X}$ = 7.33 and 7.96, respectively, for EUs in the SMSA and the non-SMSA groups (t = -1.35, df = 28, and p = .19). Exactly the opposite pattern is evident, however, in the case of economic efficiency, which, on the average, tends to be somewhat better for EUs located in non-SMSA compared to SMSA communities: $\overline{X}$ = 46.75 and 57.89, respectively, for the two groups (t = 1.20, df = 24, p = .24). Although interesting, the differences suggested by these trends do not reach statistical significance at the .05 level. Additional research would be, therefore, necessary to resolve the issue of possible association between urban/rural location and EU effectiveness more definitively. For characteristics that distinguish EUs located in SMSA areas from those located in non-SMSA areas, see Georgopoulos, Cooke, and Associates (1980).

Concerning the uncertainty of patient inputs, Argote (1979, 1982) tested the hypothesis that input uncertainty is related to organizational problem solving within EUs and also moderates the relationship between problem solving and effectiveness. Argote's (1982) findings (based on data from the project) showed that input uncertainty is, in varying degrees, directly related to the adequacy of problem solving by EUs in three areas: resource allocation, strain, and adaptation to the environment. In addition, it moderates the relationship between EU reliance on certain means for achieving coordination of activities and clinical efficiency. Specifically, programmed means of organizational coordination (for example, rules, scheduled meetings) make a greater contribution to EU effectiveness under conditions of low uncertainty than under conditions of high uncertainty, while the reverse is true in the case of nonprogrammed means of coordination (for example, staff autonomy, mutual adjustment). In areas other than coordination, however, the uncertainty of inputs was not found to moderate the relationship between organizational problem solving and EU effectiveness. Overall, then, the available evidence indicates that the relative uncertainty of patient inputs, as measured by Argote, is related to the clinical efficiency of hospital EUs only indirectly.

In summary, except for the uncertainty of inputs and possibly also median family income, the community structure variables explored in the present study show no significant relationship to either the economic or the clinical efficiency of hospital EUs. The above findings cast some doubt on the theory that differences in the environment or structural context of a system such as those explored here have an important or direct impact on the system's effectiveness. In the case of hospital EUs, at least, apparently they do not. The structural aspects of EU organization, on the other hand, as we are about to see, yield a totally different picture.

Staff-Linked Aspects of EU Organization and EU Effectiveness

The results concerning the relationship of EU effectiveness to three important structural aspects of organization are presented in this section. Reflecting the clinical structure of hospital EUs, these staff-linked aspects of organizational structure are: medical staffing pattern, medical teaching affiliation, and emergency personnel training programs.

Emergency Personnel Training Programs

Theoretically, special training programs for EU clinical personnel such as medical technicians, nurses, or physicians should enable the staff to maintain high performance standards and thus promote the quality of staff performance, thereby facilitating organizational effectiveness. This hypothesis was tested, and the findings are presented in Table 9-2.

Clearly, economic efficiency and the quality of nursing care are both significantly higher for the EUs of institutions that have emergency personnel training programs compared to those that do not. A similar though weaker trend is evident for the quality of medical care; in this case, the difference reaches statistical significance only at the .10 level. A very similar pattern emerges, moreover, from the results of correlational analysis (not shown in Table 9-2). Specifically, as a dichotomous variable, the existence of emergency personnel training programs correlates .43 ($p < .05$), .42 ($p < .05$), and .28 ($p < .10$), respectively, with economic efficiency, the quality of nursing care, and the quality of medical care across hospital EUs.

The weaker correlation with medical compared to nursing care is not easy to explain, particularly because the same number of EUs have training programs for nurses as for physicians—a total of three in each case, compared to fourteen for emergency medical technicians. Possibly, nursing care benefits more than does medical care from this particular distribution of training programs in the study sample; that is, nursing performance benefits more from the programs for physicians and technicians than medical performance benefits from the programs for nurses and technicians. It is also possible, of course, that the training programs for nurses are superior, or more effective, than those for physicians.

Table 9-2. Staff-Linked Aspects of Organizational Structure and Emergency Unit Effectiveness.

| | Emergency Unit Effectiveness | | | | | | | | |
| | Economic Efficiency | | | Quality of Nursing Care | | | Quality of Medical Care | | |
Organizational Structure Variables	Mean	SD	N	Mean	SD	N	Mean	SD	N
Medical Teaching Affiliation									
Institutions with medical teaching affiliation	53.06	19.63	16	6.81	0.91	17	6.88	1.54	17
Institutions without such affiliation	56.70	26.23	10	8.44	0.86	13	7.33	0.76	13
t:	-0.40			-4.97			-1.81		
df:	24			28			28		
p:	>.10			<.01			<.05		
Emergency Personnel Training Programs									
Institutions with training programs	44.42	24.31	12	7.03	1.18	15	6.89	1.13	15
Institutions without such programs	63.07	15.95	14	8.01	1.03	15	7.61	1.42	15
t:	-2.35			-2.43			-1.54		
df:	24			28			28		
p:	<.05			<.05			<.10		
Medical Staffing Pattern									
1. Hospital-based group on contract	39.60	12.32	5	6.63	1.03	5	6.96	1.41	5
2. Non-hospital-based group on contract	58.71	25.71	7	6.92	1.11	9	7.08	1.28	9
3. Rotating staff	49.00	27.33	6	8.56	1.10	7	7.38	1.16	7
4. All other patterns	64.13	15.08	8	7.81	0.78	9	7.48	1.57	9
All EUs combined:	54.46	21.96	26	7.52	1.20	30	7.25	1.31	30

Notes:

All means are institutional-level scores, averaged for the EUs belonging to each grouping, as indicated. In all cases, the smaller the score, the better the performance.

Medical teaching affiliation and emergency personnel training programs are not correlated ($r = .07$, $p > .10$).

The following differences between means are statistically significant: in the case of economic efficiency, pattern 1 vs. pattern 4 ($t = -3.04$, $df = 11$, $p = .01$); and in the case of nursing care, pattern 1 vs. pattern 3 ($t = -3.07$, $df = 10$, $p = .01$), pattern 1 vs. pattern 4 ($t = -2.41$, $df = 12$, $p = .03$), and pattern 2 vs. pattern 3 ($t = -2.94$, $df = 14$, $p = .01$).

Source: Adapted from Georgopoulos, 1985.

At any rate, according to the findings in Table 9-2, emergency personnel training programs at hospital EUs seem to pay off in terms of both economic and clinical efficiency (see also the results of the regression analysis presented later in this chapter). Whatever the costs of such programs may be, apparently they are offset by economic efficiency gains. Even more important, they are also offset by gains in clinical efficiency, even though (as discussed in Chapter Eight) the economic and clinical efficiency of hospital EUs are not related. Therefore, emergency personnel training programs may be strongly recommended as one major and practical means for improving both the economic and clinical performance of hospital emergency units. For a variety of descriptive differences between institutions with and without emergency personnel training programs, see Georgopoulos, Cooke, and Associates (1980).

Medical Teaching Affiliation

Other results in Table 9-2 show that, on the average, the quality of medical care is significantly better at institutions with a medical teaching affiliation than institutions lacking such affiliation. Such a difference was expected on the grounds that performance standards and staff skills, at least for the medical staff but probably also for the rest of the staff as well, would be superior at hospitals and hospital EUs which have a medical teaching affiliation. The results for both medical and nursing care are consistent with this assumption. In fact, the difference in the quality of care between institutions having and not having a medical teaching affiliation is even stronger for nursing care than it is for medical care.

It is also important to point out that these findings are basically independent of the similar results reported above concerning the relationship between training programs and clinical efficiency. One major reason for this independence is that hospital EUs with emergency personnel training programs are not significantly more likely than those without such programs also to have a medical teaching affiliation. Specifically, of the fifteen EUs in the sample which have training programs, nine also have a medical teaching affiliation; but of the other fifteen EUs which do not have such programs, eight have a teaching affiliation as well. When correlated as dichotomous variables, in fact, training programs and teaching affiliation show no relationship whatsoever ($r = .07$, $p > .05$).

Unlike its expectations concerning clinical efficiency, the study had no specific hypothesis regarding the relationship of medical teaching affiliation to economic efficiency. The obtained results, however, show no difference whatsoever in the average economic efficiency level of EUs at institutions with and without medical teaching affiliation. (See also the findings from the regression analyses discussed later in this chapter.) Finally, medical teaching affiliation as a dichotomous variable turns out to correlate .08 ($p > .05$), .68 ($p < .01$), and .32 ($p < .05$), respectively, with economic efficiency, the quality of nursing care, and the quality of medical care. These correlations confirm the results in Table 9-2.

In summary, then, medical teaching affiliation promotes the clinical efficiency of hospital EUs without affecting their economic efficiency adversely. Specifically, such affiliation seems to entail no financial burden for the EUs studied, while enhancing the quality of their medical and nursing care. Accordingly, medical teaching affiliation may also be recommended as a means for improving EU effectiveness where such affiliation is feasible. For a variety of descriptive differences between institutions with and without medical teaching affiliation, see Georgopolous, Cooke, and Associates (1980).

Medical Staffing Pattern

Not all EUs are operated by the hospitals in which they are located, even though the parent hospitals are responsible for nonmedical personnel staffing. Some institutions, apparently an increasing number, engage in contractual, franchise-like arrangements with medical groups or corporations for the operation of their emergency service; some of these groups are hospital-based, but others are not. Other institutions rely on rotating staff arrangements (with or without medical residents), the prevailing pattern in years past. Still others, usually small hospitals, rely on contracts with individual physicians, and occasionally part-time physicians only. Of the thirty EUs in the present study, five rely on a hospital-based group on contract, nine on a non-hospital-based group on contract, seven on a rotating staff arrangement, and nine on a variety of other staffing arrangements, including individual physicians on contract.

Empirical research on the significance and implications of these different medical staffing patterns for the quality and costs of the services provided by hospital EUs is badly needed. Relevant data from the present study, nevertheless, provide some very interesting though still tentative answers in this connection (see Table 9-2).

First, the results show that the medical staffing pattern of EUs is in fact associated with their economic and clinical efficiency. Such association had been anticipated, but because of the lack of any relevant past research in this area the study hypothesized no specific relationships.

Second, the results show that one particular staffing pattern, "hospital-based group on contract," ranks first among the four different patterns examined on all three indices of EU effectiveness. On the average, economic efficiency, the quality of nursing care, and the quality of medical care are all highest for this particular group of EUs.

Third, economic efficiency is highest on the average for EUs with hospital-based group arrangements, followed by rotating staff arrangements, non-hospital-based group arrangements, and all other types of staff arrangements, in that order. The difference in economic efficiency between the first and last of these patterns is statistically significant (t = 3.04, df = 11, p = .01 two-tailed), while the remaining differences among the several patterns are only directionally important. Overall, with regard to the economic efficiency of hospital EUs, the results favor the hospital-based group and rotating staff patterns (both of which score better than the sample mean), particularly the former, over the other two staffing patterns.

Fourth, the results show that the quality of nursing care on the average is best for EUs which rely on the hospital-based group pattern, followed by those with the non-hospital-based group pattern, the mixed or "all other patterns" arrangement, and the rotating staff pattern, in that order. Moreover, most of the differences in the quality of nursing care among the several medical staffing patterns are statistically significant.

Finally, concerning the quality of medical care, the results in Table 9-2 indicate that the best and second-best medical staffing patterns are the same as those for the quality of nursing care—the hospital-based and the non-hospital-based group patterns. The rotating staff pattern (which ranks second best with regard to economic efficiency but poorest of the four with regard to the quality of nursing care) ranks third in the case of medical care, followed by the mixed "all other patterns" group of EUs in last place. The differences in the quality of medical care among the several medical staffing patterns, however, are generally smaller than those found for the quality of nursing care and do not reach statistical significance by two-tailed t test at the .05 level. More research will be necessary, therefore, before a final conclusion can be reached regarding the precise relationship between particular medical staffing patterns and the quality of medical care. Still, the results from the present study are strongly suggestive that, other things being equal, the hospital-based group arrangement probably constitutes the best medical staffing pattern from the point of view of the quality of medical care, and certainly the best pattern with regard to both the quality of nursing care and the economic efficiency of EUs.

In summary, findings discussed in this section show that each of three staff-linked aspects of EU organization—medical staffing pattern, medical teaching affiliation, and emergency personnel training programs—is important to either the economic or the clinical efficiency of hospital EUs, or even to both of these components of institutional effectiveness. As expected, these aspects of structure are significantly related to EU effectiveness. Specifically, the medical staffing pattern of EUs is associated with economic efficiency, the quality of nursing care, and possibly also the quality of medical care provided by the EUs studied. Medical teaching affiliation correlates positively with the quality of medical care as well as the quality of nursing care. And the existence of emergency personnel training programs correlates positively with the quality of nursing care, probably also medical care, and with economic efficiency.

Size-Related Aspects of EU Organization and EU Effectiveness

The findings discussed in this section show how organizational size and related aspects of structure relate to EU effectiveness. Six major structural variables, measured with data from organizational records, are examined in the present series, as follows.

1. EU patient volume, represented by the number of patient visits processed at each EU.
2. Parent hospital size, measured by number of beds.
3. Breadth or scope of emergency service at each institution—a *de facto* definition of "emergency service," represented by the ratio of number of patient visits to each EU to the number of inpatient days in its parent hospital.
4. EU service specialization level, represented by the number of special facilities in the system among the following: a trauma center, poison control center, mental health center, substance abuse center, and burn center (unit, or program).
5. Institutional service complexity, represented by the number of different clinical, ancillary, and other facilities reported by each hospital in the American Hospital Association's annual *Guide to the Health Care Field.*
6. Institutional status, represented by the number of approvals granted the parent hospital by medical and other professional bodies (approvals beyond accreditation by the Joint Commission on Accreditation of Hospitals, such as approvals for residency programs), as reported in the same source.

Additional information on most of these variables was presented in Chapter Three; more detailed data on all of them, including descriptive statistics, may be found in Georgopoulos, Cooke, and Associates (1980).

The first three variables were considered to be particularly important to explaining interinstitutional variability in EU effectiveness. More generally, all six were expected to correlate significantly with either the economic or the clinical performance of EUs, and in some cases with both. Overall, the results strongly confirm this expectation. As was also expected, however, not all of these independent variables were found to correlate significantly, or even positively, with all three indices of effectiveness—economic efficiency, the quality of medical care, and the quality of nursing care. In short, as anticipated, their relative importance or potential contribution to emergency unit effectiveness was found to vary. The intercorrelations among these six variables are included in Table 9-3.

EU Patient Volume

Patient volume (the number of patient visits processed by each EU) was expected to be positively related to the quality of both medical and nursing care. First, a sufficient number of patients to constitute at least the relevant minimum "critical mass" probably would be necessary for effective clinical performance. Further, the greater the number of patients, the richer the learning experience and consequent ability of the staff would probably be and, therefore, the better their performance (unless, of course, greater patient volume meant work overload for the staff). In addition, "economies of scale" considerations suggested that patient volume would be positively related to economic efficiency. The obtained correlations provide good support for the relationship to economic efficiency but only partial support for the relationship to clinical efficiency, which is upheld with respect to the quality of nursing care but not the quality of medical care.

As anticipated, the zero-order correlation in Table 9-3 shows that the greater the patient volume of an EU, the higher the level of its economic efficiency is likely to be. Moreover, this relationship remains unaffected when partialling out the effect of parent hospital size (see Table 9-4), a variable with which EU patient volume correlates highly. Further, it remains statistically signifi-

Table 9-3. Size-Related Aspects of Organizational Structure and Emergency Unit Effectiveness.

| | Emergency Unit Effectiveness | | | |
| | Economic Efficiency | Clinical Efficiency | | |
Organizational Structure	Economic Efficiency Index (N = 26 EUs)	Quality of Nursing Care Index (N = 30 EUs)	Quality of Medical Care Index (N = 30 EUs)	
Emergency Unit Patient Volume Number of patient visits processed (or EU size)	.52**	.41*	.01	
Parent Hospital Size Number of beds	.16	.48**	.39*	
Breadth of Emergency Service Definition/Scope of Service Number of patient visits to the EU relative to the number of inpatient days in its parent hospital	.43*	-.26	-.48**	
Service Specialization Level of the Emergency Unit	.29	.34*	.22	
Hospital Service Complexity Number of different service facilities in the parent hospital	.29	.45**	.40*	
Institutional Status Number of approvals granted to the parent hospital by medical and related professional bodies	.11	.51**	.55**	

Notes:
*$p < .05$.
**$p < .01$.
All correlations shown are product-moment correlations at the institutional, or emergency unit, level.

The six independent variables are intercorrelated as follows: patient volume correlates .64, .41, .24, .41, and .43, respectively, with the variables listed below it; hospital size correlates -.28, .38, .68, and .72, respectively, with the variables below it; breadth of emergency service correlates -.17, -.26, and .24, respectively, with the variables below it; EU service specialization correlates .61 and -.23, respectively, with the variables below it; and hospital service complexity correlates .57 with institutional status. These

Table 9-4. The Relationship Between Selected Structural Variables and Emergency Unit Effectiveness, Partialling Out the Contribution of Other Structural Variables.

| | Structural Variables | | | | | | | | |
| | Zero-Order Correlations | | | EU Patient Volume Partialling Out | | Partial Correlations Parent Hospital Size Partialling Out | | Breadth of Emergency Service Partialling Out | |
Emergency Unit Effectiveness	EU Patient Volume	Parent Hospital Size	Breadth of Emergency Service	Hospital Size	Breadth of Service	EU Patient Volume	Breadth of Service	EU Patient Volume	Hospital Size
Economic Efficiency	.52**	.16	.43*	.56**	.42*	.29	.32*	.29	.50**
Clinical Efficiency									
Quality of medical care	.01	.39*	-.48**	-.36*	.25	.53**	.31*	-.53**	-.42*
Quality of nursing care	.41*	.48**	-.26	.08	.58**	.41*	.51**	-.52**	-.15

Notes:
*$p < .05$.
**$p < .01$.
All correlations are product-moment correlations at the institutional level.
Source: Adapted, with minor revisions, from Georgopoulos, 1985.

cant also when partialling out the breadth of emergency service, with which patient volume correlates positively. In this case, however, the degree of relationship between patient volume and economic efficiency becomes attenuated. It should also be noted in conjunction with these partial correlation results that parent hospital size and the breadth of emergency service do not correlate significantly ($r = -.28$, $p > .05$).

The findings on clinical efficiency are more complicated. Table 9-3 shows that patient volume correlates positively and significantly with the quality of nursing care, as hypothesized, but not with the quality of medical care. This disparity had not been expected. It is conceivable, though probably unlikely, that high-volume EUs attract better nurses but not better doctors than do low-volume EUs. It is also possible that high patient volume provides the nursing staff with valuable clinical experience and facilitates their proficiency but does not have similar benefits for the medical staff. However, when partialling out the effect of parent hospital size (see Table 9-4), the relationship of patient volume to the quality of nursing care practically disappears, the zero-order correlation of .41 being reduced to .08. Therefore, patient volume *per se* was not found to be a significant determinant of the quality of patient care, that is, of the clinical efficiency of hospital EUs.

Parent Hospital Size

The initial hypothesis of the study in the present case was that parent hospital size would probably show a curvilinear rather than a direct relationship to EU economic efficiency, with medium-sized institutions (within the 100–499-bed range) having the most efficient EUs. The small hospitals, it was theorized, might be relatively inefficient because, while they have to have reasonably adequate and properly staffed emergency facilities at all times, their facilities are likely to be underutilized considering their fixed costs. The large hospitals, on the other hand, might operate more complex or fancier, and therefore more costly, emergency services than their smaller counterparts.

An alternative expectation, based on economies-of-scale thinking, was that hospital size might show a small positive relationship to EU economic efficiency, like EU patient volume (with which hospital size correlates positively), but a weaker relationship. Finally, concerning clinical efficiency, the expectation was either a small positive relationship or no relationship at all to parent hospital size. A rather different picture emerges, however, from the empirical findings.

First, the results in Table 9-3 show no direct relationship between parent hospital size and the economic efficiency of EUs. (This finding is particularly interesting when it is recalled that EU patient volume, which correlates highly with hospital size, is significantly related to economic efficiency.) Moreover, when the scores of EUs on the two variables are plotted, the resulting scattergram shows no curvilinear relationship either. In short, parent hospital size does not have a significant effect on the economic efficiency of hospital EUs. Whether any relationship at all might exist between these two variables under particular circumstances, of course, cannot be determined from the available data.

Second, and equally unequivocally, the results show that parent hospital size correlates positively and significantly with both components of the clinical efficiency of hospital EUs, that is, with the quality of both medical and nursing care. The larger the parent hospital of an EU, the higher is the quality of patient care provided by the EU. This remains true even after partialling out the effect of patient volume and the effect of breadth of emergency service (hospital size correlates with the former but not with the latter), as may be seen in Table 9-4.

Interestingly, then, parent hospital size and EU patient volume seem to have complementary effects on the performance of the system—hospital size affects the clinical but not the economic efficiency of EUs, even when controlling for patient volume, while the latter affects only EU economic efficiency when partialling out hospital size. It would also appear, based on the relationships found, that low-patient-volume EUs in small hospitals may be inherently inefficient, although probably necessary, health service systems.

At any rate, the size of the parent system is an important correlate, if not indeed a determinant, of the clinical efficiency of hospital EUs. The larger hospitals apparently provide better clinical resources and/or a better clinical environment for their EUs than do their smaller counterparts. Moreover, the larger an institution is, the higher the probability that it can insist upon a higher level of quality in the services provided by its EU. Finally, the conclusion that hospital size is not a determinant of EU economic efficiency is also confirmed indirectly by the results involving service complexity and institutional status.

Service Complexity and Institutional Status

Institutional service complexity, represented by the number of different clinical and ancillary facilities available at each institution (including a variety of medical specialists "on call" to the EU), was also expected to correlate positively with the clinical efficiency of hospital EUs. Because EUs make extensive use of the facilities and services of their parent hospitals, EUs of hospitals which have more facilities available should enjoy a clinical advantage over EUs at institutions with fewer facilities. Accordingly, the greater the service complexity of the parent hospital, the higher the clinical (but not necessarily the economic) efficiency of its EU. A similar clinical advantage for EUs should be associated with institutional status, that is, with the number of medical-professional approvals granted the parent hospitals.

The results show strong support for these hypotheses. Moreover, the pattern of findings produced by service complexity in relation to either the clinical or the economic efficiency of hospital EUs essentially replicates that produced by hospital size (as discussed above), very likely because service complexity is a function of organizational size. The same kind of replication is evident, moreover, when the institutional status of the parent hospitals is examined in relation to either the quality of medical and nursing care or the economic efficiency of hospital EUs.

In short, all three of these structural variables—parent hospital size, service complexity, and institutional status—relate very similarly to the several indices of EU effectiveness. It is reasonable to assume that, other things being equal, these particular variables are all indicative of the richness and quality of available clinical resources—a factor which should facilitate the performance of both hospitals and hospital EUs. The findings of the present study clearly support the assumption with regard to the performance of the latter. It is also important to point out, in this connection, that the three variables apparently facilitate the clinical efficiency of hospital EUs without impairing their economic efficiency, with which they tend to correlate positively but not significantly (see Table 9-3).

Finally, since these three independent variables (1) produce very similar results in relation to each of the three indices of EU effectiveness and (2) are highly intercorrelated (institutional status correlates .72 with hospital size and .57 with hospital service complexity, and complexity correlates .68 with size), only one (hospital size) was subjected to more detailed analysis. Organizationally, parent hospital size is considered to be the most basic of these three structural variables; it also happens to be the dominant variable in the set; that is, it correlates best with each of the other two.

In all probability, both institutional status and service complexity are a function of hospital size: the larger institutions are also those which tend to possess the more complex services as well as to enjoy a better status than their smaller counterparts. Of the three, therefore, parent hospital size is regarded as the most basic variable, even though the zero-order correlations in Table 9-3 show that institutional status correlates the best with the quality of medical and nursing care. However, institutional status, as measured by number of approvals, might be an outcome instead of a determinant of institutional effectiveness (as well as a function of service complexity). This is unlikely in the case of complexity and improbable in the case of size. Parent hospital size seems to be a true "independent" variable in relation to the clinical efficiency of hospital EUs. Unlike institutional status, service complexity also may be a true independent variable. However, complexity does not correlate with clinical efficiency more highly than does size (or as highly as does institutional status), and it is a less central variable in the set than is size. For these reasons, therefore, only parent hospital size (which might also be viewed as an indicator or proxy measure of service complexity and of institutional status) is included in subsequent analyses.

EU Service Specialization

Another hypothesis tested in the study concerns the relationship between service specialization and institutional effectiveness. Some hospital EUs have special treatment facilities (trauma center, poison control center, substance abuse center, mental health center, burn center) while others do not. The existence of such facilities should indicate preparedness to deal with many patient problems in a relatively planned fashion amidst the typical uncertainty and unpredictability of patient inputs. If so, the greater the number of special treatment facilities at an EU, the better the quality of service should be.

The total number of such facilities, which was actually found to range from 0 to 4 across the EUs studied, provides a measure of the level of EU service specialization. In the present study, three levels of specialization were distinguished: "high" (three or four facilities), "moderate" (one or two facilities), and "low" (zero facilities). Correspondingly, these levels were assigned a score of 1, 2, or 3 to construct a trichotomous variable representing service specialization for analysis purposes.

Briefly, EU service specialization turns out to be the only one of the six structural variables included in Table 9-3 that fails to correlate significantly with more than one index of effectiveness. It correlates only with the quality of nursing care ($r = .34$, $p < .05$), and only weakly, the relevant correlation being the smallest of the ten statistically significant correlations in Table 9-3. Service specialization was expected to be significantly related to both components of clinical efficiency on the grounds that it would facilitate medical and nursing staff proficiency, but the study found no correlation with the quality of medical care. Nor does specialization correlate with the economic efficiency of hospital EUs, although in this case no particular relationship had been hypothesized.

Overall, these findings are also weaker than those produced by hospital service complexity, with which EU service specialization correlates fairly highly ($r = .61$). The explanation might be that some of the benefits of EU service specialization are offset by other factors, such as coordination, conflict, or integration difficulties within the system. Another possibility is that a better measure of this variable (for example, one representing more kinds of specialization) might have yielded stronger results.

Breadth, or Scope, of Emergency Service

One of the most interesting structural variables studied is the relative breadth or narrowness of "emergency service" definition at each institution. The ratio of "number of emergency patient visits" to "number of inpatient days in the parent hospital" was used in this research to represent each institution's *de facto* definition of "emergency service." The higher this ratio is, the broader an institution's conception of emergency service is considered to be. Based on data from hospital records, the mean ratio of emergency patient visits to inpatient hospital days for the thirty EUs in the study turns out to be .37. Across individual EUs, the observed ratio ranges from .09 (signifying the EU with the narrowest definition of emergency service) to .94 (signifying the EU with the greatest scope of service).

The study expected a negative relationship between the breadth of emergency service and the clinical efficiency of hospital EUs, and either a positive or curvilinear relationship between breadth and economic efficiency. The rationale for these hypotheses is not too difficult to state. Briefly, the greater the breadth of emergency service, the more nonemergency cases are probably treated by an EU—cases that, in the eyes of the staff, often are "cluttering" the unit or should have been treated at a doctor's office instead of at the EU. (See relevant data on the composition of patient inputs in Chapter Three.) A situation such as this would suggest less than optimal "emergency" service utilization and probably affect the attitudes and behavior of the staff adversely. The narrower the breadth of service, on the other hand, the more likely that the cases treated at an EU would represent actual medical emergency problems or relatively serious conditions demanding immediate attention. Such a situation would be more likely to stimulate and satisfy the clinical interests of the staff while enabling the EU to concentrate its efforts more rationally from a clinical standpoint and better utilize its capabilities. In short, other things being equal, the narrower the breadth/scope of service, the higher the clinical efficiency of an EU was expected to be; and the broader the scope of service, the lower the clinical efficiency.

An opposite pattern was expected, however, with regard to economic efficiency. In this case, greater breadth of service is likely to mean less cost per case to the system, partly due to economies-of-scale considerations, and therefore higher economic efficiency, unless, of course, such "mass-production-like" conditions led to more waste. In this latter case, a curvilinear relationship between breadth of service and economic efficiency would be more likely than a direct positive relationship, and EUs with a moderate breadth of service would probably be more economically efficient than those with either a broad or a narrow scope of emergency service.

As it turned out, the data actually show not a curvilinear but a direct positive and significant relationship. As may be seen in Table 9-3, the greater the breadth of their service, the higher the economic efficiency of hospital EUs. Table 9-3 also shows that, unlike parent hospital size but like EU patient volume, breadth of emergency service apparently promotes economic efficiency. The correlation between the latter two variables is reduced and becomes marginal, however, when partialling out the effect of patient volume, while it is strengthened when partialling out the effect of hospital size (see Table 9-4). Finally, the breadth of emergency service correlates most strongly with economic efficiency ($r = .69$, $p < .01$) for EUs located in the less affluent communities.

The results also support the hypothesis of a negative relationship between breadth of emergency service and clinical efficiency, at least with respect to the quality of medical care and possibly also in the case of nursing care as well (Table 9-3 and Table 9-4). Briefly, the quality of medical care in the EUs studied increases as the breadth of service decreases, and this negative correlation, which is statistically significant at the .05 level, remains virtually unaffected when partialling out the effects of either EU patient volume or parent hospital size. Breadth of service, as here measured, apparently impedes the quality of medical care.

The zero-order correlation obtained between breadth of service and the quality of nursing care is also negative but not statistically significant, suggesting only a marginal negative relationship in this case. This particular correlation, however, does not change appreciably when partialling out the effect of hospital size, but it increases substantially when partialling out EU patient volume. Finally, the overall negative relationship found between breadth of emergency service and the quality of patient care disappears for EUs in the less affluent communities ($r = .02$ for medical and .19 for nursing care) while increasing greatly for EUs in the more affluent communities—specifically, to -.73 for medical and -.56 for nursing care.

Based upon the results for the total sample, it would appear that a relatively narrow emergency service definition is conducive to high-quality patient care but not to economic efficiency, while a broad definition is conducive to economic but not to clinical efficiency. If so, a moderate scope of emergency service might be optimal for overall institutional effectiveness in the case of most hospital EUs.

In summary, empirical findings presented in this section show three rather distinct and partially complementary patterns of relationships between the major structural variables examined and the indices of EU effectiveness. First, parent hospital size correlates positively and significantly with the quality of medical and nursing care, and especially the latter, even after partialling out EU patient volume and the breadth of emergency service, but it is not related to the economic efficiency of hospital EUs. Second, EU patient volume correlates positively and significantly with the economic efficiency of hospital EUs, and possibly also with the quality of nursing care, but not with the quality of medical care. Third, the breadth of emergency service correlates negatively and significantly with the quality of medical care, possibly also with the quality of nursing care, but positively and significantly with the economic efficiency of EUs. Finally, EU service specialization correlates significantly only with the quality of nursing care, while hospital service complexity and institutional status yield patterns of results that closely replicate those produced by hospital size in relation to the effectiveness measures.

Effect of Selected Structural Variables on EU Effectiveness

The empirical evidence has made it clear that certain staff-linked and size-related aspects of EU organization are associated, generally as expected, with one or more of the main indices of EU effectiveness. These structural variables, in short, are significant correlates, and possibly also important determinants, of the effectiveness of hospital EUs. The question now arises as to how much of the observed interinstitutional variability in the economic and clinical efficiency of EUs can be accounted for by differences in these independent variables considered together as a set or in subsets. A related question concerns the individual contribution of particular variables to the explained variance in effectiveness when controlling for the effects of all the other variables in the set. To answer these questions, a number of multiple regression analyses (standard least squares regression) and partial least squares analyses (Wold, 1983) were performed.

Regression Analyses: Effects of Organizational Structure on Effectiveness

Regression analysis provides a reasonable tool for ascertaining both the combined and individual effects of independent, or "predictor," variables on a criterion variable. The study sample is relatively small (maximum $N = 30$ EUs in the case of clinical efficiency, 26 EUs for economic efficiency), however, and the degrees of freedom that it allows limit the legitimate number of "predictor" variables that may be simultaneously entered into the regression equation. A few predictor variables at a time, nevertheless, may be properly accommodated with a sample of this size. All things considered, in the present case it was decided that using as many as five or six predictors would be appropriate for most analyses.

The structural variables that might be used as predictors are parent hospital size, EU patient volume, breadth of emergency service, medical teaching affiliation, emergency personnel training programs, medical staffing pattern, EU service specialization, hospital service complexity, and institutional status. Of these, medical staffing pattern was not included in the regression analyses because of (1) the small number of institutions belonging to each of the four staffing patterns encountered and (2) the tentative nature of results in this case compared to other structural variables. EU service specialization was also not included, having turned out to be the weakest of the six size-related variables in relation to effectiveness. Finally, service complexity and institutional status were also omitted, (1) because of their high correlations with parent hospital size, (2) because of the greater centrality of size, and (3) to avoid problems of multicollinearity among the independent/predictor variables in the regression analyses.

In the end, therefore, the independent variables included in the regression analyses were parent hospital size, EU patient volume, breadth of emergency service, medical teaching affiliation, and emergency personnel training programs. The intercorrelations among these five variables range between –.13 and .64, the average (also median) intercorrelation being only .31, and the average N = 29 EUs. Moreover, the highest correlation coefficient among the ten in the series is that between parent hospital size and EU patient volume (r = .64)*—variables which were earlier found to behave quite differently in relation to the three indices of effectiveness. Therefore, no problem of multicollinearity exists for this set of independent variables.

*The remaining correlations are as follows: hospital size correlates –.28, .50, and .22, respectively, with breadth of service, teaching affiliation, and emergency training programs; patient volume correlates .41, .50, and .34, respectively, with the same three variables; breadth of service correlates –.01 and –.13, respectively, with teaching affiliation and training programs; and the latter two variables correlate .07. Only those correlations that are $\geq$ .34 are statistically significant ($p < .05$).

Using these five variables as predictors, regression analyses were performed with reference to the economic efficiency index and the indices of the quality of medical and nursing care. In each case, the obtained results show that: (1) as indicated by the F-ratio statistic, the systematic variance (on the criterion measure) accounted for by the five predictor variables as a set is significantly greater than the error variance; that is, the relationship between the predictors and the effectiveness criterion is a significant phenomenon and not one due to chance; and (2) as indicated by the corresponding R^2, the five variables together explain a substantial proportion of the total variance on the criterion measure. In short, organizational structure, as represented by the above variables, significantly affects the performance of the system.

More specifically, the regression results show that the five variables together account for 44 percent of the variance in the economic efficiency of hospital EUs ($R^2 = .440$, $F = 2.96$, $df = 5, 19$, and $p = .037$), 62 percent of the variance in the quality of nursing care ($R^2 = .623$, $F = 7.27$, $df = 5, 22$, and $p = .004$), and 40 percent of the variance in the quality of medical care ($R^2 = .403$, $F = 2.97$, $df = 5, 22$, and $p = .034$). A very substantial proportion of the interinstitutional variability on each of these key measures of effectiveness, in other words, can be explained by the observed differences across institutions in these five structural variables.

The regression results also show that, in terms of the partial correlations associated with the five predictor variables in each of the three regression analyses, the two most important predictors for each criterion are as follows: for economic efficiency, emergency personnel training programs (partial $r = .34$) and breadth of emergency service (partial $r = .25$); for the quality of nursing care, medical teaching affiliation (partial $r = .61$) and emergency training programs (partial $r = .37$); and for the quality of medical care, medical teaching affiliation (partial $r = .31$) and emergency personnel training programs (partial $r = .30$). Apparently, training programs are very important to both the economic and clinical efficiency of hospital EUs, and medical teaching affiliation affects the quality of both nursing and medical care.

An additional series of multiple regression analyses was performed omitting from the predictor variables both emergency personnel training programs and medical teaching affiliation. These analyses used as predictors the six structural variables included in Table 9-3: EU patient volume, parent hospital size, breadth of emergency service, EU service specialization, hospital service complexity, and institutional status (number of medical-professional approvals). The results in this case are similar to those from the regression analyses discussed above but not as strong—an anticipated result because the two strongest predictors in those analyses (training programs and teaching affiliation) were not included in the present series.

Briefly stated, the findings from these supplementary regression analyses are as follows. For economic efficiency, R^2 = .43, and F = 1.85, df = 7, 17, and p = .143. For the quality of nursing care, R^2 = .47, and F = 2.57, df = 7, 20, and p = .046. And for the quality of medical care, R^2 = .45, and F = 2.38, df = 7, 20, and p = .060. The two best predictors for each criterion, among the six independent variables in the set, are as follows: for economic efficiency, EU patient volume (partial r = .33) and service specialization (partial r = .21); for the quality of nursing care, breadth of emergency service (partial r = -.35) and EU patient volume (partial r = .32); and for the quality of medical care, institutional status (partial r = .44) and breadth of emergency service (partial r = -.30). Thus, EU patient volume and the breadth of service emerge from this supplementary series of analyses as particularly important predictors of EU effectiveness.

Overall, the regression analysis results reinforce the general conclusion from the correlational findings discussed earlier and provide additional support for the basic hypothesis that differences in EU organization such as the structural differences studied here account for a significant part of the observed interinstitutional variability in the economic and clinical efficiency of hospital EUs. As anticipated, the results from both the correlational and regression analyses indicate that in these health service systems organizational structure significantly affects performance.

Partial Least Squares (PLS) Analyses:
The Contribution of Particular Variables

An alternative method to multiple regression analysis for estimating the combined and individual effects of a set of independent variables on some criterion variable is partial least squares (PLS) analysis (see Wold, 1983). PLS is less affected than is multiple regression by sample size constraints and multicollinearity among the predictor variables. Moreover, unlike some types of regression analysis, PLS results are not affected by the order in which the predictor variables are entered in the analysis. On the other hand, PLS analysis is probably a less well-known and less used technique than is regression analysis.

In the present study, using as predictors the same five structural variables that were used in the first series of the multiple regression analyses (that is, parent hospital size, EU patient volume, breadth of emergency service, medical teaching affiliation, and emergency personnel training programs), PLS analyses were carried out with respect to each of the primary criteria of EU effectiveness and each of the nine measures of the five secondary criteria of effectiveness discussed in Chapter Eight.

The purpose of these PLS analyses was to estimate the proportion of the variance (or R^2) on each criterion measure explained by the five predictors together, and also the relative importance of the individual predictors viewed in relation to one another as indicated by the size of the partial correlation obtained for each predictor when partialling out the contributions of all other predictors. Based on the size of these partial correlations, the five predictors can be rank-ordered to indicate their relative contributions to the explained variance on a particular criterion measure. The results of the twelve PLS analyses performed are all summarized in Table 9-5. In addition to showing the partial correlations from these analyses, Table 9-5 shows the corresponding zero-order correlations between predictor variables and the criterion measures involved.

Generally, the PLS results are virtually identical to those obtained from the corresponding regression analyses. Concerning the economic and clinical efficiency indices, for example, the relevant R^2 from the PLS analysis is .47 for economic efficiency, .66 for the quality of nursing care, and .41 for the quality of medical care. Similarly, the specific structural variables which emerge as the two best predictors (among the five) of each primary criterion of EU effectiveness are the same as those identified earlier with the regression analyses, except that in the PLS analysis emergency training programs tied with breadth of emergency service as the second best predictor of the quality of nursing care.

Organizational Structure and the Secondary Criteria of EU Effectiveness

Table 9-5 also shows the correlations between the structural variables under consideration and the secondary criteria of effectiveness studied. Clearly, the proportion of the variance on each secondary criterion measure explained by the five structural variables is also very considerable for most of the nine measures (and statistically significant for all but two of them). Specifically, this proportion ranges from a low of .15 (for EU responsiveness to the community's changing needs for emergency services) to a high of .55 (for EU responsiveness in meeting community expectations regarding emergency services), and averages .35 for the nine measures.

Of the five structural variables used as predictors, parent hospital size, which correlates positively and significantly with six of the nine secondary criterion measures, is the best predictor of promptness of medical attention to incoming patients, and of patient satisfaction with the care received. EU patient volume, which correlates significantly with three of the nine measures, is the best predictor of physician satisfaction with the EU, and second best predictor of both patient satisfaction with the care received and patient satisfaction with the EU staff. The breadth of emergency service correlates (negatively) with two of the secondary criterion measures—patient satisfaction with the EU staff and parent hospital reputation. It also turns out to be the second best predictor of physician satisfaction with the EU and of RN satisfaction with the EU.

Medical teaching affiliation correlates positively and significantly with five secondary criterion measures. Moreover, it is the best predictor of EU responsiveness in meeting community expectations, EU reputation, and parent hospital reputation, and second best predictor of EU responsiveness to the community's

Table 9-5. The Relative Importance of Selected Structural Variables as Predictors of Interinstitutional Variability on Emergency Unit Effectiveness.[a]

	Correlations Between Each Predictor and Criterion Measure Partialling Out All Other Predictors[b]						
	PREDICTOR VARIABLES						
EU EFFECTIVENESS	Parent Hospital Size	EU Patient Volume	Breadth of Emergency Service	Medical Teaching Affiliation	Emergency Personnel Training Programs	Explained Variance[c] R^2	p[d]
	(Zero-Order correlations shown in parentheses)						
Primary Criteria							
Economic efficiency	.09 (.16)	.06 (.52**)	.29 (.43*)	.09 (.08)	<u>.42</u> (.43*)	.47	.04
Clinical efficiency							
Quality of medical care	.24 (.39*)	.22 (.01)	-.07 (-.48**)	.32 (.32*)	.31 (.28)	.41	.03
Quality of nursing care	.16 (.48**)	.21 (.41*)	-.33 (-.26)	<u>.64</u> (.68**)	<u>.33</u> (.42*)	.66	.00
Secondary Criteria							
Promptness of medical attention to incoming patients	.30 (.23)	.20 (.01)	-.11 (-.22)	.13 (-.07)	.23 (.19)	.17	.35
Physician satisfaction with EU	.03 (.45**)	.23 (.41*)	-.19 (-.13)	.15 (.16)	.13 (.37*)	.32	.11

Criterion measure						
Satisfaction of RNs with EU	.23 (.12)	.17 (.17)	-.24 (-.19)	.20 (.22)	.35 (.49**)	.33	.17
Patient satisfaction with care received	.40 (.36*)	.38 (.12)	-.28 (-.18)	.34 (.34*)	.37 (.24)	.32	.11
Patient satisfaction with EU staff	.45 (.36*)	.47 (.04)	-.28 (-.32*)	.41 (.33*)	.50 (.33*)	.45	.05
EU responsiveness in meeting community expectations	.02 (.33*)	.03 (.42*)	-.05 (-.02)	.61 (.62**)	.46 (.45**)	.55	.01
EU responsiveness to community's changing needs	.11 (.19)	.08 (.24)	.13 (.05)	.16 (.22)	.28 (.30*)	.15	.72
Reputation of emergency unit	.05 (.32*)	.07 (.33*)	-.04 (-.08)	.48 (.52**)	.40 (.41*)	.41	.05
Reputation of parent hospital	.25 (.42*)	.26 (.08)	-.03 (-.43*)	.49 (.48**)	.33 (.27)	.48	.00

Notes:
*$p < .05$.
**$p < .01$.
For underlined partial correlations, $p < .05$.

[a] The number of emergency units in the analyses varies between 26 and 30 EUs.

[b] Obtained from partial least squares analyses: a separate PLS analysis was performed for each criterion measure, using the same five structural variables as the predictors or independent variables. (For a discussion of PLS, see Wold, 1983.)

[c] This shows the proportion of the total variance on each criterion measure explained by the five structural variables as a set.

[d] These are two-tailed p values, obtained from corresponding regression analyses in which the predictor variables were entered in the order shown here.

changing needs for emergency services. Finally, like parent hospital size, the presence of emergency personnel training programs correlates positively and significantly with six of the nine secondary criterion measures. Moreover, it is the best predictor of RN satisfaction with the EU, patient satisfaction with the EU staff, and EU responsiveness to the community's changing needs, and second best predictor of the same three criterion variables for which medical teaching affiliation is the best predictor.

As was the case for the primary criteria of EU effectiveness, therefore, emergency personnel training programs and medical teaching affiliation turn out to be major explanatory variables also in the case of the secondary criteria of effectiveness. Overall, as expected, the results of both the PLS and regression analyses provide strong support for the hypothesis that system structure affects the effectiveness of hospital EUs to a very substantial degree. The importance of organizational structure variables to the performance of this system, in short, has been empirically demonstrated.

Summary

The findings discussed in this chapter clearly show that the structural aspects of organization studied have important implications for institutional effectiveness. Not all of these independent variables, of course, are directly or equally strongly related to every criterion of effectiveness. Nearly all of them, however, correlate significantly with one or more of the indices representing the principal criteria of effectiveness. These indices themselves, it will be recalled from Chapter Eight, do not correlate highly. It is not surprising, therefore, to find that the organizational correlates of the two components of clinical efficiency overlap only in part. The same is true concerning the correlates of economic and clinical efficiency. Not unexpectedly, then, the study finds that different subsets of the independent variables under consideration account best for the observed interinstitutional variability on the different criteria of effectiveness.

According to the findings, the economic efficiency of hospital EUs is significantly related to several of the structural variables studied, including medical staffing pattern, training programs for emergency personnel, breadth of emergency service, and EU patient volume. This last variable correlates positively with economic efficiency, even when controlling for parent hospital size or for the breadth of emergency service. Likewise, the latter variable correlates positively with economic efficiency even when controlling for hospital size and possibly also patient volume. Economic efficiency also tends to be somewhat higher, on the average, for EUs located in non-SMSA compared to SMSA communities. Medical teaching affiliation, on the other hand, is not related to the economic efficiency of hospital EUs. Nor is the size of the parent hospitals, which had been expected to show either a curvilinear or a small positive relationship to this criterion.

EU patient volume correlates positively and significantly with the quality of nursing care but not the quality of medical care. However, its relationship to the quality of nursing care disappears after partialling out the effect of parent hospital size. The latter variable correlates positively with both aspects of clinical efficiency, even after partialling out the breadth of emergency service and EU patient volume. In contrast, the breadth of emergency service is negatively and significantly related to the quality of medical care, even when controlling for patient volume and hospital size; scope of service also appears to be negatively related to the quality of nursing care. Hospital service complexity and institutional status, both of which correlate highly with hospital size, show very similar patterns of relationships to the economic and clinical efficiency indices as the patterns produced by hospital size. Finally, the medical staffing pattern most closely associated with high-quality patient care, nursing as well as medical, and also with high economic efficiency is the hospital-based group pattern.

Of the structural variables considered, emergency personnel training programs turn out to be especially important to both economic and clinical efficiency. Medical teaching affiliation apparently enhances the quality of both nursing and medical care without adversely affecting the economic efficiency of hospital

EUs. Training programs and teaching affiliation probably reflect high levels of clinical staff competence and/or high clinical performance standards. Parent hospital size, service complexity, and institutional status (measured by number of medical approvals), all of which are probably indicative of the richness of available clinical resources, also emerge as important correlates of the quality of patient care across hospital EUs. The several community structural variables explored in the study, on the other hand, apparently have no significant effect on either the quality of patient care or the economic efficiency of hospital EUs.

The overall conclusion from the results in this chapter is that organizational structure, represented by the above variables, significantly affects the performance, or effectiveness, of the system. Most of the structural variables specified were found to be important direct correlates of the primary, as well as of some of the secondary, criteria of EU effectiveness. In addition, some of these structural variables may well affect institutional performance also indirectly, namely by facilitating (or impeding) problem solving within the system. The results concerning the relationship between organizational problem solving in certain major areas and the effectiveness of hospital EUs, the second major hypothesis of this research, are discussed next.

Chapter Ten

Organizational Problem Solving and Effectiveness

In large measure, differences in the economic and clinical performance of hospital emergency units (EUs), and in other criteria of institutional effectiveness as well, were expected to be accounted for by differences in organizational structure and problem solving. The results testing the hypothesized relationships between organizational structure and EU effectiveness were discussed in Chapter Nine. The second major hypothesis investigated was that the adequacy, or relative success, of internal organizational problem solving in the areas of resource allocation, coordination of efforts, integration, strain, and adaptation to the environment will be directly related to the effectiveness of the system.

Previous organizational research in the hospital field and elsewhere (for example, see Cheng, 1977; Cooke and Rousseau, 1981; Georgopoulos, 1975; Georgopoulos and Mann, 1962; Georgopoulos and Matejko, 1967; Hage, 1974; Longest, 1974; Money, Gilfillan, and Duncan, 1976; Shortell, Becker, and Neuhauser, 1976; Sutton and Ford, 1982) has yielded a great deal of empirical evidence supporting the existence of important relationships between various aspects of problem solving in these key areas and the effectiveness of organizations. The theoretical bases and rationale for such relationships have also been discussed in the organizational literature, both by the author and others (see, especially, Georgopoulos, 1972; Georgopoulos and Mann, 1962; Katz and Georgopoulos, 1971; March and Simon, 1958; Mintzberg, 1979; Shortell and Kaluzny, 1983; Thompson, 1967). In the present investigation, the relationship of organizational problem solving to effectiveness has occupied a prominent place (Georgopoulos, 1978; Georgopoulos and Cooke, 1979; Georgopoulos, Cooke, and Associates, 1980). The principal findings of the study concerning this relationship are discussed in this chapter.

Presented first are the results on organizational strain and its relationship to the various criteria of EU effectiveness. Strain is viewed both as a problem area in itself and as an indicator of problems in other areas of organizational functioning. Discussed next are certain indicators of the adequacy of organizational problem solving in the different areas and their interrelationships. These indicators are then examined in relation to prevailing strain in the system and to organizational structure. Shown next are the relationships between organizational problem solving and the primary and secondary criteria of institutional effectiveness. These are followed by findings regarding the relative importance of particular problem-solving variables to effectiveness. Finally, regression analysis results showing the combined effects of organizational structure and problem solving on EU effectiveness are considered.

Organizational Strain and EU Effectiveness

A good indicator of unresolved problems and prevailing difficulties in organizations is the level of strain (tension, friction, conflict) in the system. In particular, the level of tension within and between interacting groups whose cooperation is essential to achieving the organization's objectives, such as clinical and economic efficiency in the present case, is an important factor to consider.

A certain amount of strain, such as intergroup tension, probably is inevitable under the best of organizational circumstances. Some "error," noise, and entropy are always present in a complex social system (Georgopoulos and Matejko, 1967; Miller, 1965, 1978). Associated or resulting strain, therefore, is a problem endemic to the system, and no organization is ever completely strain-free. But, in addition, strain may stem from structural deficiencies, poor performance, or inadequate problem solving in the organization. Therefore, some of the strain prevailing in an organization is derived rather than generic or inherent to the system (Georgopoulos, 1972; Georgopoulos and Cooke, 1979). In practice, of course, it is extremely difficult if not impossible to separate the two components of strain. The particular source of strain, however, is less consequential for organizational functioning than is the total amount of strain.

Some strain is a normal fact of organizational life and is probably not detrimental to the effectiveness of the system. In hospitals, for example, intergroup tensions are fairly widespread but not necessarily high (Georgopoulos and Matejko, 1967). In some cases, strain may even serve as a catalyst for innovation or as a precondition for desirable change (for example, see Coser, 1956). But beyond some point—some unknown threshold which may be fairly low for many organizations—tensions and conflicts between closely interdependent groups and members are likely to affect performance adversely, particularly in complex organizations where behavior is highly constrained, controlled, and contractual.

Relatively high levels of tension that remain unchecked and unresolved eventually are likely to be dysfunctional for the system. Such tensions can affect performance (or the motivation to perform) not only directly but also indirectly, by impairing organizational problem solving in other important areas, such as the areas of adaptation, integration, and coordination (for example, see Georgopoulos and Mann, 1962; Georgopoulos and Matejko, 1967; Wieland, 1965). Consequently, organizations must constantly deal with the problem of resolving, reducing, and managing the tensions and conflicts which arise in the system. Not all tensions, however, can be best managed by the same type of leadership. In hospital EUs, for example, Peterson (1979) found that tension between doctors and nurses is more likely to be minimized by physician than nursing leadership, while tension between EU staff and others outside the unit is more likely to be minimized by the leadership of supervising nurses than of physicians.

Since strain is both a major organizational problem and a likely indicator of difficulties in other problem areas, in this research it was examined not only in relation to EU effectiveness but also in relation to organizational structure and problem solving in other major areas. The measures of strain are based on data from EU physicians (MDs) and registered nurses (RNs) and hospital administrators (HAs). They include three measures of tension among staff within the EU, two measures of tension between EU staff and hospital administration, and two measures of tension between the EU and the outside community.

All of the measures of strain are based on responses to the following question: "All things considered, how much *tension* (friction, strain, or conflict) would you say is there between _____ and _____?" Response alternatives ranged from 1 = "a high level of tension" to 5 = "no tension at all."

Measures of Organizational Strain and Their Interrelationships

The first measure of strain within the EU is a three-item index of tension among the clinical staff. This index is based on data from RNs reporting, on a five-point scale, the amount of tension existing at their respective EUs among doctors, among nurses, and between doctors and nurses. The index correlates highly and significantly with each of its three components (.68, .84, and .72, respectively; $p < .01$ in all cases), and its Cronbach alpha is .61. Tension among the nurses correlates significantly with both tension among the doctors ($r = .37$, $p < .05$) and tension between doctors and nurses ($r = .43$, $p < .01$). The latter measure also correlates positively, but not significantly, with tension among the doctors ($r = .23$, $p > .01$), and this explains why the Cronbach alpha for this index is not higher. The F and η^2 values for the three component measures of this index are all satisfactory (see Table 10-1).

The second measure of strain within the EU is also a composite measure, combining the amount of tension between doctors and nurses in the EU which is reported by MDs with that which is reported by RNs. The F and η^2 values of the two items, shown in Table 10-1, are methodologically satisfactory. The third measure of strain within the EU represents the amount of tension that exists among the MDs, according to themselves. The amount of self-reported tension by MDs, however, correlates positively but not significantly with the amount of tension among the doctors that is reported by RNs (r = .24, p > .05), even though the F and η^2 values of both measures are acceptable.

Also included in the analysis are two measures of strain between the EU and hospital administration, one representing tension as reported by RNs and the other tension as reported by MDs. Both of these measures have satisfactory F and η^2 values, and they correlate positively and significantly. A third measure, based on corresponding data from HAs, was also obtained but omitted from further consideration because it turned out to be statistically defective (F = 0.96 and p = .44, and six of the thirty EUs showed zero variance in the responses of HAs).

The last two measures in the series concern the level of tension between the EU and the outside community, respectively as assessed by HAs and MDs. These too are methodologically acceptable and significantly correlated measures. A similar measure, representing tension between EU staff and the selected community respondents (CRs) as reported by the latter, was also considered but eliminated when it was found to be statistically defective (F = 0.82, p = .73, and η^2 = .13). The omitted measure, incidentally, correlates positively and significantly with the level of tension between the EU and the community as assessed by the HAs (r = .33, p < .05) but not as assessed by the MDs (r = .01, p > .05). It is also interesting to note that, in addition, it is significantly related both to the index of tension among the clinical staff (r = .35, p < .05) and to the level of tension between doctors and nurses (r = .45, p < .01) prevailing at the various EUs.

EU scores on these seven measures of strain show that, on the average, the highest level of reported tension is that which prevails between EU staff and hospital administration, according to both RNs and MDs (Measures 4 and 5 in Table 10-1), and the lowest level is that which prevails between the EU and the outside community as reported by MDs (Measure 7 in Table 10-1). On the five-point scale used, EU means on this last measure range from 3.25 (signifying "a low level of tension") to 4.80 (signifying "almost no tension at all"), the grand mean being 4.01 (which corresponds exactly to "a very low level of tension") and the standard deviation being .41. At the other extreme, EU scores on the level of tension between EU and hospital administration, as reported by the RNs, range from 2.08 (signifying "a moderate level of tension") to 4.00 and average 3.20 (which corresponds to "a low level of tension") with a standard deviation of .53.

Table 10-1. Selected Aspects of Organizational Strain in the Emergency Units Studied and Their Interrelationships.

Aspect of Strain	Measure						
	1	2	3	4	5	6	7
Tension Within the EU							
1. Tension among the clinical staff, according to RNs (three-item index, $\alpha = .61$)[a]	--	.59**	.15	.02	.33*	.12	.08
2. Tension between doctors and nurses, according to MDs and RNs (for MDs: $F = 1.83$, $p < .01$; $\eta^2 = .24$; for RNs: $F = 2.44$, $p < .01$; $\eta^2 = .23$)		--	.37*	.30*	.07	.08	.22
3. Tension among doctors, according to MDs ($F = 2.25$, $p < .01$; $\eta^2 = .29$)			--	.64**	.00	.15	.54**
Tension Between EU and Hospital Administration							
4. As reported by MDs ($F = 1.96$, $p < .01$; $\eta^2 = .16$)				--	.31*	.27	.71**
5. As reported by RNs ($F = 2.02$, $p < .01$; $\eta^2 = .21$)					--	.25	.13
Tension Between the EU and the Outside Community							
6. According to hospital administrators (HAs) ($F = 2.42$, $p < .01$; $\eta^2 = .66$)						--	.32*
7. According to MDs ($F = 1.23$, $p = .17$; $\eta^2 = .19$)							--

Notes:
*$p < .05$.
**$p < .01$.
Product-moment correlations are shown. $N = 30$ EUs in each case.
[a]The three-item index that makes up Measure 1 includes tension among doctors ($F = 2.25$, $p < .01$; $\eta^2 = .22$), tension among nurses ($F = 2.77$, $p < .01$; $\eta^2 = .26$), and tension between doctors and nurses ($F = 2.44$, $p < .01$; $\eta^2 = .23$).

The interrelationships among the seven measures of organizational strain retained in the analysis are shown in Table 10-1. As already pointed out, the two measures of tension between the EU and the outside community correlate positively and significantly, but not highly, and the same is true of the two measures of tension between EU staff and hospital administration. Similarly, the index of tension among the clinical staff is significantly related to the other two measures of tension within the EU (that is, the level of tension between doctors and nurses and the level of tension among doctors), while the latter two measures show no statistically significant relationship. The twenty-one correlation coefficients in the series are all positive, ranging from .00 to .71, and nine of them are statistically significant. Further, every measure in the series, except tension between the EU and the community as assessed by HAs, correlates significantly with at least two other measures. Overall, the results in Table 10-1 show that the aspects of strain measured in this study tend to be positively interrelated and possibly mutually reinforcing, but also considerably more heterogeneous than might have been expected. Organizational strain in hospital EUs is not a unidimensional or simple phenomenon.

The Relationship of Strain to Economic and Clinical Efficiency

Table 10-2 shows the relationships between the measures of organizational strain and the economic and clinical efficiency of hospital EUs. First, neither tension within the EU nor tension between it and either hospital administration or the outside community correlates significantly with the economic efficiency of EUs. Apparently, organizational strain within the range of prevailing levels at the various EUs during the period of data collection (for descriptive data in this connection, see Georgopoulos, Cooke, and Associates, 1980) did not affect the economic performance of these health service systems. Regardless of the specific measure considered, EUs with higher levels of strain were neither more nor less likely than EUs with lower levels of strain to be economically inefficient or efficient.

Table 10-2. Relationship Between Organizational Strain and Emergency Unit Effectiveness.

| | Emergency Unit Effectiveness (Primary Criteria) | | |
| | Economic Efficiency | Clinical Efficiency | |
Organizational Strain	Economic Efficiency Index (N = 26 EUs)	Quality of Nursing Care Index (N = 30 EUs)	Quality of Medical Care Index (N = 30 EUs)
Tension Within EU			
Among clinical staff	.17	-.06	-.38*
Between MDs and RNs	.10	-.02	-.24
Among MDs	.21	-.37*	-.44**
Tension Between EU and Hospital Administration			
As reported by MDs	-.20	-.43**	-.30*
As reported by RNs	-.13	-.35*	-.26
Tension Between EU and Outside Community			
According to HAs	.05	-.28	-.17
According to MDs	-.05	-.50**	-.40*

Notes:
*$p < .05$.
**$p < .01$.
All correlations are product-moment correlations at the EU level.

The picture with respect to clinical efficiency is very different. All seven measures of tension correlate *negatively* with the quality of both nursing and medical care, and the majority of these relationships are statistically significant. In fact, three of the measures—tension among EU doctors, tension between EU and hospital administration according to MDs, and tension between the EU and the outside community also as reported by MDs—are negatively and significantly related to both medical and nursing care. In addition, tension among the clinical staff (the index based on data from RNs) correlates significantly with the quality of medical but not nursing care, while tension between the EU and hospital administration as reported by RNs shows a reverse pattern (its correlation with medical care, however, approaches statistical significance at the .05 level). Generally, clinical efficiency is higher in those EUs which have lower levels of organizational strain.

Clearly, the pattern of results in Table 10-2 supports the hypothesis that organizational strain at the observed levels adversely affects the clinical performance of hospital EUs, being negatively related to both components of clinical efficiency. It does not, however, affect their economic performance. At the same time, additional findings show that strain is dysfunctional with regard to several other criteria of EU effectiveness.

Organizational Strain and the Secondary Criteria
of EU Effectiveness

The seven measures of strain were also examined in relation to the nine measures of the secondary criteria of EU effectiveness discussed in Chapter Eight. The results are presented in Table 10-3. With respect to every criterion measure, the emerging pattern is one of a negative relationship between organizational strain in the EUs and the effectiveness of the system. In all, fifty-three of the sixty-three correlation coefficients in the series are negative, ranging from –.01 to –.62, and twenty-four of them are statistically significant ($p < .05$) in addition. Further, the ten positive coefficients are small, ranging from .01 to .17, and none of them approaches significance even at the .10 level.

Table 10-3. Relationships Between Organizational Strain and the Secondary Criteria of Emergency Unit Effectiveness.

	EU Effectiveness (Secondary Criteria)							
		Staff Satisfaction with EU		Patient Satisfaction with	EU Staff Expectations	EU Responsiveness to Community Needs	Reputation of	
Organizational Strain	Promptness of Medical Attention to Patients	MDs	RNs	Care			EU	Hospital
Tension Within EU								
Among clinical staff	-.24	.01	-.47**	.04	-.15	-.13	-.07	-.14
Between MDs and RNs	-.44**	.03	-.19	.03	-.09	-.13	-.01	-.01
Among MDs	-.30*	-.49**	-.15	.13	-.13	-.21	.15	-.31*
Tension Between EU and Hospital Administration								
As reported by MDs	-.23	-.40*	-.31*	.07	-.22	-.52**	-.07	-.32*
As reported by RNs	-.07	-.06	-.62**	-.37*	-.45**	-.50***	-.48**	-.40*
Tension Between EU and Outside Community								
According to HAs	-.22	-.23	-.52**	-.12	-.21	-.31*	-.14	-.05
According to MDs	-.39*	-.42*	-.30*	.17	-.04	-.43*	-.02	-.26

Notes:
*p < .05.
**p < .01.
All correlations shown are product-moment correlations. N varies between 27 and 30 EUs.

Of the several aspects of strain examined, tension between the EU and hospital administration shows the strongest pattern of negative relationships with the secondary criteria; nearly two-thirds of the relevant correlations (eleven of eighteen) are statistically significant. The next strongest pattern involves the level of tension between the EU and the outside community; nearly half of the correlations with the criterion measures (eight of eighteen) are statistically significant in this case. It is also interesting, though far from surprising, that four of these eight significant correlations involve the criterion of EU responsiveness to community expectations and needs concerning emergency medical services. This particular criterion also seems to be adversely affected by the level of tension between EU and hospital administration.

Of the five secondary criteria of effectiveness, staff satisfaction with the EU, which reflects the social efficiency of the system, appears to be the most severely affected by organizational strain. More specifically, all but two of the measures of tension are negatively and significantly related to the satisfaction of RNs with their respective EUs. Especially dysfunctional in this connection appear to be tension between the EU and hospital administration as perceived by RNs, and tension between the EU and the outside community as reported by HAs. Similarly, three of the measures of tension are negatively and significantly related to the satisfaction of MDs with their respective EUs, the strongest relationship in this case involving the tension among EU doctors. On the other hand, patient satisfaction, either with the care received or with the EU staff, correlates significantly only with one of the measures of organizational strain—namely, with tension between the EU and hospital administration as reported by the RNs.

The promptness of medical attention to incoming patients at the various EUs is significantly related, again negatively, to three of the measures of strain: level of tension between doctors and nurses, level of tension among the doctors, and level of tension between EU and the outside community according to the doctors.

Finally, institutional reputation in the community also correlates negatively with certain aspects of organizational strain. Specifically, the reputation of the parent hospitals correlates significantly with both measures of tension between the EU and hospital administration and with the level of tension among EU doctors; and the reputation of EUs is negatively related to the tension prevailing between the EU and hospital administration according to the RNs.

In summary, the relationships found in this study between organizational strain and the secondary criteria of EU effectiveness are consistently negative and often significant as well. In terms of these criteria, at least, organizational strain is dysfunctional for the system. On the whole, moreover, the relationships between strain and the secondary criteria of effectiveness are similar to the relationships found between strain and clinical efficiency. With the exception of economic efficiency, the results confirm the expectation of an inverse relationship between organizational strain and the effectiveness of hospital EUs.

Adequacy of Organizational Problem Solving

Other major problem areas, in addition to that of strain, which received special attention in this research are those of organizational resources, coordination, integration, and adaptation. These areas are of central importance to effective organizational functioning according to the research model which has guided this study and which views organizations as complex work-performing and problem-solving systems. The conceptual and theoretical bases of the model were discussed in Chapter One and are further elaborated in Appendix A and elsewhere (see, especially, Georgopoulos, 1972, 1975, 1978; Georgopoulos and Cooke, 1979; Georgopoulos, Cooke, and Associates, 1980; Georgopoulos and Mann, 1962; Georgopoulos and Matejko, 1967). In this section, the interest is in various indicators (measures and indices) of the relative adequacy of organizational problem solving in these key areas, their interrelationships, and their relationships to EU effectiveness. Such indicators constitute the second major set of independent variables studied in relation to the different criteria of EU effectiveness, the first set comprising the aspects of organizational structure discussed in Chapter Nine.

The present set of independent variables includes: (1) certain aspects of organizational resources which reflect the availability of important resources to the EU as well as the nature of EU-parent hospital relations; (2) certain aspects of organizational coordination (that is, of the functional articulation of the system) which reflect the nature of work relations within the EU; (3) certain aspects of organizational integration (that is, of the social-psychological articulation of the system), including reciprocal understanding by the medical and nursing staff of their work situation, and identification with the system; and (4) certain aspects of organizational adaptation to the external environment which represent the nature of interinstitutional and EU-community relations.

Two or more indicators of organizational problem solving were developed from the data for each of these problem areas, as follows: one index and one measure in the area of resources, two indices and one composite measure in the area of coordination, one composite and two single measures in the area of integration, and two indices in the area of adaptation. All of these indicators of the adequacy of internal organizational problem solving involved data aggregation to the EU level. These basic indicators of organizational problem solving are here examined in relation to one another, in relation to the measures of organizational strain and organizational structure previously discussed, and in relation to the primary and secondary criteria of EU effectiveness.

Organizational Resources: EU-Hospital Relations

In this area, one measure of problem solving at the various EUs was developed using data provided by MDs in response to the following questions: *"When you request services or support* from others in the hospital outside the emergency unit (for example, ancillary services, administrative support, cooperation from other medical units), on the whole, *how satisfactorily* are your requests met? *Are most of these requests* met completely satisfactorily, very satisfactorily, fairly satisfactorily, not so satisfactorily, or not satisfactorily at all?" This question, included in the personal interview completed by MDs, yielded EU means ranging from 1.56 (best-scoring unit) to 2.75 and a grand mean of 2.08 (with a standard deviation of .29), suggesting "very satisfactory" problem solving on the average. Analysis of variance of the data from this item, however, shows borderline results ($F = 1.19$, $p > .05$, and $\eta^2 = .14$), indicating that the obtained measure is statistically weak at the organizational level; however, because the measure reflects the MDs' assessments of how well the hospital fulfills their requests, it was retained in the analysis.

The five-item index in this area, which is based on data provided by the RNs, is a much stronger measure. These data were collected using the tabular-form question shown in Exhibit 10-1.

Results from the one-way analysis of variance performed on the data pertaining to each of the five kinds of requests show a statistically significant F in every case ($p < .05$), the specific F values ranging from 1.70 to 3.02. The corresponding η^2 values also exceed the established standard in every case, ranging from .21 to .27. Accordingly, data aggregation to the EU level produces good measures for the organizational variables represented by all five items. Moreover, the intercorrelations among the resulting five measures are all positive and statistically significant ($p < .05$), the ten coefficients in the series ranging from .33 to .86 and the average correlation being .55. These findings suggest considerable differences among EUs on how well EU requests for services or assistance are fulfilled by their parent hospitals.

Finally, when the five measures corresponding to the items in the above tabular-form question are combined (with equal weights), the resulting index correlates highly with each of the five component measures (.81, .86, .82, .71, and .81, respectively) and has a Cronbach coefficient alpha of .86, or high reliability. Obviously, this indicator of the adequacy of organizational problem solving in the area of resources is superior to the measure that is based on the data from MDs, with which it correlates significantly ($r = .55$, $p < .01$). EU scores on the obtained index range from 1.72 to 2.93, and they average 2.30 with a standard deviation of .30.

Organizational Coordination

The adequacy of organizational problem solving in this area was measured separately for programmed coordination

Exhibit 10-1. Responsiveness of Other Hospital Departments in Meeting EU Requests.

When you request the services, assistance, or support of others in the hospital (outside the emergency unit), on the whole, how satisfactorily are your requests met for each of the following? (Check one for each item.)

Usually, Most of These Requests Are Met:

Requests for:	Completely satisfac-torily (1)	Very satisfac-torily (2)	Fairly satisfac-torily (3)	Not so satisfac-torily (4)	Not satisfac-torily at all (5)
The services of medical specialists from the hospital who are "on call"	☐	☐	☐	☐	☐
Ancillary services from various units in the hospital (outside the emergency unit)	☐	☐	☐	☐	☐
The cooperation or assistance of the in-patient medical services or departments in the hospital	☐	☐	☐	☐	☐
The cooperation or assistance of the *non-emergency outpatient clinics* (if any) of the hospital	☐	☐	☐	☐	☐
Administrative service or support from the hospital	☐	☐	☐	☐	☐

(Georgopoulos and Mann, 1962; March and Simon, 1958), nonprogrammed coordination (Georgopoulos and Mann, 1962), and coordination by mutual adjustment (Thompson, 1967).

Programmed Coordination. Programmed coordination was assessed with data from MDs, using two measures originally developed in another study of hospitals by Georgopoulos and Mann (1962). The two measures represent the extent to which the work assignments of EU staff are well planned and the extent to which interdependent tasks and activities in the unit are well timed. The specific questionnaire items were: "In general, how well planned are the work assignments of the different people who have to work together in this emergency unit?" with response alternatives ranging from 1 (extremely well planned) to 5 (not well planned at all); and "To what extent are the various interrelated tasks and activities *well timed* in the everyday work of this emergency unit?" For this question, the response alternatives ranged from 1 (extremely well timed) to 5 (not well timed at all).

The data from these two items were aggregated to the EU level, and the resulting measures, which correlate positively and significantly ($r = .40$, $p < .05$), were combined into a single index. The two components correlate highly, .83 and .84, respectively ($p < .01$), with the index, which has a Cronbach alpha of .57. EU scores on this index of programmed coordination at the various EUs range from 1.60 (best-scoring EU) to 2.83, averaging 2.37 with a standard deviation of .25.

The obtained index of programmed coordination is also related to certain measures which provide at least inferred support for its validity. More specifically, it correlates positively and significantly with (1) the extent to which authority arrangements are used in the EU to solve work problems, according to the RNs ($r = .42$, $p < .05$); (2) the degree to which corrective efforts in handling problems that arise in the work relations of people in the unit are effective, according to the MDs ($r = .59$, $p < .01$); (3) the extent to which MDs and RNs feel that they can rely on others whose work is related to theirs to do their jobs right ($r = .39$, $p < .05$); and (4) the degree to which people in the unit make an effort to avoid creating problems or interferences with each other's duties and responsibilities according to the MDs ($r = .47$, $p < .01$).

Coordination by Mutual Adjustment. Data on the adequacy of coordination of work efforts by mutual adjustment were obtained from the MDs and RNs with two questions asked of these respondents in their personal interviews. The two groups were asked complementary questions, the MDs responding about the adjustments made by nurses and the RNs about the adjustments made by MDs. Specifically, the MDs were asked: "Generally, to what extent do the nurses in this emergency unit *make adjustments in their work activities* in order to facilitate the work of the medical staff? *Would you say* that they make adjustments to a very great extent, a fair extent, a small extent, or to a very small extent or not at all?" The question asked of RNs was the same except for substituting "doctors" for "nurses" and "nursing staff" for "medical staff" in the stem.

Using the five-point scale indicated, the data from each question were aggregated to the EU level in the usual manner. For the resulting measure based on the data from RNs, $F = 3.10$, $p < .01$, and $\eta^2 = .27$; and for that based on the data from MDs, $F = 1.10$, $p = .34$, and $\eta^2 = .13$. Although the latter is only a marginally adequate measure, it constitutes the essential complement of the former. The two measures in question also correlate positively and significantly ($r = .39$, $p < .05$). Apparently, the work adjustments made by nurses at the various EUs to facilitate the work of doctors are reciprocated to a degree by medical staff adjustments to facilitate the work of nurses, and vice versa.

The two measures finally were combined, by multiplying each EU's score on the MDs measure by its score on the RNs measure, to develop a single measure of coordination by mutual adjustment. EU scores on this rather unique indicator of coordination by mutual adjustment, which has moderate statistical reliability ($R = .56$), range from 2.13 (for the best-scoring EU) to 6.27 and average 3.97 with a standard deviation of 1.17.

Nonprogrammed Coordination. An index of the adequacy of nonprogrammed coordination also was developed, using interview and questionnaire data from MDs, RNs, and patients (PATs) who participated in the study. In their personal interviews, the MDs and RNs were asked to respond to this question: "Overall, how well do the *different jobs and activities around the patient fit together* in this emergency unit? (I mean the activities of the different people who are working in the emergency unit.) *Do they fit together* extremely well, very well, fairly well, not so well, or not well at all?" The same two groups also responded to the following questionnaire item: "How frequently do the people in this emergency unit do their jobs in a way that their joint efforts and activities will fit together smoothly?" The response alternatives, forming a five-point scale, ranged from 1 (always or nearly always) to 5 (infrequently). Finally, the PATs answered a similar question shortly after visiting the EU: "How *smoothly* did the staff seem to work together while you were there (that is, in the emergency unit)?" Response alternatives in this case ranged from 1 (they seemed to work together extremely smoothly) to 5 (not smoothly at all).

By aggregating the data (to the EU level) from each of the above questions and groups of respondents, a total of five specific measures of nonprogrammed coordination were derived. The statistical quality of these measures in terms of corresponding F and η^2 values from an analysis of variance is lowest for the measure based on the responses to the MD questionnaire item ("How frequently do the people . . .") and the measure based on the data from PATs; it is highest for the measure based on the interview data from MDs (how well jobs and activities fit together) and the measure based on the questionnaire data from RNs ("How frequently do the people . . ."). The five measures correlate positively with one another, but not significantly in all cases, the ten coefficients in the series ranging from .05 to .38 (four of them are statistically significant at the .05 level, and another three are significant at the .10 level).

When the five measures are combined, equally weighted, into a single index of nonprogrammed coordination, the index correlates significantly with each of the measures (r = .54 to .67, depending on the particular component measure considered, and p < .01).* The Cronbach alpha for this index is .65, suggesting

---

*In contrast, only two of the five component measures of the nonprogrammed coordination index correlate significantly (p < .05) with

moderate reliability. EU scores on this index of the adequacy of nonprogrammed coordination in hospital EUs range from 1.61 (best-scoring EU) to 2.44 and average 2.07 with a standard deviation of .17.

The nonprogrammed coordination index is also related to a number of measures which support its validity. First, it is significantly related ($p < .05$) to all four of the correlates of programmed coordination specified above, the corresponding product-moment correlations in this case being .35, .51, .40, and .40, respectively. All but one of these coefficients are smaller than their counterparts in the case of programmed coordination, very probably because most of the variables in question are particularly important to programmed coordination while also being relevant to nonprogrammed coordination.

Second, and more important, the adequacy of nonprogrammed coordination at the EUs studied, as represented by the developed index, correlates positively and significantly with (1) the degree to which, according to the MDs, EUs rely on "the autonomy and discretion of the professional staff to ensure that everyone contributes properly to the work and operation of the unit" ($r = .54$, $p < .01$); (2) the degree to which, also according to the MDs, EUs rely on the "existing standards of clinical practice and clinical decision making" for the same purpose ($r = .36$, $p < .05$); (3) "how well the work activities of the various staff fit together when work procedures or the procedures of the unit are neither clear-cut nor well established," according to both RNs ($r = .60$, $p < .01$) and MDs ($r = .46$, $p < .01$); and (4) the extent to which the different people who have to work together in the EU "take into account each other's work problems and needs," again according to both RNs ($r = .39$, $p < .05$) and MDs ($r = .46$, $p < .01$).

---

the programmed coordination index—the two measures based on the data from MDs. Conversely, the two components of the programmed coordination index correlate considerably more highly with this index than they do with the nonprogrammed coordination index (.83 versus .40 in the case of the planning component and .85 versus .42 in the case of the timing component), as they should on both theoretical and methodological grounds.

It should be noted that the variables in this last series are especially relevant to nonprogrammed coordination, or more indicative of the adequacy of nonprogrammed than of programmed coordination. In fact, all except one of the corresponding correlations between these same variables and programmed coordination are smaller, and only half of them are statistically significant (the specific coefficients in that case being .33; .20; .11 and .45; and .21 and .53, correspondingly). Thus, the findings in the present section also support the conceptual-theoretical distinction between programmed and nonprogrammed coordination.

Finally, of the three indicators of coordination just discussed, the one which best represents the overall adequacy of organizational coordination in hospital EUs is that of nonprogrammed coordination. This index of coordination correlates significantly both with the measure of coordination by mutual adjustment ($r = .52$, $p < .01$), which could be viewed as a special form of nonprogrammed coordination, and the programmed coordination index ($r = .49$, $p < .01$). The latter two measures also correlate positively but less strongly ($r = .37$, $p < .05$).

Organizational (Social-Normative) Integration

The problem of integration, like those of coordination and strain, is a multifaceted one. As pointed out in Chapter One, organizational integration refers to the social-psychological articulation of an organization (see Georgopoulos, 1965, 1972; Georgopoulos and Cooke, 1979; Georgopoulos and Matejko, 1967; Katz and Georgopoulos, 1971; Katz and Kahn, 1966, 1978). Generally, it involves both the psychological incorporation of individual members into the system, which is essential to their loyalty and support, and the social-psychological articulation of subsystems, which ensures that the different groups will support both the system and one another to mutual advantage.

At least three important aspects of organizational integration may be usefully distinguished: member integration, normative integration, and structural integration. Member integration concerns the degree of personal identification with the system on the part of individual members, a variable that reflects their organizational commitment, interest, and involvement. Normative integration concerns the nature of intergroup and interpersonal relations in the system, and especially the degree to which different but interdependent groups (and members) develop common understandings and share the same or congruent frames of reference in their interactions. Structural integration, not examined in the present study, concerns the articulation of the basic structures of a social system (authority and control structure, role structure, normative structure)—that is, the degree of compatibility and complementarity characterizing these structures, which presumably relates to the likelihood that the different structures will be mutually supportive and reinforcing.

Among other things, good integration is expected to facilitate organizational coordination, and poor integration is expected to impede it while also generating strain for the system and its members. Good integration may also promote staff satisfaction, that is, the social efficiency of the system. In addition, integration could affect performance, directly by promoting and reinforcing organizationally relevant behavior on the part of all concerned, and indirectly by facilitating coordination and strain resolution in the system. Member integration and normative integration in particular are likely to affect individual and group performance directly. Accordingly, both of these aspects of organizational integration were considered in this research.

Normative Integration. The adequacy of normative integration at the various EUs is represented by an indicator of the level of reciprocal/mutual understanding between doctors and nurses, that is, between the two principal groups in the system. The relevant data were obtained with the following pair of questions: "On the whole, to what extent does the *nursing staff understand and appreciate* the work problems and needs of the *medical staff* in this emergency unit?" (asked of the MDs) and "On the whole, to what extent does the *medical staff understand and appreciate* the work problems and needs of the *nursing staff* in this emergency unit?" (asked of the RNs). The response alternatives, forming a five-point scale, were the same for both questions and ranged from 1 (they have an excellent understanding) to 5 (they have a rather poor understanding). The two questions were included in the structured questionnaire forms that the MDs and RNs working at the various EUs completed.

Based on these data, the required EU means were computed and then summed (separately for each EU) to develop an overall indicator of the adequacy of normative integration for each EU. More specifically, the obtained indicator is a composite measure that represents the degree to which the nursing and medical staffs (of each EU as a group) understand and appreciate each other's work problems and needs.

Across EUs, the degree to which the nursing staff understands the work problems and needs of the medical staff according to the MDs ranges from 1.56 (midway between "excellent" and "very good") to 3.00 (exactly "good") and averages 2.11 (nearly "very good") with a standard deviation of .34. And the degree to which the medical staff understands and appreciates the work problems and needs of the nursing staff according to the RNs ranges from 2.27 (nearly "very good") to 4.10 (signifying only a "fair understanding") and averages 3.08 (nearly "good") with a standard deviation of .43. These two measures (and the corresponding data from the other group of respondents in each case as well) also show that EU physicians and registered nurses are in agreement that the nursing staff in hospital EUs has a better understanding of the work problems and needs of the medical staff than the medical staff has of the work problems and needs of the nursing staff. The medical staff, therefore, may be particularly responsible for inadequacies in this area.

The measure based on the data from MDs is somewhat problematic because it is statistically marginal at the aggregate level ($F = 1.03$, $p > .05$; $\eta^2 = .14$), but it is also the essential complement of the measure based on the data from RNs, which fully meets the usual criteria ($F = 1.57$, $p < .05$; $\eta^2 = .16$). The two measures, only in combination and as a pair, are conceptually necessary and sufficient to represent normative integration. EU scores on the composite indicator of normative integration, which was constructed by summing up the scores of EUs on these two measures, range from 4.02, which signifies a "very good" level of reciprocal/mutual understanding between the two groups, to 6.17, which signifies almost a "good" level of understanding. The grand mean of the thirty EUs on this particular indicator is 5.19, and the standard deviation of the distribution of EU scores is .54.

The obtained indicator of normative integration correlates significantly with both of the components that it subsumes (r = .78 with the RNs' data measure, and .61 with the MDs' data measure, $p < .01$ in both cases). EU scores on the two components, however, are unrelated (r = -.02, $p > .05$). It also correlates positively and significantly with the degree to which the medical staff understands and appreciates the work problems and needs of the nursing staff according to the MDs (r = .54, $p < .01$), and the degree to which the nursing staff understands the work problems and needs of the medical staff according to the RNs (r = .59, $p < .01$). These last two measures, however, are not significantly related (r = .19, $p > .05$). It is also interesting, though perhaps not surprising, to find that, according to the data from MDs, the degree to which the medical staff understands the nursing staff's problems correlates significantly with the degree to which the nursing staff understands the medical staff's problems (r = .75, $p < .01$), and the same holds true according to the data from RNs (r = .71, $p < .01$).

Other results show that the level of normative integration at the various EUs, as represented by the composite indicator developed, correlates highly (r = .88, $p < .01$) with the degree to which the medical staff understands and appreciates the work problems and needs of the nursing staff (of the two groups, it will be recalled, the former generally has the poorer understanding) according to the responses of MDs and RNs combined. In addition, it correlates significantly with the extent to which the various people working together in the EU take each other's work problems and needs into account according to both MDs (r = .38, $p < .05$) and RNs (r = .42, $p < .01$). Finally, the level of normative integration in hospital EUs is positively and significantly related to organizational coordination (see Table 10-4).

Member Integration. Two measures of member integration, one for nurses and the other for doctors, were also developed. Both are based on questionnaire data obtained from RNs and MDs, respectively, in response to the following item: "Personally, how strongly *identified with* or how strongly committed do you feel you are to this emergency unit?'' The response alternatives provided were 1—extremely strongly, 2—very strongly, 3—moderately strongly, 4—fairly strongly, and 5—not strongly.

Although, strictly speaking, personal identification is an individual-linked concept and not an organizational variable (such as normative or structural integration), it is not inappropriate to aggregate the data to the EU level, since the specific referent of identification in the present case is the EU. Accordingly, the data were aggregated, and the usual analysis of variance was performed.

The results show that the member integration measure for MDs is stronger statistically than that for RNs, the latter being somewhat marginal as an aggregate-level measure. With respect to the latter, $F = 1.28$, $p > .05$, and $\eta^2 = .14$; with respect to the former, $F = 1.44$, $p < .05$, and $\eta^2 = .19$. EU scores (means) on the identification of RNs with the EU range from 1.40 (for the unit with the strongest member identification) to 2.83 on the above scale, yielding a grand mean of 2.12 and a standard deviation of .38. The corresponding figures concerning the identification of MDs with the EU are 1.50 to 3.83, 2.58 (which signifies an average level of identification intermediate between "moderate" and "strong"), and .60.

Obviously, as a group and on the average, RNs identify more strongly with their respective units than the MDs do. In other words, hospital EUs generally have a more strongly identified, or more committed, staff of registered nurses than they have medical staff. Across hospital EUs, the identification of RNs with the system tends to correlate positively but not significantly with the identification of MDs with the system ($r = .25$, $p > .05$). Finally, irrespective of the specific measure, member identification is not significantly related to the normative integration measure (Table 10-4).

Organizational Adaptation: EU-Community Relations

All of the problem areas considered thus far focus on the internal organizational situation of hospital EUs. The remaining area to be examined, organizational adaptation, concerns relationships of the system to its relevant external environment. Organizational adaptation, which is sometimes considered as a criterion of organizational effectiveness, focuses on the two-way interchange between organization and environment. Therefore, it should not be confused with the characteristics of the environment (such as those discussed earlier in Chapter Nine, which were found not to be related to EU effectiveness). The adequacy of organizational problem solving in the area of adaptation, which is expected to relate both to the adequacy of problem solving in other major areas and to EU effectiveness, is reflected in the relative success with which the system handles its external affairs problems and in the reputation that it enjoys in the outside community. Here, it is represented by two indices: an index of collaboration with other institutions and an overall "emergency unit adaptation index."

Institutional Collaboration Index. This is a three-item index which is based on questionnaire data from the EU supervising nurses (SRNs) and hospital administrators (HAs) who participated in the research. These respondents were asked: "At the present time, to what extent is this hospital or emergency unit collaborating with other hospitals, emergency units, or other relevant service agencies for the following purposes?" The response alternatives that were provided ranged from 1 (to a very great extent) to 5 (to a very small extent or not at all). The specific purposes of collaboration included (1) "to provide better or less costly emergency medical services to the community"; (2) "to facilitate or improve the work of this emergency unit"; and (3) "to share useful information about the emergency medical needs of the community." Following the usual aggregation to the EU level, three measures were developed from the obtained data, one for each of these purposes, and then combined into an index.

For the measure of collaboration to provide better or less costly emergency services, $F = 2.02$, $p < .01$, and $\eta^2 = .43$; for collaboration to facilitate/improve the work of the EU, $F = 1.11$, $p > .05$, and $\eta^2 = .30$; and for collaboration to share information, $F = 1.96$, $p < .05$, and $\eta^2 = .43$. The three measures turned out to be highly interrelated. The first one correlates .72 ($p < .01$) with the second and .76 ($p < .01$) with the third, and the latter two correlate .86 ($p < .01$). Accordingly, the scores of EUs on the three measures were summed and averaged (separately for each EU) to construct an index of institutional collaboration. The scores of the 30 EUs on this index range from 1.00 (best-scoring unit) to 4.33 on the five-point scale used, suggesting great interinstitutional differences in the extent of collaboration, and average 2.96 (which corresponds almost exactly to "a fair extent") with a standard deviation of .65. All three of its component measures correlate very highly with the index: .91, .92, and .94, respectively. Moreover, the index has a Cronbach coefficient alpha of .91, which indicates high reliability.

Finally, certain evidence relevant to the validity of this index is also available. This evidence involves the relationship between the obtained index and an index of how satisfactory the contacts of EU staff are with certain key outside groups with which it has frequent interactions. These key groups are sheriff's department personnel, police department personnel, fire department personnel, and private ambulance services personnel. The relevant data concerning contacts with each of these groups were obtained, also from HAs and SRNs, in response to this questionnaire item: "Considering all of the work-related contacts that the staff of the emergency unit have with each of the following, *how satisfactory* would you say are their contacts from the standpoint of accomplishing the work of the emergency unit?"

Briefly, these data too were aggregated to the EU level in the usual manner, and the resulting EU scores concerning the four groups were summed and averaged to construct a single index of how satisfactory EU staff contacts with these important groups are. This index has a Cronbach alpha of .81, indicating high reliability, and correlates very highly ($r = .89$, $p < .01$) with the index of institutional collaboration for the purposes specified. It also correlates significantly but not as highly with the adaptation index described below.

Emergency Unit Adaptation Index. The last and final indicator of the adequacy of organizational problem solving at the EUs studied is an index of organizational adaptation. This index incorporates three component measures that partially overlap with two of the secondary criteria of EU effectiveness previously discussed (see Chapter Eight)—namely, the criteria of EU responsiveness to community expectations and needs and institutional reputation. Of the three component measures, one is a single-item measure and the other two are two-item indices.

The first component of the EU adaptation index consists of a rating by the selected community respondents (CRs) of how well their respective EUs have been able to respond to the community's changing needs for emergency medical services. For this measure, $F = 1.45$, $p < .05$, and $\eta^2 = .21$. The second component consists of similar ratings by MDs and RNs of the responsiveness of EUs in meeting community expectations regarding emergency medical services. For the ratings provided by the MDs, $F = 2.12$, $p < .01$, and $\eta^2 = .25$; and for those provided by the RNs, $F = 1.78$, $p < .05$, and $\eta^2 = .18$. These two ratings correlate positively and significantly ($r = .47$, $p < .01$), and when they are combined the resulting composite measure has a Cronbach alpha of .63. The third component of the adaptation index, which is also a two-item measure, consists of ratings by hospital administrators (HAs) and the selected hospital physicians (HMDs) of the reputation of their respective EUs in the outside community. For the ratings provided by the HAs, $F = 3.10$, $p < .01$, and $\eta^2 = .70$; and for those provided by the HMDs, $F = 2.02$, $p < .01$, and $\eta^2 = .26$. These two measures also correlate positively ($r = .57$, $p < .01$), and when they are combined to form the component in question the resulting measure has a Cronbach alpha of .67.

The first component correlates .42 ($p < .01$) with the second and .13 ($p > .05$) with the third, and the latter two measures correlate .53 ($p < .01$). The scores of EUs on the three components ultimately were combined (summed and averaged) to construct the emergency unit adaptation index. The obtained index correlates fairly highly with all three of its components (.65, .78, and .82, correspondingly, and $p < .01$ in all cases) and has satisfactory reliability ($R = .67$). EU scores on this index range from 1.53 to 3.01, suggesting considerable interinstitutional differences in this area, and average 2.29 (indicating almost a "very good" adaptation level) with a standard deviation of .34. Finally, the emergency unit adaptation index correlates positively and significantly, though not highly, with the institutional collaboration index ($r = .33$, $p < .05$).

Table 10-4. Indicators (Measures or Indices) of Organizational Problem Solving and Their Interrelationships.

Problem Area	1	2	3	4	5	6	7	8	9	10
Organizational Resources										
1. Responsiveness of other departments in meeting EU requests for services or assistance (five-item index, α = .86)	--	.55**	.26	.34*	.25	.32*	-.30	.00	.34*	.19
2. Fulfillment by hospital of EU physician requests for services or support, according to MDs (F = 1.19, $p > .05$; η^2 = .14)		--	.43*	.33*	.21	.35*	-.14	.15	.18	.16
Organizational Coordination										
3. Adequacy of programmed coordination in the EU (two-item index, α = .57)			--	.49**	.37*	.54**	.05	.11	.43*	.37*
4. Adequacy of nonprogrammed coordination (five-item index, α = .65)				--	.52**	.48**	.14	.09	.28	.56**
5. Mutual adjustment by RNs and MDs to facilitate each other's work (a special two-item measure, R = .56)					--	.31*	.21	.36*	.23	.15

Measure or Index

Organizational Integration

6. Normative integration: level of reciprocal/mutual understanding between MDs and RNs (a composite two-item indicator)	--	-.07	.23	.36*	.26
7. Member integration (MDs): degree MDs identify with the EU ($F = 1.44$, $p < .05$; $\eta^2 = .19$)		--	.25	-.01	.19
8. Member integration (RNs): degree RNs identify with the EU ($F = 1.28$, $p < .10$; $\eta^2 = .14$)			--	.23	.15

Organizational Adaptation

9. Collaboration with other institutions re: emergency services (three-item index, $\alpha = .91$)				--	.33*
10. Emergency unit adaptation index (incorporates three measures, $R = .67$)					--

Notes:
*$p < .05$.
**$p < .01$.
All correlations shown are product-moment correlations at the EU level. $N = 30$ EUs in all cases.

Interrelationships Among Problem-Solving Indicators

The measures and indices of the adequacy of organizational problem solving discussed in the preceding pages are, of course, not unrelated. Successful/unsuccessful organizational performance in any of the areas examined to some degree also affects performance in the rest, since the problem areas in question are interdependent (Cooke and Rousseau, 1981; Georgopoulos, 1972; Georgopoulos and Cooke, 1979; Georgopoulos and Matjeko, 1967; Sutton and Ford, 1982). The effects may be direct or indirect, strong or weak, and even negative in some cases, although for most organizations most of the time successful problem solving in one area will probably facilitate rather than impede problem solving in the other major areas specified. Similarly, the effects may vary from one hospital EU to another, as well as for the same EU over time, and the various problem areas are not necessarily equally consequential in terms of mutual impact. Generally, however, in terms of successful problem solving, interrelationships among the problem areas will tend to be positive. The results presented in Table 10-4, together with those in Table 10-5 (which shows the relationships of organizational strain to the other problem areas), confirm this expectation for the thirty hospital EUs in the sample.

Table 10-4 shows the interrelationships among the different measures developed, both within and between problem areas, for the areas of organizational resources, coordination, integration, and adaptation. The correlations between measures within each area have been presented above. To summarize, all except one of the relevant correlations, which range from -.07 to .55 and average .35, are positive, as was expected. Moreover, the majority of them are statistically significant as well. In fact, for each of the problem areas except that of integration the correlations between measures are positive and significant. Perhaps integration is a more heterogeneous area internally than are the others, or has been least well measured among the four, and/or is associated with uneven or inconsistent organizational problem solving. It must be also noted, however, that, even when the area of integration is excluded, the average intercorrelation among measures within areas is not high ($r = .46$)—all of the problem areas are multifaceted and relatively heterogeneous internally.

The remaining correlations in Table 10-4 show whether the relative adequacy of organizational problem solving in any one area is associated with the adequacy of problem solving in any other area (concerning the area of strain, see Table 10-5). Overall, as anticipated, the findings show that this tends to be the case. The general pattern is one of positive though only weak-to-moderate association. More specifically, all but three of the thirty-seven correlation coefficients in Table 10-4 which are relevant to this issue (the others show within-area relationships) are positive, and fourteen of the thirty-three positive correlations are statistically significant. The significant correlations range in size from .33 to .56, suggesting moderate rather than strong interrelationships across the problem areas.

The results shown in Table 10-4 also reveal the critical importance of organizational coordination for hospital EUs. Specifically, when the several areas are compared, the adequacy of coordination turns out to correlate best overall with the adequacy of problem solving in the other areas (nearly half of the relevant correlations are statistically significant in this case). Least strongly related to the other areas is that of organizational adaptation, which involves the external affairs of the system (nearly one-third of the correlations being significant in this case). The areas of organizational resources and organizational integration occupy intermediate positions in this respect.

Organizational Strain and Problem Solving

The centrality of coordination becomes even greater when the relationships between the above problem areas and organizational strain are also taken into account. Two-thirds of the correlations between coordination and the other four areas (including organizational strain) are statistically significant and in the expected direction. These relationships are shown in Table 10-5. As hypothesized, strain, represented by the seven measures of tension discussed earlier, is inversely related to the adequacy of

Table 10-5. Organizational Strain in Hospital Emergency Units and Organizational Problem Solving in Key Areas.

| | Organizational Problem Solving | | | | | | | | | |
| | Resources | | Coordination | | | Integration | | | Adaptation | |
Organizational Strain	Responsiveness of Other Departments	Fulfillment of EU Physician Requests	Programmed Coordination	Non-programmed Coordination	Mutual Adjustment by RNs and MDs	Normative Integration	Member Integration MDs	Member Integration RNs	Collaboration with Other Institutions	EU Adaptation Index
Tension Within the EU										
Among clinical staff	-.29	-.22	-.12	-.15	-.06	-.25	-.51**	-.16	-.08	-.16
Between MDs and RNs	-.13	-.05	-.32*	-.34*	-.38*	-.47**	-.34*	-.13	-.25	-.24
Among MDs	-.16	-.21	-.33*	-.29	-.37*	-.24	-.16	-.26	-.16	-.24
Tension Between EU and Hospital Administration										
As reported by MDs	-.05	-.41*	-.58**	-.52**	-.38*	-.40*	-.26	-.10	-.26	-.54**
As reported by RNs	-.28	-.50**	-.42*	-.35*	.01	-.16	.09	-.07	-.25	-.51**
Tension Between EU and Outside Community										
According to HAs	.07	.01	-.09	-.36*	-.14	-.15	.03	.01	-.13	-.22
According to MDs	-.14	-.29	-.69**	-.49**	-.53**	-.39*	-.31*	-.11	-.33*	-.39*

Notes:
*p < .05.
**p < .01.
All correlations shown are product-moment correlations at the EU level. N = 30 EUs in all cases.
The measures of organizational problem solving are the same as those included in Table 10-4.
The measures of organizational strain are the same as those included in Tables 10-1 and 10-2.

problem solving in the other major areas. All but five of the seventy correlation coefficients are negative and twenty-six of them are statistically significant as well. The specific correlations range from .09 to –.58, the majority being of small to moderate size.

Of the several aspects of strain examined, the level of tension between the EU and hospital administration appears to be particularly dysfunctional for the system, since it correlates most strongly (inversely) with the adequacy of organizational problem solving in the other areas. And of the specific measures of strain, the level of tension between doctors and nurses in the EU, between the EU and hospital administration (as reported by MDs), and between the EU and the outside community (also as assessed by MDs) produce the largest number of significant relationships, each correlating negatively and significantly with at least half of the measures of the adequacy of organizational problem solving in the areas of resources, coordination, integration, and adaptation combined.

Strain correlates least well with problem solving in the area of organizational resources, a finding which suggests that for the most part it is not linked to resource problems. Nor does it seem to be of structural origin, since, when examined in relation to the eight measures of organizational structure discussed in Chapter Nine, the seven measures of strain produce relatively few significant relationships: A total of only six of the resulting fifty-six correlations (which range between .28 and –.40, and thirty-six of which are negative) are statistically significant at the .05 level. Nevertheless, these particular correlations show that some measures of strain are significantly related to certain aspects of structure.* Based on the results in Table 10-5, the prevailing strain

---

*The significant relationships obtained from this analysis are as follows: tension between the EU and the outside community, as reported by MDs only, correlates –.40 with medical teaching affiliation and –.34 with emergency personnel training programs; tension between the EU and hospital administration, as reported by RNs only, correlates –.36 with personnel training programs and –.32 with EU service specialization; tension among the clinical staff correlates –.31 with parent hospital size; and tension among EU doctors correlates –.32 with institutional status as measured by number of professional approvals.

in hospital EUs appears to be associated mainly with coordination problems, replicating findings from some earlier hospital studies (Georgopoulos and Matejko, 1967; Wieland, 1965) in this respect.

Organizational Structure and Problem Solving

In Chapter Nine, it was pointed out that the structure of the system may affect EU effectiveness not only directly (as shown in that chapter) but also indirectly through its impact on organizational problem solving. Therefore, it might be instructive at this point to examine briefly the relationships between structure and problem solving in areas other than that of strain, before considering the relationship of organizational problem solving to EU effectiveness. The relevant findings are presented in Table 10-6.

The adequacy of organizational problem solving in areas other than that of strain shows a number of relationships to organizational structure. In fact, all but one of the structural variables considered, that of parent hospital size, are significantly related to some of the indicators of organizational problem solving. Of the various aspects of structure, medical teaching affiliation shows the most relationships. Specifically, it correlates positively and significantly with programmed coordination, the two measures of member integration, and the EU adaptation index. The remaining structural variables correlate significantly with two or three of the measures of organizational problem solving, as shown in Table 10-6.

One-fourth of the correlations obtained between structure and problem solving are statistically significant, indicating the importance of the former to the latter. Of the various areas of problem solving, that of coordination seems to depend the least on the structure of the system (shows the fewest relationships), probably because most of the coordination of efforts that takes place in hospital EUs is nonprogrammed—the type that depends mainly on voluntary and spontaneous staff adjustments and on informal feedbacks. At the other extreme, organizational adaptation as measured by the EU adaptation index correlates significantly with all but two of the measures of organizational structure,

Table 10-6. System Structure and Organizational Problem Solving.

| | Resources | | Organizational Problem Solving in Key Areas | | | | | | | | |
| | | | Coordination | | | Integration | | | Adaptation | | |
Aspect of Structure	Responsiveness of Other Departments	Fulfillment of EU Physician Requests	Programmed Coordination	Non-programmed Coordination	Mutual Adjust-ment by RNs and MDs	Normative Integration	Member Integration MDs	RNs	Collaboration with Other Institutions	EU Adaptation Index
Medical Teaching Affiliation	.08	.13	.23	.35*	.29	.02	.47**	.35*	.19	.50**
Emergency Personnel Training Programs	.14	.03	.35*	.22	.13	.16	.04	.00	.11	.43*
EU Patient Volume	-.12	-.26	.08	.04	.28	.11	.46**	.49**	.14	.32*
Parent Hospital Size	.19	.09	.11	.12	.14	.14	.22	.28	.18	.28
Breadth/Scope of Emergency Service	-.34*	-.40*	-.17	-.19	.28	-.13	.24	.35*	-.13	-.14
EU Service Specialization	.30*	.18	.01	.06	-.01	.26	.06	.22	.43*	.34*
Service Complexity	.36*	.25	.21	.13	.02	.11	.16	.21	.41*	.43*
Institutional Status (Number of Approvals)	.32*	.04	-.04	.25	.18	.00	.16	.14	.10	.35*

Notes:
*p < .05.
**p < .01.
All correlations shown are product-moment correlations. N varies between 28 and 30 EUs.
The measures of organizational problem solving are the same as those included in Tables 10-4 and 10-5.
The structural variables used here are discussed in Chapter Nine.

and the responsiveness of other hospital departments in meeting EU requests for services or assistance correlates significantly with half of the structural variables. Normative integration, like coordination, shows no relationship to organizational structure, in contrast to member integration, which is related to medical teaching affiliation, EU patient volume, and the breadth/scope of emergency service. Other details may be seen in Table 10-6.

Adequacy of Problem Solving in Specific Areas and Institutional Effectiveness

The results testing the hypothesis that the adequacy of organizational problem solving in the areas specified will be directly related to the effectiveness of hospital EUs are discussed in this section. In part, this hypothesis was already tested above with reference to one problem area—organizational strain (see Tables 10-2 and 10-3). It was found to be supported in relation to clinical efficiency (according to most measures of strain) and several of the secondary criteria of EU effectiveness (according to some of the measures), but not in relation to economic efficiency. In this section, it will be tested with reference to the problem areas of resources, coordination, integration, and adaptation. The results concerning the primary criteria of effectiveness are summarized in Table 10-7 (for all of these areas) and those concerning the secondary criteria in Table 10-8.

Organizational Resources and EU Effectiveness

The findings in this area show strong support for the above hypothesis in relation to the clinical efficiency of hospital EUs, particularly the quality of medical care, moderate support in relation to most of the secondary criteria, and no support in relation to economic efficiency.

More specifically, the responsiveness of other departments in meeting EU requests for services or assistance (the principal indicator of problem solving in the area of resources) turns out to be important not only to the quality of medical care, with which

Table 10-7. Relationships Between Organizational Problem Solving and Emergency Unit Effectiveness.

| | EU Effectiveness (Primary Criteria) | | |
| | Economic Efficiency | Clinical Efficiency | |
Problem Area	Economic Efficiency Index (N = 26 EUs)	Quality of Nursing Care Index (N = 30 EUs)	Quality of Medical Care Index (N = 30 EUs)
Organizational Resources			
Responsiveness of other departments	-.07	.37*	.69**
Fulfillment of EU physician requests	-.09	.32*	.46***
Organizational Coordination			
Adequacy of programmed coordination	.02	.41*	.30*
Adequacy of nonprogrammed coordination	-.12	.58**	.50**
Mutual adjustment by RNs and MDs	-.01	.47**	.39*
Organizational Integration			
Normative integration	.12	.36*	.30*
Member integration (MDs)	.20	.28	-.16
Member integration (RNs)	.34*	.42*	.15
Organizational Adaptation			
Collaboration with other institutions	.06	.42*	.28
EU adaptation index	.19	.61**	.52**

Notes:
*$p < .05$.
**$p < .01$.
All correlations shown are product-moment correlations at the EU level.

Table 10-8. Relationships Between Organizational Problem Solving and the Secondary Criteria of Emergency Unit Effectiveness.

Problem Area	Promptness of Medical Attention to Patients	Staff Satisfaction with EU		Patient Satisfaction with Care	EU Staff Expectations	EU Responsiveness to Community Needs	Reputation of	
		MDs	RNs				EU	Hospital
Organizational Resources								
Responsiveness of other departments	.40*	.10	.08	.33*	.17	.24	.13	.40*
Fulfillment of EU physician requests	.13	.09	.20	.19	.22	.27	.07	.31*
Organizational Coordination								
Adequacy of programmed coordination	.21	.39*	.22	.06	.18	.31*	.17	.41*
Adequacy of nonprogrammed coordination	.52**	.33*	.37*	.35*	.50**	.52**	.25	.31*
Mutual adjustment by RNs and MDs	.58**	.28	.13	.12	.10	.36*	.09	.12
Organizational Integration								
Normative integration	.38*	.26	.33*	-.17	-.10	.28	.03	.04
Member integration (MDs)	-.18	.12	.02	-.15	-.03	.23	.01	-.13
Member integration (RNs)	.09	.10	.34*	.12	.17	.23	.10	-.03
Organizational Adaptation								
Collaboration with other institutions	.22	.12	.25	.10	.17	.36*	.07	.07
EU adaptation index	.16	.20	.61**	.42*	.41*	.85**	.71**	.56**

EU Effectiveness (Secondary Criteria)

Notes:
*$p < .05$.
**$p < .01$.
All correlations shown are product-moment correlations. *N* varies between 27 and 30 EUs.
Secondary criteria and their interrelationships are discussed in Chapter Eight.

it correlates most strongly ($r = .69$), but also to the quality of nursing care, the promptness of medical attention given to patients, and the satisfaction of patients with their care. Apparently, however, it is of no direct consequence to the economic performance of hospital EUs (which in Chapter Nine was shown to be related to organizational structure differences). Fulfillment by the hospital of EU physician requests for services or support also correlates significantly with clinical efficiency, again better with the quality of medical than the quality of nursing care, though less strongly than does the responsiveness index. Further, it is significantly related to one of the secondary criterion measures, that of hospital reputation. It, too, however, shows no relationship to economic efficiency.

Clearly, the adequacy of organizational problem solving in the area of resources is directly related to the clinical efficiency of hospital EUs, but not to their economic efficiency. In addition, it is positively related to some of the secondary measures of institutional effectiveness, as shown in Table 10-8. Finally, it is interesting to note that resource availability at the EUs studied, measured in terms of the quantity, quality, and/or stability of certain specific resources (including physical facilities, the budget, information, and personnel), is also related to certain aspects of EU effectiveness, as well as to the adequacy of organizational problem solving in hospital EUs (D'Aunno, 1984). As might be expected, in other words, successful organizational problem solving and resource availability are both interrelated and associated with the effectiveness of the system.

Organizational Coordination and EU Effectiveness

Of all the problem areas, coordination is the most consistently associated with the measures of institutional effectiveness, and the adequacy of nonprogrammed coordination clearly emerges as a particularly important independent variable in this connection.

First, as anticipated, nonprogrammed coordination is positively related to both components of clinical efficiency—that is, to the quality of both medical and nursing care. Second, it correlates significantly with all five of the secondary criteria of EU effectiveness. In other words, promptness of medical attention to patients, staff satisfaction, patient satisfaction, responsiveness to community expectations and needs, and parent hospital reputation are all higher in those hospital EUs which have better nonprogrammed coordination. In fact, the only criterion measures with which the adequacy of nonprogrammed coordination fails to correlate significantly are EU reputation ($r = .25$) and economic efficiency ($r = -.12$).

Coordination by mutual adjustment (a special form of nonprogrammed coordination, for which the measure is not included in the nonprogrammed coordination index) shows a similar though weaker pattern. Briefly, it is related to the clinical but not economic efficiency of hospital EUs, to the promptness of medical attention, and to the responsiveness of EUs to community expectations. The adequacy of programmed coordination also correlates significantly with the quality of medical and nursing care but less strongly than coordination by mutual adjustment or nonprogrammed coordination. In addition, programmed coordination is positively related to medical staff satisfaction, EU responsiveness to community expectations, and the parent hospital's reputation.

Because of the relative unpredictability of workload and patient requirements associated with the uncertainty and heterogeneity of patient inputs, organizational and clinical planning and programming are severely constrained in hospital EUs. This probably accounts for the greater importance of nonprogrammed over programmed coordination in this system, and also in hospitals more generally (Georgopoulos and Mann, 1962; Georgopoulos and Matejko, 1967). In fact, results from another analysis, by Argote (1982), of some of the data from the study reinforce this interpretation. Specifically, Argote found that programmed means of coordination (for example, rules, scheduled meetings) make a greater contribution to organizational effectiveness under conditions of low rather than high input uncertainty, and nonprogrammed means of coordination make a greater contribution under conditions of high uncertainty. But Uhlaner (1980) further showed that nonprogrammed means of coordination are the most likely to promote good overall coordination in hospital EUs under most conditions. Argote (1979) also found that input uncertainty is directly related to organizational problem solving in the areas of resources, strain, and adaptation, impeding problem solving in each case.

In summary, the findings of this research underscore the great importance of coordination to virtually all aspects of effective organizational functioning, the sole exception being economic performance. Thus, for the most part, they substantiate similar conclusions from earlier organizational research in hospital settings (for example, see Georgopoulos and Mann, 1962; Georgopoulos and Matejko, 1967; Hage, 1974; Shortell and Kaluzny, 1983; Wieland, 1965, 1981). Finally, they are consistent with the central place of coordination in the research model which guided this study as well as with prevailing theoretical expectations in the organizational research literature (see, for example, Georgopoulos, 1972; Georgopoulos and Mann, 1962; Hage, 1974; Likert, 1967; Mintzberg, 1979; Shortell and Kaluzny, 1983; Thompson, 1967) concerning the significance of coordination for the effectiveness of modern organizations.

Organizational Integration and EU Effectiveness

Normative integration, represented by the level of reciprocal understanding between doctors and nurses working at the various EUs, correlates positively with clinical efficiency, but not as highly as coordination. Like the latter, it is not related to the economic efficiency of EUs. Normative integration also seems to facilitate the promptness of medical attention to patients and RN satisfaction with the EU but is unrelated to the other secondary criteria of institutional effectiveness.

Physician integration into the system shows no direct relationship to either the primary or the secondary criteria of EU effectiveness. On the average, in other words, the strength of the doctors' personal identification with (or commitment to) the EU does not affect the clinical or economic efficiency of the unit directly, nor does it affect the secondary criteria of institutional effectiveness. Similarly, it is not directly related to organizational problem solving in other areas (see Table 10-4). The same variable, however, may affect EU performance indirectly. Earlier, for example, it was found that physician integration is inversely related to the levels of prevailing tension among the clinical staff, between MDs and RNs, and between the EU and the outside community (see Table 10-5). These three measures of tension, in turn, were shown to be negatively related to several criteria of effectiveness (see Tables 10-2 and 10-3) as well as to the adequacy of organizational coordination (Table 10-5), which correlates with effectiveness very strongly.

Unlike physician integration, the integration of RNs (who, unlike the physicians, are employees of the hospital) is directly related to the quality of nursing care, to RN satisfaction with the EU as a place to work, and to economic efficiency. In fact, of all aspects of the adequacy of organizational problem solving measured in the study, only the integration of RNs turns out to be significantly related to the economic efficiency of hospital EUs (r = .34, $p < .05$). The same variable, however, is not directly related to either the quality of medical care or the secondary criteria of effectiveness (except RN satisfaction), behaving much like the physician integration measure in this respect.

In view of these results, and with the notable exception of its relationship to economic efficiency, it appears that organizational integration is not related to the effectiveness of hospital EUs as strongly as the other problem areas studied. This is particularly evident in regard to the various secondary criteria of effectiveness (only three of the twenty-seven correlations between the integration measures and the secondary criterion measures shown in Table 10-8 are statistically significant). With regard to the primary criteria of EU effectiveness, on the other hand, the results in Table 10-7 show a much stronger pattern; four of the relevant correlations are statistically significant and in the expected direction. In addition, of course, integration may facilitate organizational problem solving in other areas (see Tables 10-4 and 10-5). Finally, it is possible that the relationships between organizational integration and institutional effectiveness would have been stronger had the adequacy of integration been better measured than it was.

Organizational Adaptation and EU Effectiveness

The results in Tables 10-7 and 10-8 also show the relationships between adaptation to the external environment and the effectiveness of hospital EUs. First, collaboration with other institutions on emergency care matters apparently facilitates the quality of nursing care provided by the various EUs ($r = .42$, $p < .05$), but it is only marginally related to the quality of medical care ($r = .28$, $p < .10$). A stronger relationship to the quality of medical care, however, has been reported by Uzun (1980), who, based on her analysis of related data from the study, concluded that interorganizational collaboration is strongly associated with improved intrasystem processes and patient care quality.

Second, the more hospital EUs engage in such collaboration, the more successful they are in meeting community expectations and needs concerning emergency medical services. On the other hand, interinstitutional collaboration is not directly related to economic efficiency, promptness of medical attention, staff or patient satisfaction, or institutional reputation. However, institutional collaboration is significantly related to the second and more inclusive indicator of adaptation (see Table 10-4), the EU adaptation index, which shows more and stronger relationships to EU effectiveness.

As measured by this index, adaptation to the environment, like collaboration, is not related to economic efficiency, promptness of medical attention to incoming patients, or physician satisfaction with the EU as a place to work. But, unlike collaboration, it correlates strongly with the quality of both medical and nursing care, with RN satisfaction with the EU, and with the reputation of the parent hospital in the community. In addition, it correlates positively and significantly, though less highly, with patient satisfaction—both with the care received at the different EUs and with the staff providing that care.

Further, as measured by the same index, adaptation correlates highly with the secondary criterion measures of EU responsiveness to community expectations and needs and EU reputation. But these particular relationships are in part artificial and inflated because of overlap between components of this index (see description earlier in this chapter) and components of these particular criterion measures (see Chapter Eight). Since adaptation concerns the nature of organization-environment relations and external affairs of the system, however, it would not be inappropriate for researchers to use EU responsiveness and reputation as indicators of organizational adaptation (similar to institutional collaboration) instead of treating them as secondary criteria of effectiveness. Nor would it be inappropriate, depending upon one's research model and objectives, to view adaptation to the environment as a criterion of organizational effectiveness instead of treating it as a major organizational problem area.

For present purposes, at any rate, the three correlation coefficients in Table 10-8 that are affected by the overlap in question could even be disregarded without altering the basic pattern of relationships found between adaptation and most of the primary and secondary criteria of EU effectiveness. The data show that, regardless of the specific indicator of adaptation that might be used, the relative adequacy of organizational problem solving in this area is positively and significantly related to the clinical efficiency of hospital EUs as well as some of the secondary criteria of effectiveness that have been examined (see Tables 10-7, 10-8, and 8-2).

Apparently, adaptation does not affect the economic efficiency of hospital EUs, according to the available measures, with one possible exception that involves one of the secondary criterion measures. The specific exception consists of a direct and significant relationship between economic efficiency and EU responsiveness to the community's changing needs for emergency medical services ($r = .39$, $p < .05$), which was reported in Chapter Eight—specifically, Table 8-2.

Overall, the results of this research support the hypothesis that the better their adaptation to the external environment, the higher the effectiveness of hospital EUs, and vice versa. These findings concerning the relationship of organizational adaptation to EU effectiveness, moreover, are in sharp contrast to the general absence of direct relationships between the structural characteristics of the communities being served and the effectiveness of hospital EUs, discussed earlier in Chapter Nine. It therefore appears that successful organizational problem solving on the part of the system concerning external affairs problems is much more important to EU effectiveness than are various major characteristics of the relevant external environment.

Summary of Results on Problem Solving and Effectiveness

Clearly, for every major problem area (including that of strain) and by most measures, the hypothesis of a direct relationship between the adequacy of organizational problem solving and the clinical efficiency of hospital EUs is well supported by the data (see Table 10-7). Moreover, in most cases this holds true for both components of clinical efficiency, that is, for the quality of both medical and nursing care. In fact, all but one (MD integration) of the ten basic indicators of successful organizational problem solving included in Table 10-7 were found to correlate positively and significantly with the quality of nursing care provided at the various EUs, the specific correlations ranging from a low of .28 to a high of .61 and averaging .43. And, similarly, all but two of the nine indicators showing a significant relationship to the quality of nursing care are also related to the quality of medical care. The correlations concerning the latter average .41; and, if the single negative but not significant correlation of –.16 is excluded from the series, they range from .15 to .69. The measures in the area of organizational resources show stronger relationships to the quality of medical care than to the quality of nursing care, the reverse being the case for the measures in the areas of coordination, integration, and adaptation (Table 10-7). Lastly, the findings concerning the relationship of organizational strain to clinical efficiency discussed earlier (see Table 10-2) also support the hypothesis under study, strain being dysfunctional to clinical efficiency.

The results are equally clear, however, that the adequacy of organizational problem solving in the areas investigated is not directly related to the economic efficiency of hospital EUs (see Tables 10-7 and 10-2). Of all the specific indicators examined, only one integration measure turns out to be significantly related to this criterion of effectiveness: the identification of registered nurses with the EU correlates positively with economic efficiency ($r = .34$, $p < .05$). Either the aspects of organizational problem solving studied or the behavior and activities of the clinical staff are not directly linked to the financial and economic performance of hospital EUs. Given the role structure and authority arrangements of the system, the large majority of the staff at most EUs were probably neither responsible for nor concerned with the organization's economic matters. Related data from the study on the goal priorities of hospital EUs (see chap. 3 in Georgopoulos, Cooke, and Associates, 1980) provide support for this interpretation by showing that, on the average, "Keeping the costs of emergency service down" was not regarded as a high priority by either the physicians (MDs) or the registered nurses (RNs) working at the various EUs at the time of data collection. Since the time of data collection, of course, the situation may have changed in this respect.

On the other hand, as shown in Chapter Nine, the economic efficiency of hospital EUs is directly related to certain aspects of organizational structure. It is probably also affected by broader market conditions. In terms of the present research objectives, however, the main conclusion from the findings is that the economic efficiency of these health service systems depends upon their organizational structure but probably not their internal organizational problem solving, whereas their clinical efficiency depends upon both organizational structure and problem solving. For the most part, interinstitutional differences in economic and clinical efficiency alike are significantly affected by organizational structure differences, while only the differences in clinical efficiency apparently are affected by organizational problem solving.

Concerning the five secondary criteria of EU effectiveness—promptness of medical attention, staff satisfaction, patient satisfaction, responsiveness to community expectations and needs, and institutional reputation—the results again show varying degrees of support for the hypothesis that the effectiveness of the system is directly related to the adequacy of internal organizational problem solving.

In the area of organizational strain (see Table 10-3), this hypothesis is best supported with reference to staff satisfaction, or the social efficiency of EUs, and especially RN satisfaction, and it is least supported with reference to patient satisfaction. Especially dysfunctional in relation to the several secondary criteria viewed as a set is the level of prevailing tension between EU staff and hospital administration.

In the area of organizational resources (see Table 10-8), the hypothesis is supported to some extent with reference to every criterion except staff satisfaction, but mainly according to one of the two indicators of problem solving.

The hypothesis receives the strongest support in the area of nonprogrammed coordination, being supported in relation to every criterion and all nine criterion measures used except one— that of EU reputation (see Table 10-8). Programmed coordination, on the other hand, is significantly related to only three of the same criterion measures: physician satisfaction, responsiveness to the community's expectations, and parent hospital reputation.

Overall, the hypothesis is least supported in the area of organizational integration. Of the three measures in this area, normative integration (level of reciprocal understanding between nurses and physicians) correlates positively with the promptness of medical attention to incoming patients and with the satisfaction of registered nurses; in addition, the latter variable is significantly related to member integration, but only in the case of RNs.

Lastly, in the area of adaptation, the hypothesis is supported with reference to most criteria and criterion measures when the EU adaptation index is used as the indicator of adaptation, but only with reference to the criterion of responsiveness to community expectations and needs when the narrower index of institutional collaboration is used.

Considering finally the relationships of each particular criterion of effectiveness to the specific measures of organizational problem solving, the results show that the quality of medical care relates especially well to the responsiveness of other hospital departments in meeting EU requests for services or assistance, the adequacy of nonprogrammed coordination within the EU, adaptation to the environment as measured by the EU adaptation index, the fulfillment of physician requests by other hospital units, and (inversely) the level of prevailing tension among the doctors working in the EU. The quality of nursing care (which correlates .61 with the quality of medical care) is especially well related to adaptation (EU adaptation index), the adequacy of nonprogrammed coordination, the level of mutual adjustment between doctors and nurses, and the level of prevailing tension between EU staff and hospital administration. The economic efficiency criterion correlates significantly with only one of the member integration measures, the identification of RNs with the system.

Of the secondary criteria of effectiveness, promptness of medical attention to incoming patients relates best to the level of mutual adjustment between doctors and nurses and (inversely) to the level of prevailing tension between MDs and RNs. Physician satisfaction correlates best (negatively) with the level of prevailing tension among the doctors working in the EU, and nursing staff satisfaction has the strongest negative correlation with the level of prevailing tension between EU staff and hospital administration. Patient satisfaction with the care received correlates best with the EU adaptation index, while patient satisfaction with the staff correlates best with nonprogrammed coordination. Responsiveness to community expectations correlates especially well with nonprogrammed coordination and the level of tension between the EU and hospital administration, and responsiveness to the community's changing needs for emergency services correlates best with nonprogrammed coordination (both of these criterion variables correlate most highly with the EU adaptation index, whose components include responsiveness). Finally, parent hospital reputation is best related to organizational adaptation (the EU adaptation index), and EU reputation correlates best with the same index (but one of the components of this index includes a measure of EU reputation) and the level of prevailing tension between the EU and hospital administration.

Relative Importance and Joint Contribution of Selected Problem-Solving Variables

The overall conclusion from the research findings just summarized is that successful organizational problem solving in every one of the above areas facilitates the effectiveness of hospital EUs to a significant degree, particularly the quality of patient care and the secondary criteria of effectiveness. The contribution of problem solving in the different areas to EU effectiveness varies, of course, from one criterion of effectiveness to another. Further, to some extent the level of contribution associated with each area also varies depending upon the particular indicator of problem solving (that is, the specific independent variable) considered. The relative importance and joint contribution of six indicators (selected from the ten available indicators discussed in this chapter to represent the areas studied) to each criterion of effectiveness are summarized in Table 10-9. Organizational coordination, having emerged as the dominant area in relation to EU effectiveness, is represented by two indicators, and all the other problem areas—organizational resources, strain, integration, and adaptation—are represented by one indicator each.

Included in this set of selected indicators are the following: responsiveness of other departments in meeting EU requests for services or assistance, tension among EU doctors, programmed coordination, nonprogrammed coordination, normative integration, and collaboration with other institutions on emergency services matters. The average intercorrelation among these six indicators of the adequacy of organizational problem solving at the EU level is statistically significant ($p < .05$) but of modest size (average $r = .35$, and median $r = .33$), and the fifteen product-moment correlations generated in this series range from $-.24$ to $.54$ (all of the negative coefficients involve the tension indicator, as expected). As a set, therefore, these independent or predictor variables (in relation to effectiveness) present no significant multicollinearity problem.

The zero-order correlations between each of the selected independent variables and each of the primary and secondary criteria of EU effectiveness (shown in parentheses in Table 10-9) have already been discussed. Table 10-9 summarizes the results of partial least squares analyses, which show the correlation of each predictor variable to each criterion measure, partialling out the contribution of all other predictors in the set. Based upon the partial correlations associated with the six predictors, therefore, it

Table 10-9. Relative Importance of Selected Organizational Problem-Solving Variables as Predictors of Interinstitutional Differences in Emergency Unit Effectiveness.

| | Correlations Between Each Predictor and Criterion Measure Partialling Out All Other Predictors[a] | | | | | | | |
| | PREDICTOR VARIABLES | | | | | | | |
EU Effectiveness	Responsiveness of Other Departments	Tension Among EU Doctors	Programmed Coordination	Nonprogrammed Coordination	Normative Integration	Collaboration with Other Institutions	Explained Variance[b] R^2	p^c
Primary Criteria								
Economic efficiency	-.10 (-.07)	-.25 (.21)	.05 (.02)	-.22 (-.12)	.19 (.12)	.06 (.06)	.12	.84
Clinical efficiency								
Quality of nursing care	.14 (.37*)	-.22 (-.37*)	.03 (.41*)	.42 (.58**)	-.01 (.36*)	.25 (.42*)	.45	.02
Quality of medical care	.66 (.69**)	-.41 (-.44**)	-.05 (.30*)	.33 (.50**)	-.07 (.30*)	.00 (.28)	.64	.00
Secondary Criteria								
Promptness of medical attention to patients	.24 (.40*)	-.19 (-.30*)	.20 (.21)	.39 (.52**)	.17 (.38*)	.04 (.22)	.38	.06
Staff satisfaction with EU								
MDs	-.05 (.10)	-.40 (-.49**)	.20 (.39*)	.13 (.33*)	.02 (.26)	-.08 (.12)	.32	.15
RNs	-.12 (.08)	-.03 (-.15)	-.07 (.22)	.26 (.37*)	.18 (.33*)	.15 (.25)	.19	.49
Patient satisfaction with								
Care received	.35 (.33*)	.27 (.13)	.06 (.06)	.47 (.35*)	-.46 (-.17)	.05 (.10)	.40	.07
EU staff	.05 (.17)	-.02 (-.13)	.06 (.18)	.57 (.50**)	-.30 (-.10)	.14 (.17)	.42	.07
EU responsiveness to community								
Expectations	.00 (.24)	-.05 (-.21)	-.01 (.31*)	.41 (.52**)	-.03 (.28)	.24 (.36*)	.33	.13
Needs	.14 (.32*)	.11 (-.03)	-.12 (.18)	.32 (.40*)	.01 (.24)	.31 (.39*)	.28	.22
Reputation of								
EU	.09 (.13)	.27 (.15)	.16 (.17)	.25 (.25)	-.15 (.03)	-.03 (.07)	.16	.64
Parent hospital	.42 (.40*)	-.20 (-.31*)	.43 (.41*)	.13 (.31*)	-.36 (.04)	-.22 (.07)	.42	.06

Notes:

*p < .05.

**p < .01.

For underlined partial correlations, $p < .05$. Zero-order correlations are shown in parentheses.

The number of emergency units in the analyses varies between 26 and 30 EUs.

[a] Correlations were obtained from partial least squares analyses: a separate PLS analysis was performed for each criterion measure, using the same six problem-solving variables as the predictors or independent variables.

[b] This column shows the proportion of the total variance on each criterion measure explained by the six predictor variables as a set.

[c] These are two-tailed p values, obtained from corresponding regression analyses in which the predictor variables were entered in the order shown here.

is possible to estimate the relative contribution of the different variables to any given criterion and also identify the one or two most important predictors among them.

In the case of economic efficiency, of course, none of the selected problem-solving variables produced a significant zero-order correlation. Accordingly, the partial correlations in Table 10-9 simply affirm the absence of a relationship with this criterion (the highest partial correlation obtained in this case, $r = -.25$, involves the tension variable). In the case of the quality of nursing care, the best predictor variable is nonprogrammed coordination (partial $r = .42$); in the case of the quality of medical care, the responsiveness of other departments is the single most important predictor (partial $r = .66$), followed by the level of tension among EU doctors (partial $r = -.41$). The results from the partial least squares analyses also show that the six problem-solving variables specified together explain 12 percent of the variance in economic efficiency (not statistically significant),* 45 percent of the variance in the quality of nursing care, and 64 percent of the variance in the quality of medical care among hospital EUs. Corresponding regression analyses, incidentally, yield identical results regarding the proportion of explained variance on each criterion measure.

Clearly, as was hypothesized, the adequacy of organizational problem solving in the areas studied accounts for a very substantial portion of interinstitutional variability in both components of clinical efficiency. With reference to economic efficiency, however, the data do not support the hypothesis. The five selected organizational structure variables discussed in Chapter Nine, on the other hand, were shown to account for 47 percent of the variance in economic efficiency. They were also found to account for 66 percent of the variance in the quality of nursing care but only 41 percent of the variance in the quality of medical care. Organizational structure differences, therefore, are more important to economic efficiency than are differences in the adequacy of organizational

---

*It should be noted, however, that the only problem-solving indicator found to correlate positively and significantly with economic efficiency—the integration of RNs into the EU—is not included among these six predictor variables.

problem solving. It is also obvious from the findings that organizational structure accounts for more of the variance in the quality of nursing than the quality of medical care, the reverse being true of organizational problem solving. Apparently, structure affects the performance of nurses more than it does the performance of physicians (nurses typically are employees of the institution, and physicians are not), while problem solving affects medical performance more than it does nursing performance. Although both are very important to explaining differences in both components of clinical efficiency, structure and problem solving have differential (and in a sense complementary) effects on medical and nursing performance.

Explained Variability in the Secondary Criteria. The results summarized in Table 10-9 also show the individual and combined contribution of the selected problem-solving indicators to each secondary criterion of effectiveness. Briefly, these six independent variables as a set have no appreciable effect on three of the nine secondary criterion measures: the satisfaction of RNs with their respective EUs, the reputation of EUs, and EU responsiveness to the community's changing needs. They also appear to have only a small effect on physician satisfaction and EU responsiveness to community expectations regarding emergency services. (Concerning the responsiveness criterion, it should be remembered that the EU adaptation index is not included among the six predictors in the present analysis.) The same variables, however, account for a significant proportion of the variance in promptness of medical attention to patients (38 percent of the variance), patient satisfaction with the care received (40 percent) and with the EU staff (42 percent), and parent hospital reputation (42 percent).*

The single most important predictor among the six problem-solving variables in relation to the promptness criterion is nonprogrammed coordination. This particular variable also

---

*With reference to these findings, incidentally, it should be noted that the *p* values shown in Table 10-9 are two-tailed, although only one-tailed tests are required to test the hypothesis of a significant relationship between the adequacy of organizational problem solving and EU effectiveness.

turns out to be the best predictor of patient satisfaction with the care received, patient satisfaction with the EU staff, and EU responsiveness to community expectations. For physician satisfaction with the EU, the most important predictor is the level of tension among the doctors. And for parent hospital reputation, the best predictor is programmed coordination, followed very closely by the responsiveness of other departments in meeting EU requests.

Joint Effects of Organizational Structure and Problem Solving on Effectiveness

It is clear from these findings that the observed interinstitutional differences in the effectiveness of hospital EUs may be accounted for to a great extent by differences in the adequacy of internal organizational problem solving in the areas specified. A similar conclusion was reached in Chapter Nine about organizational structure differences and EU effectiveness. Further, the combined effects of a selected set of five structural variables (parent hospital size, patient volume, breadth/scope of emergency service, medical teaching affiliation, and emergency personnel training programs) on the different criteria of effectiveness were estimated, as were the combined effects of the six organizational problem-solving variables discussed in the previous section. In both cases, the effects in question were found to be considerable.

The final series of analyses performed in this study regarding the hypothesized relationship between EU organization and EU effectiveness provide similar estimates of the joint effects of organizational structure and problem solving on effectiveness. These are regression analyses using as independent/predictor variables a set of three structural and three problem-solving variables. The former include parent hospital size, medical teaching affiliation, and emergency personnel training programs; and the latter include the responsiveness of other departments in meeting EU requests for services or assistance, the level of prevailing tension among doctors in the EU, and nonprogrammed coordination. Each of these variables, it will be recognized, was shown not only to be significantly related to more than one criterion of institutional effectiveness but also to be "best predictor" within its respective set of structural or problem-solving variables in relation to at least one criterion measure. It should be also pointed out that, on the average, these particular variables do not correlate significantly with one another to pose a multicollinearity problem.*

Using the six independent variables just specified as predictors, standard multiple regression analyses (least squares regression) were performed for each criterion measure representing the primary and secondary criteria of effectiveness. These analyses were performed primarily to ascertain the magnitude and statistical significance of the joint effects, or contribution, of these particular independent variables. Secondarily, they were performed with the expectation that the proportion of variance on each criterion measure explained by this set of six structural and problem-solving variables will in most cases exceed the proportion earlier explained by either of the above-mentioned sets of structural or problem-solving variables alone—that is, the sets of five structural variables and six problem-solving variables earlier examined (see Table 9-5 for the former and Table 10-9 for the latter). The obtained regression results are summarized in Table 10-10.

Considering first the primary criteria of EU effectiveness, the joint effects of the selected organizational structure and problem-solving variables are most impressive in the case of the quality of nursing care. Together, the six variables specified account for three-fourths of the observed interinstitutional differences in nursing care quality. This exceeds the proportion of the variance explained earlier by either the five structural variables (.66) or the six problem-solving variables (.45) in the analysis. The joint effects of structure and problem solving on the quality of medical care are nearly as impressive. At least two-thirds of the observed variance in

---

*The average intercorrelation among the six variables is only .24 ($p > .05$), and the median correlation is .19 ($p > .05$). In fact, of the fifteen correlation coefficients in the series, which range from -.33 to .50, only three are statistically significant ($p < .05$). These involve the relationships between hospital size and medical teaching affiliation ($r = .50$), training programs and nonprogrammed coordination ($r = .35$), and tension among EU doctors and nonprogrammed coordination ($r = -.33$).

Table 10-10. Combined Effects of Selected Organizational Structure and Problem-Solving Variables on the Effectiveness of Hospital Emergency Units (EUs).

| EU Effectiveness | Multiple Regression Analysis Results Showing Combined Effect of Six Independent Variables[a] | | | |
| | Proportion of Explained Variance R^2 | Statistical Significance | | |
		F	df	p[b]
Primary Criteria				
Economic efficiency	.32	1.43	6, 19	.25
Clinical efficiency				
Quality of nursing care	.75	11.31	6, 23	.00
Quality of medical care	.69	8.48	6, 23	.00
Secondary Criteria				
Promptness of medical attention to patients	.52	4.17	6, 23	.01
Staff satisfaction with EU				
Physicians	.52	4.14	6, 23	.01
Registered nurses	.34	1.95	6, 23	.12
Patient satisfaction with				
Care received	.34	1.78	6, 21	.15
EU staff	.34	1.76	6, 21	.16
EU responsiveness to community				
Expectations	.62	6.16	6, 23	.00
Needs	.26	1.35	6, 23	.28
Reputation of				
EU	.50	3.87	6, 23	.01
Parent hospital	.39	2.10	6, 20	.10

Notes:

[a]Included in the selected set of independent variables are three organizational structure and three organizational problem-solving variables. The former include parent hospital size, medical teaching affiliation, and emergency personnel training programs (see Chapter Nine); and the latter include responsiveness of other departments in meeting EU requests for services or assistance, tension among EU doctors, and adequacy of nonprogrammed coordination of work efforts within the EU. The six variables were entered in the regressions in the following order: hospital size, responsiveness of departments, coordination, tension, teaching affiliation, and training programs.

[b]The values shown in the p column are two-tailed values.

the quality of medical care across hospital EUs (specifically, .69 of
the variance) can also be accounted for by the selected structure
and problem-solving variables jointly—a proportion that is again
higher than that explained earlier by either the problem-solving
(.64) or the structural variables (.41) alone.

In short, the hypothesis that organizational structure and
problem solving significantly affect the clinical efficiency of
hospital EUs is strongly supported by the findings, and supported
most strongly when structure and problem solving are considered
jointly. The results concerning economic efficiency show a
different pattern. Specifically, the combined effects of structure and
problem solving on this criterion are not stronger than the effects
of structure alone: Whereas five structural variables were shown to
account for .47 of the observed interinstitutional differences in the
economic efficiency of hospital EUs (see Chapter Nine), the three
structural and three problem-solving variables in Table 10-10
together account for .32 of the variance, and the problem-solving
variables alone are not significantly related to economic efficiency.
With regard to economic efficiency, therefore, only the hypothesis
that organizational structure differences affect institutional
effectiveness is supported by the data.

Other results, associated with but not included among those
presented in Table 10-10, show that the specific variables (from
among the six structural and problem-solving variables in the set)
contributing significantly to the explained variance on each
criterion individually are as follows: for economic efficiency,
emergency personnel training programs (partial $r = .48$, $p = .03$);
for the quality of nursing care, medical teaching affiliation (partial
$r = .61$, $p = .00$), training programs (partial $r = .48$, $p = .02$), and
nonprogrammed coordination (partial $r = .38$, $p = .07$); and for the
quality of medical care, responsiveness by other hospital departments (partial $r = .67$, $p = .00$) and tension among EU doctors
(partial $r = -.39$, $p = .05$).

Combined Effects on the Secondary Criteria of EU Effectiveness

Turning to the secondary criteria of effectiveness, the results
in Table 10-10 also generally provide support for the relationship

between the organization and effectiveness of hospital EUs. First, the proportion of the variance on each criterion measure that can be jointly explained by the six structural and problem-solving variables specified ranges from .26 (for EU responsiveness to the community's changing needs) to .62 (for EU responsiveness to community expectations) and averages .43 for the nine criterion measures involved. Moreover, the variance accounted for is not statistically significant (at least at the .10 level one-tailed) for only one of these measures—EU responsiveness to the community's changing needs (the same and only measure for which, earlier, neither the structural nor the problem-solving variables as a group proved important).

Second, for five of these secondary criterion measures— promptness of medical attention, physician satisfaction, RN satisfaction, EU responsiveness to community expectations, and EU reputation in the community—the proportion of explained variance exceeds that explained earlier by either the structural or the problem-solving variables alone. Further, in the case of four of these same measures (RN satisfaction constituting the exception), the structural and problem-solving variables in question together explain half or more of the observed variance across EUs. Concerning the remaining criterion measures, the problem-solving variables account for a greater proportion of the variance on patient satisfaction with the care received than do the structural variables as a group, and the structural variables account for a somewhat greater proportion of the variance on patient satisfaction with the EU staff and parent hospital reputation. Moreover, in these particular cases, the amount of variance accounted for by structure or by problem solving alone, correspondingly, is not smaller than that accounted for by the combined set of the selected structural and problem-solving variables.

Finally, with reference to the same five measures of the secondary criteria of effectiveness for which the variance explained by this combined set of independent variables exceeds that explained by either structural or problem-solving variables alone, it is also possible (based on obtained regression results, not shown in Table 10-10) to identify the particular independent variables in the set which were found to contribute significantly to the explained variance individually. Regarding the promptness of medical attention to incoming patients, for example, the most important independent variables in the combined set are nonprogrammed coordination (partial $r = .56$, $p = .00$), medical teaching affiliation (partial $r = .50$, $p = .01$), and parent hospital size (partial $r = .39$, $p = .06$). For physician satisfaction with the EU, the corresponding variables include tension among EU doctors (partial $r = -.49$, $p = .01$) and hospital size (partial $r = .47$, $p = .02$). For RN satisfaction, only one independent variable shows a statistically significant contribution individually—emergency personnel training programs (partial $r = .47$, $p = .02$). Regarding EU responsiveness to community expectations, the most important independent variables are medical teaching affiliation (partial $r = .56$, $p = .00$) and emergency personnel training programs (partial $r = .49$, $p = .01$). Lastly, concerning EU reputation, the significant independent variables include medical teaching affiliation (partial $r = .52$, $p = .01$), emergency personnel training programs ($r = .44$, $p = .03$), and tension among EU doctors (partial $r = -.39$, $p = .05$).

In conclusion, with the few exceptions noted, the joint effects of organizational structure and problem solving on the effectiveness of hospital EUs, reflected only partially in the combined set of the six independent variables included in the regression analyses summarized in Table 10-10, are generally both statistically significant and large. Once again, therefore, the hypothesis that the effectiveness of hospital EUs depends on the organization of these health service systems, and specifically on differences in organizational structure and internal problem solving, is amply confirmed by the empirical evidence.

Summary

Discussed in this chapter were the results of the study concerning the relationship of internal organizational problem solving to the effectiveness of hospital EUs. Briefly, it was shown that the clinical performance or efficiency of these health service systems is directly related to the relative success of the system in providing solutions to the problems that it encounters in the areas of organizational resources, coordination, integration, strain, and adaptation to the environment. Successful problem solving relates positively to the quality of both medical and nursing care. The economic efficiency of these organizations, on the other hand, which previously was found to be affected by organizational structure differences (Chapter Nine), is not directly dependent on the adequacy of problem solving in these areas. Relationships similar to those concerning clinical efficiency were also found between organizational problem solving and the secondary criteria of institutional effectiveness (promptness of medical attention, patient satisfaction, staff satisfaction, responsiveness to community expectations and needs regarding emergency care services, and institutional reputation), the strength of relationship depending upon the specific criterion measure and problem-solving variable considered.

Of the problem areas, organizational coordination emerged most salient overall in relation to the secondary criteria of EU effectiveness, as well as in relation to the quality of patient care. The adequacy of nonprogrammed coordination, in particular, proved to be especially important. Similarly, in the area of resources, the response of other hospital departments in meeting EU requests for services or assistance was found to be very important to the quality of medical care. The hypothesis of a direct positive relationship between organizational problem solving and institutional effectiveness was least well supported in the area of integration. On the whole, except with reference to economic efficiency, this hypothesis received strong support from the data.

In part, the findings also show that interinstitutional differences in problem solving are, in varying degrees, related to differences in organizational structure. These relationships, however, do not involve all measures of problem solving, and each aspect of structure is associated with some but not all aspects of problem solving. Jointly, differences in organizational structure and problem solving were found to account for more than half of the variance in the quality of medical and nursing care provided by hospital EUs, and also in promptness of medical attention, physician satisfaction, and responsiveness to community expectations. In addition, differences in organizational structure, but not problem solving, were found to account for nearly half of the variance in the economic efficiency of EUs. On the other hand, differences in organizational problem solving were shown to affect the quality of medical care more than do differences in organizational structure. Together, however, organizational structure and problem solving have greater effects on the quality of both medical and nursing care, and on some of the secondary criteria of effectiveness as well, than either of them has alone.

Chapter Eleven

Conclusions and Implications

The basic question addressed by the research discussed in this book concerns the relationship between the organization and effectiveness of hospital emergency services. Specifically, which organizational factors, both structural and social-psychological, facilitate or hinder the effectiveness of these important health care delivery systems, and how significant are these factors in explaining interinstitutional differences in effectiveness? This question was approached using an open-system theory perspective and a methodology relying on a comparative organizational research design. The results are based on data obtained from a probability sample of thirty hospitals and nearly 1,500 individuals associated with them, including physicians and nurses responsible for the emergency service; physicians and administrators from the parent hospital; patients; and selected respondents from the community.

Conceptually and theoretically, hospital emergency units (EUs) were viewed as complex work-performing and problem-solving systems that function within a complex organizational environment. Their effectiveness was considered to be a joint (but not equally weighted) outcome of the economic, clinical, and social performance, or efficiency, of the system—three kinds of efficiency that correspond to three distinct and only partially congruent kinds of organizational rationality. Interhospital differences in effectiveness were expected and found to be determined, to an important extent, by differences in organization. Two major aspects of organization were considered particularly significant in this connection: (1) the basic structure of the system and (2) the system's response to problems of resource acquisition and allocation, coordination of work efforts, internal strain, integration, and adaptation to the environment. Both proved to be extremely important to an explanation of differences in the effectiveness of hospital EUs.

Two principal sets of empirical findings were discussed in the book: one concerning the concept, criteria, and measurement of EU effectiveness, and the other concerning the organization of hospital EUs and its relationship to effectiveness. Some of the findings are methodological, though most are substantive or mainly substantive. In their entirety, the results clearly demonstrate the great potential of comparative organizational methodology for the study of complex systems such as the hospital EU, the theoretical utility and analytical power of the conceptual-theoretical model employed in the research, and the value and promise of the approaches used to assess institutional effectiveness, as well as the importance of organizational structure and problem solving to effectiveness.

One major conclusion from the research is that the economic, clinical, and social efficiency of hospital EUs can be assessed validly and reliably, and with a great deal of precision, using the methodology discussed in this book. Corresponding interinstitutional differences can be ascertained rigorously and quantitatively (not only for the participating institutions but for any sample or population of hospital EUs, including the EUs of multihospital systems and for-profit hospitals). In this respect, the results generally show very substantial, and often great, differences in EU performance across hospitals, regardless of the particular criterion, or even measure, of effectiveness examined. More specifically, the variability found to characterize EUs in the economic efficiency area is great, and so is the variability in the clinical efficiency area, which includes the quality of medical and nursing care separately assessed. This means that some EUs clearly are doing a very good job, while others function at a low level of effectiveness.

Clinical efficiency was assessed at the institutional level using several independent sources of data and measurement techniques, including the quasitracer patient conditions approach and the patient visit staging approach that were developed for this purpose. The results that they yielded justify a great deal of confidence in these new approaches, both of which appear to be promising tools (on financial as well as technical grounds) for evaluating the quality of care that patients on the aggregate receive at different institutions. Economic efficiency was assessed using financial, personnel, and patient visit data.

The Nature of Institutional Effectiveness

Generally, the results show considerable variability across institutions, not only with respect to clinical and economic efficiency but also with respect to the secondary criteria of effectiveness that were used to supplement, and in part also validate, these major criteria. The secondary criteria include patient satisfaction, staff satisfaction or social efficiency, promptness of medical attention to incoming patients (the reverse of patient waiting time), responsiveness to community expectations and needs regarding the provision of emergency medical care, and institutional reputation (for both the EU and its parent hospital) in the community.

The specific measures used to represent the various criteria of effectiveness are positively interrelated in the large majority of cases, but not always significantly. The relevant intercorrelations range greatly in size, and some of them are very close to zero or even negative. None of the negative correlations, however, is statistically significant. Accordingly, even though the different measures of effectiveness do not turn out to be mutually reinforcing in all cases, or even in the large majority of cases, they are never conflicting in a statistically significant way. This is a finding of considerable practical importance because it suggests that rational organizational actions aimed at improving some major criterion of effectiveness or increasing the overall effectiveness of the system are not inherently precluded by the nature of institutional effectiveness and in principle could produce positive results, at least up to a point, without the risk of contradictory criterion outcomes or trade-offs.

Concerning the clinical and economic efficiency of the system, the results are generally but not always as anticipated.

First, as expected, the quality of medical care provided to patients at the various EUs is positively and significantly related to the quality of nursing care given to the same patients, and vice versa. The relationship is far from perfect, however, since only about 37 percent of the variability in the quality of medical care can be accounted for by differences in the quality of nursing care, and vice versa. Consequently, it is not surprising to find that not all of the factors which facilitate one of these major components of clinical efficiency also facilitate the other (although in most cases they do), or facilitate the other to a similar degree. Thus, for example, while EU patient volume correlates positively and significantly with the quality of nursing care (and with economic efficiency), it shows no relationship to the quality of medical care. Nevertheless, certain aspects of organizational structure and problem solving did turn out to correlate positively with the quality of both medical and nursing care as hypothesized.

Equally important, the findings show that neither the quality of medical nor the quality of nursing care correlates significantly with the economic efficiency of hospital EUs, even after controlling statistically for such major variables as EU patient volume (number of patient visits), parent hospital size, or community complexity. For the organizations studied, in short, there is no relationship, either positive or negative, between the costs and quality of service; a small but significant relationship had been expected. Hospital EUs which provide high-quality patient care, nursing or medical, may show any level of economic efficiency—high, moderate, or low—and vice versa.

Consequently, the criteria of clinical and economic efficiency cannot be combined into a single and convenient index of overall effectiveness. On the other hand, both criteria correlate positively with the social efficiency of the system. Even more significantly, many important aspects of organizational structure and problem solving turn out to correlate positively and significantly with both economic and clinical efficiency, the principal components of EU effectiveness. Accordingly, to some extent it would probably be feasible for many EUs to improve both of these major criteria simultaneously.

It should also be pointed out that, although clinical and economic performance generally are not significantly related, some of the EUs in the sample did score better than average (than the median) on both economic efficiency and the quality of medical care. This shows that some EUs in fact are successful in providing care of relatively "high" quality (higher than median quality) at relatively "low," and possibly reasonable, cost (better than median economic efficiency). Obviously, then, it should be possible for particular EUs to achieve at least moderately high levels of both clinical and economic efficiency. Furthermore, for most institutions there is probably considerable room for improvement in this connection—that is, for genuine improvement through better organization or better performance and not merely contrived "improvement" through artificial manipulations of costs by such mechanisms as the filtering of patient inputs to keep costly cases out.

On the other hand, beyond some upper limit, an EU would probably be unable to keep raising the quality of care while lowering the cost, or even holding cost constant, as it would be unable to control costs without affecting the quality of care adversely. Similarly, in the short run, an EU might be unable to improve both its clinical and economic efficiency simultaneously or to the same degree. In some institutions sequential improvement may be more feasible, or trade-offs among the interests and goals of relevant constituencies may be necessary.

Improving both criteria of effectiveness will probably require that practitioners in the field learn to consider the two criteria in conjunction with one another. Thus, those primarily concerned with quality should also learn to take costs into account, seriously and systematically, while those concerned primarily with costs should learn to take quality into account. Increased cost-consciousness on the part of the medical and nursing staff together with increased concern for the quality of service on the part of administrative and managerial personnel might well contribute not only to improved effectiveness but also to the eventual emergence of a significant positive relationship between the economic and clinical efficiency of hospital EUs—a relationship not existing at the time of the study.

Factors Contributing to Institutional Effectiveness

Overall, the research showed that differences in the organization of hospital EUs strongly affect the effectiveness of these health care delivery systems. Both independently and jointly, organizational structure and problem solving explain a substantial proportion of the variance in effectiveness across institutions. (Additionally, certain aspects of organizational structure also appear to affect the adequacy of problem solving in the system.) As might be expected, however, the amount of explained variance differs from one criterion to another and depends upon the particular predictor variables examined, but overall it turns out to be higher for clinical than for economic efficiency. Some of the independent variables, however, are significantly related to both of these criteria of institutional effectiveness.

Generally, organizational structure variables are better predictors of economic efficiency than is adequacy of internal organizational problem solving. This suggests that the economic efficiency of hospital EUs is affected more strongly by the structure of the system than by problem solving. In addition, organizational structure is more important to explaining differences in the quality of nursing care than in the quality of medical care, while the reverse is true for organizational problem solving. Many of the structural variables, however, would probably be more difficult for the system to alter than the problem-solving variables, at least in the short run.

It is also important, both pragmatically and theoretically, to point out that the separate, or independent, effects of structure and problem solving on the quality of patient care, though significant, are smaller than the joint contributions of structure and problem solving. Thus, the amount of explained variance in the quality of both medical and nursing care increases substantially (to 69 percent of the variance in medical and 75 percent of the variance in nursing care) when the combined effects of structure and problem solving are considered, and specifically when using the following variables as predictors: emergency personnel training programs, medical teaching affiliation, parent hospital size, the responsiveness of other hospital departments in meeting EU requests for services or assistance, tension among EU doctors, and the adequacy of nonprogrammed coordination within the EU.

Aspects of Organization Facilitating Both Economic and Clinical Efficiency

One of the most important findings of the research is that the economic and clinical efficiency of hospital EUs are both higher for those institutions which have emergency personnel training programs than for those which do not. Moreover, regression analyses show that the effects of such programs on effectiveness are strong. In addition to promoting the quality of medical and nursing care (especially the latter), training programs are associated with higher economic efficiency levels at the institutions studied. Apparently, not only do they constitute a sound economic investment, and pay for themselves, they also constitute a potentially important as well as feasible organizational mechanism for increasing the effectiveness of hospital EUs. Institutions now lacking such programs should consider introducing them, and those having them might consider strengthening them and/or expanding them to include personnel (for example, EMTs, nurses, doctors) not now participating in the programs.

From a practical standpoint, there are at least three basic reasons for the importance of emergency personnel programs to effectiveness. First, such programs can impart useful knowledge to the participants that would increase their technical and/or organizational skills. Second, they can enhance the level of understanding that participants have about their own jobs and contributions to the organization. And, third, they can improve the appreciation that participants have of their interdependence and of each other's work problems and needs, thus making it easier for all concerned to coordinate their activities and cooperate.

The medical staffing pattern of hospital EUs provides another potential mechanism for increasing the effectiveness of these institutions. This research shows that economic efficiency and the quality of both medical and nursing care are all highest, on the average, for those EUs which rely on a hospital-based group on contract as their medical staffing pattern. All other staffing patterns show mixed performance. Non-hospital-based group arrangements, for example, are associated with higher clinical but lower economic efficiency than are rotating staff arrangements. The hospital-based group pattern, which in principle should be feasible for a great many EUs, ranks higher than either of these two patterns on both criteria. It appears that EUs relying on hospital-based groups enjoy the clinical and economic benefits of group practice along with the organizational benefits of a direct medical staff linkage to the parent hospitals. Because the sample of EUs with each staffing pattern is rather small, however, additional data will be required to establish the superiority of the hospital-based group pattern more definitively.

Medical teaching affiliation is another important factor that contributes to institutional effectiveness. On the average, the quality not only of medical but also of nursing care is significantly higher at those institutions which have some medical teaching affiliation than those which do not. Further, mean economic efficiency is slightly better for the former than for the latter, although the difference is not statistically significant in this case. Clearly, teaching affiliation enhances the clinical efficiency of hospital EUs without in any way impeding their economic efficiency, and possibly may even facilitate economic efficiency. Medical teaching affiliation is likely to promote clinical efficiency, without increasing the cost of care, by enabling the medical and nursing staff of EUs to keep up to date with developments in emergency medicine and the health services field, and by enabling the system to establish, maintain, and adhere to high standards of patient care and professional performance. In addition, it is positively related to the reputation of EUs and their responsiveness to community expectations. Therefore, where some form of affiliation is possible, it probably should be pursued as another major means for improving institutional effectiveness.

Also to be included among the major variables which turned out to facilitate both the clinical and economic efficiency of hospital EUs is staff satisfaction with the EU as a place to work. (Patient satisfaction correlates with clinical efficiency only.) Staff satisfaction, which is an indicator of the social efficiency of the system, is one of the five secondary criteria of effectiveness examined in this research, and the only one among the five which in organizational theory has been viewed both as an outcome variable in its own right and as an "independent variable" in relation to system performance. In the present case, when treated as an independent variable, medical staff satisfaction correlates positively and significantly with the economic as well as the clinical efficiency of hospital EUs, and the same is true of nursing staff satisfaction (medical and nursing staff satisfaction, incidentally, themselves do not correlate significantly, although their relationship is a positive one and approaches statistical significance). To a certain extent, therefore, the social efficiency of the system appears to promote both economic and clinical efficiency.

Similarly, like staff satisfaction, the strength of commitment to the EU, or identification with the EU, reported by registered nurses correlates positively and significantly both with the quality of nursing care (but not medical care) and with economic efficiency. In the long run, staff commitment to the organization, which is an indicator of member integration into the system, and staff satisfaction are probably mutually reinforcing variables that are likely to facilitate economic and clinical performance while themselves being enhanced by better performance. In effect, the relationship of nursing satisfaction and commitment to nursing staff performance is likely to be not only positive but also circular. If so, hospital EUs could increase their effectiveness by improving nursing staff satisfaction and commitment. Such improvement, however, in many cases will require modifications to existing rewards, incentives, and opportunities for nursing staff members.

Finally, it is also interesting to point out that medical staff identification with the EU, unlike medical staff satisfaction or nursing staff satisfaction and identification, is not significantly related to either the clinical or the economic efficiency of hospital EUs. The diversity of medical staffing patterns (several of which involve only outside physicians who, unlike the nurses, are not on the staff of the parent hospitals) which characterizes the EUs in the study sample is probably responsible for the absence of a relationship in the case of the medical staff.

Aspects of Organization Facilitating One Major Criterion of
Effectiveness Without Impeding the Other

Most of the remaining aspects of organization affect the
clinical but not economic efficiency of hospital EUs. In the
majority of cases, they promote the former while being unrelated
to the latter. The converse applies, however, to one of the major
independent variables studied—patient volume, which turns out to
enhance economic efficiency without hindering clinical efficiency.
Moreover, the greater the patient volume, the higher the economic
efficiency of an EU is likely to be, even after controlling for
breadth of emergency service definition (which correlates positively
with but behaves differently than patient volume) and parent
hospital size (which is unrelated to EU economic efficiency). Not
all EUs, of course, would be able to increase the number of patient
visits or accommodate a larger patient volume as a means to
greater economic efficiency, but some might find it feasible to
accomplish.

Patient volume also correlates positively with the quality of
nursing care (but not medical care), possibly because EUs with a
high patient volume have a more experienced nursing staff than
do other EUs. But the obtained zero-order correlation disappears
(reduces from .41 to .08) when partialling out the effect of parent
hospital size. Since, in addition, patient volume is not significantly
related to the quality of medical care, it must be concluded that it
only affects the economic efficiency of hospital EUs.

Among the aspects of organization which promote clinical
efficiency without affecting economic efficiency adversely are a
great many social-psychological variables that represent the
relative adequacy, or success, of internal organizational problem
solving in certain major areas, as well as a few structural variables.
The most important among the latter are parent hospital size and
service complexity.

Hospital size is positively and significantly related to the
quality of both medical and nursing care at the EUs studied, even
after partialling out the effects of patient volume and scope of
service. Of interest also is the fact that, while hospital size (which
correlates positively with EU patient volume) is not significantly

related to the economic efficiency of EUs (patient volume is), it shows a small positive correlation with economic efficiency. Accordingly, it does not impede economic efficiency. Hospital size, of course, is not a readily manipulable variable to be used as a mechanism for improving EU effectiveness. Nevertheless, EUs in the larger hospitals provide better patient care than their counterparts in the smaller hospitals while also being at least equally cost-efficient.

Compared to a smaller institution, a larger hospital probably facilitates the clinical efficiency of its EU because it is more able to provide needed services or support to the EU and because it possesses richer clinical and organizational resources on which the EU might draw. In fact, institutional service complexity, which is a better indicator of the number and variety of available facilities than size (with which complexity correlates highly), shows the same pattern of relationships with the clinical and economic efficiency of EUs as does size. The same is true, moreover, of the number of approvals granted the parent hospital by various professional bodies, another structural variable that correlates highly with both service complexity and hospital size. Service complexity and the number of approvals, of course, may also vary among hospitals of the same size, with corresponding implications for the clinical efficiency of their EUs.

Contributions of Organizational Problem Solving. Of all the independent variables that were found to facilitate clinical efficiency without any adverse effects for economic efficiency, nonprogrammed coordination of activities within the EU is the most powerful. Nonprogrammed coordination contributes significantly not only to the quality of both medical and nursing care but also to three of the five secondary criteria of EU effectiveness examined in this research—namely, to patient satisfaction (both with the care received and with the EU staff), promptness of medical attention to incoming patients, and EU responsiveness in meeting community expectations and needs regarding emergency medical care.

Nonprogrammed coordination within an organization takes place on the basis of mutual staff adjustments, informal feedback among members, and reciprocal understanding of one another's work problems and needs by the participants. It requires good work relations and spontaneous cooperation among the people who have to work together. In contrast, programmed coordination takes place on the basis of formal work plans, schedules, and procedures, and formally required communication. And although the two kinds of organizational coordination correlate positively, both with each other and also with the quality of medical and nursing care, only nonprogrammed coordination shows strong positive effects on clinical efficiency. Programmed coordination at hospital EUs is of severely limited utility as a means of improving clinical efficiency because of the unpredictability, heterogeneity, and uncertainty of patient inputs which determine the work of this system.

On the other hand, good programmed and nonprogrammed coordination alike appear to contribute significantly to the reduction of organizational strain. They both correlate negatively with the levels of prevailing tension within the EU, between the EU and hospital administration, and between the EU and the outside community. These aspects of strain, in turn, generally correlate negatively with the quality of patient care (as well as with some of the secondary criteria of effectiveness) provided by the various EUs.

In the area of resources, the responsiveness of other hospital departments in meeting EU requests for various services or assistance (which correlates positively with nonprogrammed coordination within the EU and negatively with the level of prevailing tension between the EU and hospital administration) strongly affects the clinical efficiency of hospital EUs, and especially the quality of medical care.

The responsiveness of other hospital departments is higher at institutions having a higher level of EU service specialization, greater service complexity, and more professional approvals than at other institutions. This important independent variable, as might be expected, also correlates positively with the fulfillment by parent hospitals of EU physician requests—another indicator of successful organizational problem solving in the area of resources which itself correlates positively and significantly (though not as highly as does responsiveness) with the quality of both medical and nursing care. Good relationships between EUs and the parent hospitals, therefore, would be essential to foster as another major means for improving institutional effectiveness.

Internal organizational strain, as reflected in the levels of existing tension among EU physicians, between the EU and hospital administration, and between the EU and the outside community, generally appears to undermine both components of the clinical efficiency of the system, but not its economic efficiency. In addition, nearly all of the measures of strain are negatively related to the secondary criteria of EU effectiveness, with more than one-third of the obtained relevant correlations being statistically significant. Especially dysfunctional in this connection is the level of prevailing tension between the EU and hospital administration, as reported by the doctors and registered nurses working at the various EUs. The results also show that, for the most part, existing strain does not appear to be of structural origin. Accordingly, improvements in staff relations and interpersonal relations, possibly through such factors as training programs and better coordination of activities, are likely to reduce the levels of prevailing strain in hospital EUs while also improving the levels of staff satisfaction (which, as might be expected, correlate negatively with organizational strain).

The ability of the system to adapt to its relevant environment is also important to institutional effectiveness. Hospital EUs have a dual environment. First, the parent hospitals constitute the immediate environment of EUs, since the latter are organizational subsystems of the former, and we have already seen that good EU-hospital relations are critical to EU effectiveness. In addition, EUs interact directly with the outside community, receiving from it and returning to it patients and information, and engaging in various transactions with health system agencies, city health departments, ambulance services, police and fire departments, and the like. In short, EUs have a variety of direct work contacts and organizational relationships with parts of the environment beyond the confines of their parent hospitals. How well they handle such contacts and relationships is a good indicator of the system's adaptation to the environment. Successful organizational problem solving in this area should provide the system with useful information and also enhance its potential for control over its work inputs, a potential which is generally very low.

The findings in this area show that collaboration with other institutions for the purpose of providing or improving emergency services, and the degree to which contacts with health service agencies and relevant individuals in the community are satisfactory, correlate positively and significantly with the clinical efficiency of hospital EUs (especially with the quality of nursing care) without affecting economic efficiency adversely. EU adaptation to the environment, as measured by an index developed for this purpose, is also positively related to patient satisfaction, nursing staff satisfaction, and institutional reputation. The results further show that EU adaptation to the environment is affected not only by organizational problem solving but also by the system's structure. Specific aspects of structure significantly related to adaptation include EU service specialization, institutional service complexity, EU patient volume (but not parent hospital size), medical teaching affiliation, and emergency personnel training programs. Therefore, adaptation to the environment could be improved by means of appropriate structural changes as well as by means of better organizational problem solving.

Anomalous or Surprising Findings

Clearly, most aspects of organizational structure and problem solving that might be altered in order to enhance one major criterion of institutional effectiveness (for example, economic or clinical efficiency) in the great majority of cases are not likely to affect another such criterion adversely. In fact, the research identified only two variables which failed to show similar, complementary, or at least noncontradictory relationships with economic and clinical efficiency. These are EU location and breadth of emergency service.

Briefly, EUs located in SMSA communities on the average tend to show slightly higher economic efficiency than EUs in non-SMSA communities, while the latter tend to show slightly higher clinical efficiency than the former. But these differences do not even approach statistical significance.

Secondly, EUs with a relatively broad definition or scope of "emergency service" show higher levels of economic efficiency than EUs with a more narrow definition, but also lower levels of patient care quality, especially medical care quality. This holds true, moreover, even after partialling out the effects of patient volume and parent hospital size. In short, a narrow definition of emergency service appears to facilitate the quality of medical care while impeding economic efficiency, the reverse being true of a broad definition (which suggests a high proportion of nonemergency cases and/or medically uninteresting cases). The obtained relationships, however, are not especially strong.

Moreover, as a potential mechanism for improving EU effectiveness, an institution's breadth of emergency service definition would be both more difficult and less suitable to alter than most of the structural or problem-solving variables studied. The same applies to EU location even more strongly. The corresponding practical implications associated with these two variables, therefore, are minimal.

Apart from these relatively anomalous findings, only the community structure variables that were explored in the research yielded clearly surprising results in relation to EU effectiveness. Unlike the impact of organizational structure, the effects of internal organizational problem solving, and the importance of adaptation to the environment as reflected in the nature of EU-community relations, the structural characteristics of the community do not appear to affect either the clinical or the economic efficiency of hospital EUs. With one minor exception, aspects of community structure such as population stability, formal education level, economic status, and community heterogeneity and complexity show no significant relationship to the quality of medical care or to economic efficiency, both when examined individually and as a set. The exception involves median family income in the community, which correlates positively with the quality of nursing care provided by hospital EUs. Overall, however, regression analyses show that community structure has no significant effect on the performance of hospital EUs. This unanticipated finding contrasts sharply with the results concerning the relationships between organizational problem solving in the area of adaptation to the environment, that is, in the area of EU-community relations, and EU effectiveness.

The tentative conclusion from these findings is that successful adaptation to the external environment is not, and should not be, as difficult a problem for hospital EUs as some researchers and practitioners in the field would contend. Concerning the effectiveness of these health service systems, the parent hospital environment (that is, the immediate suprasystem) is much more critical, both structurally and in terms of organizational problem solving, than is the structure of the external community environment within which they function. And, additionally, good EU-community relations are more consequential for EU effectiveness than are the structural characteristics of the community.

Suggestions for Future Research

Since organizational research in emergency medical care has been minimal, the possibilities for additional work along the lines of the research discussed in this book are numerous. Some of the more interesting possibilities are suggested by theoretical and methodological issues which were encountered in this research and by the findings.

First, additional research might be fruitfully undertaken to examine more intensively community structure differences in relation to the effectiveness of hospital EUs (and of hospitals), and also to determine whether the above findings relating to institutional location and scope of service will be affirmed.

Second, the results obtained in the area of organizational integration are not only the weakest when compared to those involving the other problem areas studied but are also mixed. For example, the integration of nurses and of physicians into the system yielded dissimilar outcomes in relation to EU effectiveness, while normative integration appears to contribute little to effectiveness. Additional research in this area, perhaps with more and/or better measures, should help clarify the picture.

In the case of physician and nurse integration, the dissimilarity of outcomes may well be attributable to the diverse medical staffing arrangements of hospital EUs (which contrast sharply with the more uniform nursing staff arrangements), and a study of more institutions with each of the staffing patterns distinguished should help resolve the issues. In addition, and perhaps more importantly, because of the increased N, such a study would make possible more rigorous statistical analyses and thus yield more definitive findings concerning the relationship between medical staffing pattern and institutional effectiveness.

Third, it would be both interesting and important to determine whether the absence of a significant relationship between clinical and economic efficiency revealed in this research continues to hold for hospital EUs under current conditions, which are marked by steadily increasing cost-consciousness, clear pressures toward cost control, and actual cost-containment efforts based on prepayment for medical service. Further, it would be important to know whether the lack of relationship between clinical and economic efficiency also exists in multihospital systems, including for-profit institutions, in the case of free-standing emergency centers, and on a nationwide basis. Appropriate replications and extensions of the present research, therefore, would be very useful to undertake.

Fourth, in light of the actual empirical findings, possible adjustments that had been contemplated for the indices developed to measure economic efficiency and the quality of medical care proved unnecessary. Concerning the latter index, for example, which provides a valid and reliable measure of quality that takes into account both patient volume and case-mix, the initial intention was to adjust it further through the introduction of case severity scores based on certain indicators and thus construct also an adjusted index of the quality of medical care. As it turned out, however, severity indicators, such as the proportion of patients who arrived at the EU by ambulance or the proportion of patients who were sent by the EU to an intensive care unit or operating room of the parent hospital, yielded results that did not warrant any adjustment to the original medical care index. The quasitracer patient conditions measure included in the medical care index appears to provide sufficient adjustment for case severity. Furthermore, the results demonstrated that using fewer than the ten quasitracers which were actually included in the measure (for example, using only the six with the largest patient volume) statistically could yield a nearly identical measure of the quality of medical care at the EU level.

Future methodological work, nevertheless, should investigate the relevance and potential of other severity adjustors and also examine the value of using alternative sets, and sets with varying numbers, of quasitracer patient conditions in assessing the quality of medical care. In addition, it should investigate more fully and more intensively the usefulness and promise of the patient visit staging approach for assessing clinical efficiency at the institutional level. Similar methodological work, moreover, might address the problem of developing alternative indices of economic efficiency, as well as issues involved in considering possible adjustors for such indices. Additional and/or improved measures of both economic and clinical efficiency, more generally, should be of continuing concern to the health services field for researchers and practitioners alike.

Fifth, the findings suggest that the secondary criteria of EU effectiveness developed and used in the present research, mainly to supplement and validate the primary criteria, should receive more research attention in the future, both in relation to economic and clinical efficiency and as important dependent variables in their own right. Patient satisfaction and its determinants, in particular, should be carefully and rigorously studied, as should its relationship to the economic, clinical, and social efficiency of hospital EUs.

Sixth, although no significant relationship was found between economic efficiency and the quality of medical care, some hospital EUs scored better than the median on both indices, and a few of these scored considerably better than the median. Intensive case studies of such "stars" would help to further illuminate the structural, managerial, and social-psychological determinants of overall institutional excellence, as well as the nature of superior effectiveness.

Finally, future organizational students of hospital EUs, hospitals, and other human service organizations (for example, academic institutions, government agencies) might consider implementing, and possibly also refining, the conceptual-theoretical model which guided the present research. The research model employed, it will be recalled, is an open-system theory model which views complex organizations as work-performing and problem-solving systems. Comparative organizational analyses relying on this or similarly tested and equally general models for theory-based empirical research appear to hold significant promise, both scientifically and pragmatically. Judging from the results of the present research, at any rate, such analyses have great potential for contributing to organizational knowledge; therefore, they should be supported and undertaken with much greater frequency than in the past, both in the health services and in other fields.

Summary

Using a conceptual-theoretical model based on open-system theory and a new methodology for assessing the effectiveness of hospital EUs at the institutional level, the research discussed in this book investigated the relationship of EU organization to EU effectiveness. Observed interinstitutional differences for most criteria of effectiveness, including economic and clinical efficiency, and for most aspects of organizational structure and problem solving are considerable. Differences in structure and problem solving explain much, if not most, of the variance in effectiveness across institutions. Moreover, structure and problem solving have both independent and synergistic effects on institutional effectiveness.

The research also shows certain relationships between organizational structure and problem solving. Moreover, it demonstrates that the different aspects of structure examined are interrelated, as is the adequacy of organizational problem solving across certain areas, but not necessarily strongly or in a simple manner. The specific relationships vary considerably in magnitude and do not encompass all aspects of either structure or problem solving.

Successful organizational problem solving, particularly in the areas of coordination and resources, is essential to enabling hospital EUs to provide medical and nursing care of high quality.

It also affects institutional effectiveness by promoting the system's performance on the various secondary criteria examined, including patient satisfaction and staff satisfaction. However, although it also influences the economic efficiency of EUs indirectly, problem solving in the areas studied does not directly affect it to any significant degree. The structure of the system, on the other hand, does affect economic efficiency, in addition to having direct and significant effects on clinical efficiency.

In addition to good nonprogrammed coordination and good EU-hospital relations in the area of resources, effective handling of intraorganizational strain and organization-environment relations are important contributing factors to institutional effectiveness. Accordingly, administrators and other concerned practitioners should periodically assess, and monitor, the state of their organizations in all these important areas and then take appropriate steps, as needed, for effecting improvements. Emergency personnel training programs, medical teaching affiliation, and a medical staffing pattern that relies on hospital-based group arrangements also contribute importantly to effectiveness. In short, as expected on theoretical grounds, the effectiveness of hospital EUs depends very greatly upon their organization, and specifically the structure of the system and the adequacy of its internal organizational problem solving.

The kind of organization that fosters high institutional effectiveness in the case of these health service systems involves considerable yet flexible structuring of activities and work relations, coupled with a great deal of reliance on professional autonomy and discretion, nonprogrammed coordination, and informal mutual understandings, cooperation, and adjustment among the people doing the work. Additionally, it requires satisfactory linkages and work relations with the parent hospital. Such organization fits neither the rational bureaucratic/mechanistic model nor the organic/human relations model. Instead, it is a curious mixture of elements from both of these contrasting models that can be better understood in open-system theory terms, and specifically by means of the research model employed in the present comparative study. Hospital EUs are specialized professional organizations. They are also complex work-performing and problem-solving systems which are quasi-organic and quasi-mechanistic, which are functioning within a dual organizational environment (involving the parent hospital and the external community), and whose work inputs are very heterogeneous and largely unpredictable. In large measure, differences in the effectiveness of these interesting social systems can be explained by differences in their organization.

Underlying
Conceptual-Theoretical
Framework

Presented here is a conceptual-theoretical framework for the analysis of complex organizations, as applied in a comparative study of hospital emergency units (EUs).* The hospital EU can be viewed conceptually as a complex work-performing and problem-solving subsystem of the hospital. This subsystem functions under a variety of constraints imposed by the nature of its work and work inputs, its relationships to the parent hospital, and the character of the relevant external environment. Although the EU is a subsystem of the hospital, here it is treated as a "system" in order to facilitate discussion.

Note: This appendix is an abbreviated and slightly modified version of the paper *Conceptual-Theoretical Framework for the Organizational Study of Hospital Emergency Services*, by Basil S. Georgopoulos and Robert A. Cooke, which first appeared under this title in the Working Paper Series of the Institute for Social Research (article 8011, Jan. 1979). A similar version of the paper was also presented at the 40th Annual Meeting of the Academy of Management, as part of the symposium "A Problem-Solving Approach to Studying the Effectiveness of Health Care Organizations" (B.S. Georgopoulos, Chairman), Detroit, Aug. 1980. The material is used with the Institute's permission.

*This framework draws heavily on the organization research model proposed previously by Georgopoulos (see especially 1972). That particular model is here augmented and refined in an important way with the incorporation of certain contributions from March and Simon (1958) and Thompson (1967). Secondly, the framework builds on the

The EU, like other complex organizations, is characterized by certain basic system properties, such as internal continuity, interdependence, and constancy relative to the external environment. These and other properties, together with the work requirements of the system (that is, the nature of the task or work to be done) and the characteristics of its members, give rise to a set of interrelated major problems that are encountered at various points along the organization's work cycle (that is, the input-transformation-output cycle of the system). These system problems, which concern such things as the coordination of interdependent activities and maintenance of orderly behavior patterns, are not amenable to total or permanent solution. They are relatively enduring, or open-ended and recurring, so that they can never be regarded as completely or conclusively solved. Yet the effectiveness of the EU, as an organization, depends precisely upon the system's ability to deal with and adequately "solve," at least temporarily and for the most part, these major problems.

System Properties and Organizational Problem Areas

The basic system properties of organizations themselves are complexly interrelated and have important implications for the nature and resolution of the problems that EU systems will face. In our view, the most important of these properties are differentiation, interdependence within the system, patterning, internal continuity, equifinality, constancy relative to the environment, openness, system-environment interdependence, and performance potential.

---

discussion included in the original research proposal for the present study of hospital emergency services (DHHS-USPHS, National Center for Health Services Research, Research Grant 3 RO1 HS-02538) and on preliminary working documents from the project which amplify the research model. Finally, it incorporates selected open-system theory contributions from Katz and Kahn (1966) and Miller (1971), and certain other contributions from the organization theory literature, as cited.

One basic property is differentiation of structures and functions. Open systems typically move in the direction of increased elaboration of internal structures and components, and diffuse global patterns are replaced by specialized ones (Parsons and Shils, 1952; Katz and Kahn, 1966; Miller, 1971; Hage, 1974). Particular organizations, however, may vary considerably as to the level of their internal differentiation.

A second basic property is that of interdependence among the components of the system: work roles are carried out by members, and groups of members, who possess different characteristics but who interact with one another and who relate themselves in various ways to their respective roles and groups, to each other, and to the total system (Georgopoulos, 1972; Thompson, 1967). In short, components function not unilaterally but interdependently, and interdependence (called "conditionality" by Ashby, 1960) reflects the contingencies governing work performance and problem solving in an organization.

Patterning is another fundamental property of "organization" for all systems; it represents the degree of order and underlying regularity (nonrandomness) of organizational structures and activities (Georgopoulos, 1972). A related property is internal system *continuity:* The patterns of articulation and interdependence among the subsystems and components of an organization are not transient or ephemeral but, rather, exhibit certain continuity over time (Georgopoulos, 1972). Organizational systems are also characterized by *equifinality*. This property refers to the fact, and the likelihood, that the same final system outcome can be attained from different initial conditions, including different inputs and different structures and processes (von Bertalanffy, 1956; Katz and Kahn, 1966).

Open systems, including complex organizations such as the EU, are further characterized by certain properties which reflect their relation to, and dependence upon, the larger environment. These properties are critical because all open systems, as a condition of their survival, must import (in a continuous or recurring fashion) various forms of energy and information from the external environment, and then export some "finished" product, service, or information into the environment (Georgopoulos, 1972; Miller, 1971). The property of *constancy* represents the relative stability of the system-environment configuration and reflects the organization's regular and more or less predictable interchange with the external environment (Georgopoulos, 1972; Weiss, 1959). Additionally, as an organization, the EU is characterized by *openness*, the relative permeability of its boundaries through which inputs enter the system and outputs leave it, and *interdependence* with the environment, the mutual dependence between the system and its relevant external environment.

Finally, organizations are characterized by a property representing the *performance potential* or *problem-solving capacity* of the system (Georgopoulos, 1972). This important property represents the composite capacity of the system's components that inheres in their qualifications. The components of all systems possess certain qualifications and information. Their particular qualifications endow the components with certain individual and collective performance potential that can be used to solve work problems and attain effective work performance. The qualifications of components, however, provide only the *potential* for work performance and problem solving. This potential may or may not be fully realized in a given system. The extent to which it is harnessed will, among other things, depend on the way in which system components are ordered and interconnected—that is, on how the organization is structured. Disorder and inappropriate ordering will constrain release of the performance potential of components (viewed both individually and collectively). Accordingly, a system may be relatively ineffective even if its components are highly qualified. On the other hand, experience of success in dealing with the major problems of the system will probably increase the likelihood that the performance potential of individual components will materialize.

The basic system properties are related to one another in various ways, both directly and indirectly. For example, the properties of continuity and constancy are alike in that they both imply a degree of stability and order. Similarly, interdependence (organizational-environment) and openness are alike in that both properties are related to the importation of energy and the character of inputs from the external environment. Other properties, however, may be inversely related and seem to be, at least superficially, inconsistent or even opposing. For example, differentiation implies a centrifugal force, while continuity implies a centripetal force. High internal continuity implies low equifinality, and vice versa. Similarly, openness seems to be in opposition to continuity and constancy, but positively related to equifinality. The specific system properties, therefore, may be either mutually reinforcing or antithetical. They are interrelated, either directly or indirectly, but not necessarily in a simple positive or mutually enhancing manner.*

This constellation of system properties, in conjunction with the differentiated character of components and the nature of work to be done, gives rise to various basic problems which must be "solved" by the EU if the organization is to continue functioning as a system at some level of effectiveness. More specifically, as a complex organizational system, the EU must be able to:

1. *Allocate* resources, authority, information, and rewards among various groups and members (components) whose expectations may differ but whose work roles are interdependent (for a conceptual definition of allocation, see Georgopoulos, 1975, p. 144).
2. *Coordinate* the diverse activities and contributions of members, so that they function according to each other's work needs, and so that the efforts of all concerned are properly articulated (in time and space) to converge toward the solution

---

*From the preceding discussion, it should be obvious that the different properties may vary, in degree or value, from one system to another and for the same system at different points in time. In every ongoing system, however, each of these basic properties has a greater than zero value. High values are not necessarily desirable from the point of view of system effectiveness, however, nor are low values. It is not unlikely that unusually high and unusually low values may both be dysfunctional (this applies even to the property of performance potential, for high potential may be indicative of underutilization of talent by the system). From the standpoint of the research model here discussed, moreover, the various system properties could be treated either as "independent" or as "exogenous" variables.

of work problems and the attainment of organizational objectives (Georgopoulos, 1975, p. 163).

3. *Integrate* the various structures encompassed by the system (role, authority, normative, communication structures), and also integrate member aspirations and goals with group objectives and organizational goals so as to ensure member involvement, cooperation, compliance, and the like, with organizational requirements (Georgopoulos, 1975, p. 163).

4. *Maintain* the character of the system (the existing configuration of structures and work arrangements) and structural stability and orderly—if not entirely predictable—behavior patterns (Georgopoulos, 1975, p. 130).

5. *Ameliorate* the strains arising from the preceding, from the characteristics of members, and also from the subsystem's relationships with the external environment (Georgopoulos, 1975, p. 144).

6. *Adapt* to instability, change, and uncertainty in the environment within which the subsystem functions and from which it obtains the requisite energy and resources to do its work; and, more generally, respond to and influence the environment (Georgopoulos, 1975, p. 130).

In the case of EUs, the problems of adaptation, coordination of efforts, and resource allocation are considered to be especially critical to the effectiveness of the system.

Although the entire range of system properties implies the need for problem solving in each of these major problem areas, particular subsets of properties most directly generate, or are associated with, particular problems. For example, continuity and constancy give rise to maintenance problems, while openness and organization-environment interdependence generate problems of adaptation. Because the EU is an internally differentiated system that must import needed energy and information—must obtain scarce and costly resources of relatively limited quantity and quality—the problem of allocation arises. Systems develop toward multiplication and elaboration of roles as they grow, and this gives rise to opportunity (or necessity) for differentially allocating resources, information, and the like among their various components in order to do their work efficiently. Furthermore, internal differentiation generates the problem of integration (Parsons and Shils, 1952).

The differentiation of the system's structures (for example, role, normative, and communication structures), together with the need for internal continuity, generates the problem of structural integration—that is, how to render the various structures congruent, complementary, or mutually reinforcing, so that the total configuration is internally consistent and unified. Furthermore, as members perform tasks associated with specialized roles or particular organizational subunits, the objectives directly relevant to these roles and subgroup goals may displace or supersede the organization's objectives. This implies a need to bring the organization together by integrating members' goals with the objectives of the larger system. Openness has similar implications for integration. The EU is open not only in terms of the permeability of its boundaries but also in the sense that some of its components (members) are only "partially included" in the system (Allport, 1933). The members are not only components of the system but are also components of the larger environment and have their own personal needs and goals (whether or not they are viewed as members of the system). Consequently, the EU is faced with an additional integration problem apart from that of structural integration—the problem of integrating the goals and aspirations of the members with the objectives of the system.

The basic system property of interdependence among component elements, which is an outcome of differentiation and work specialization (see Thompson, 1961), gives rise to the problem of coordination (see Georgopoulos and Mann, 1962). Additionally, interdependence—both among the components and between the EU and the environment—generates problems of strain. First, a lack or excess of matter-energy or information from the environment can force system variables beyond their range of stability (stress) and produce strain (Miller, 1971). Similarly, conflicts and confrontations between interdependent groups within the EU can produce strain that must be ameliorated. Demands on the components beyond their capacities, errors in the system, and fluctuations in ambiguity and uncertainty may also create strains (Georgopoulos and Matejko, 1967). Finally, strain may be generated from imperfect solutions to the other major system problems, and, in this sense, it can be a derived or "second-order" problem.

In considering the relevant system properties which are associated with the various problems, it becomes evident that the problems themselves also are interrelated in systematic though complex ways. First, the properties most involved in a particular problem area may imply forces that are inconsistent with the forces entailed by the properties which are most involved in the case of other problem areas. Continuity and openness, for example, imply forces which are at least superficially in opposition. This suggests that solving a problem in one area (for example, maintenance) could exacerbate a problem in another area (for example, adaptation). Second, certain properties may give rise to, or at least complicate, different problems simultaneously. Differentiation, for example, may render both the allocation and coordination problems more difficult to solve. Third, the resolution of certain problems may facilitate the resolution of other problems—even when the problems involved are not directly generated by the same system properties. Integration, for example, may make it possible for coordination to be achieved with less transmission of information (Miller, 1971).

The approach taken thus far assumes that the system properties, together with the characteristics of the components of the system and the nature of work to be done, give rise to various problems in the above major areas. An alternative, but consistent, approach would propose that the problem areas themselves could be formulated in the sense of maximizing corresponding system properties in a facilitative or positively reinforcing manner. Adaptation, for example, could be viewed as the system's problem of maximizing facilitative system-environment interdependence and achieving adequate constancy in relation to the external environment. Similarly, coordination could be viewed as the system's problem of maximizing facilitative (or promotive) interdependence and minimizing hindering interdependence among the different components and their work efforts.

These two approaches to viewing the problem areas are consistent and complementary. Thus, while the property of interdependence may generate problems of coordination, successful resolution of these problems may in turn enhance facilitative interdependence among interacting components of the system. Similarly, continuity may give rise to maintenance problems, but the amelioration of maintenance problems will, at least temporarily, promote internal system continuity. This line of reasoning suggests feedback loops; the properties are related to the problem areas, and the problem areas are related to the properties. Such feedback, however, implies that system problems are dealt with properly or are temporarily solved, at least for the most part. Whether or not this is actually the case, in turn, depends on whether the EU has the appropriate structures and programs to address the problems.

Organizational Structures, Bases, and Problem Solving

The organizational structure of EUs or, more precisely, the various structures encompassed by this organization—such as the role structure, normative structure, authority structure, and communication structure—constitute the basic problem-solving framework of the system. Structures make it possible for the system not only to control work performance and regulate members' behavior on an organization-wide basis but also to deal with the problems faced by the system. These basic structures serve as the main base and principal point of departure for system problem solving and actually constitute the system's core *organization*.

> Organization involves information, but it also involves ordering and coupling, or interconnectedness, among elements (components); it implies structure and form. Each of a number of elements carrying certain information or qualifications is connected to other elements, and the various elements involved are arranged in some particular order according to some controlling or "organizing" principle [Georgopoulos, 1972, p. 14].

The elements of a system can be interconnected, arranged, or interrelated with respect to more than one variable (Blalock and Blalock, 1959) and according to several different principles and composition rules (Feibleman and Friend, 1945). Members of an EU, for example, are interconnected in terms of authority, communication, norms, and roles. These structures are juxtaposed and coexist in the system but typically are imperfectly correlated. Additionally, they have both formal and informal aspects which are not necessarily well matched or mutually reinforcing. Associated inconsistencies, both within and between structures, undoubtedly suppress the performance potential of the system and its components, while resulting in strain that must be dealt with by the organization.

Perhaps the most fundamental aspect of organizational structure is patterning. Order plus information constitutes patterning, and patterning is a core aspect of "organization"—a basic system property that represents the level of structuring within an organization (Georgopoulos, 1972). Patterning, together with coupling or connectedness, represents organization in the generic sense and at the most fundamental level: individual elements with particular qualifications which are patterned and coupled comprise a structured *set* of component elements, which constitutes what is meant by the concept of "organization."

Figure A-1 illustrates that elements, with particular information and qualifications, which are placed in relation to one another in some orderly manner (for example, vertically and horizontally) and coupled (that is, connected to each other and to the system as a whole) on the basis of some controlling principle (such as the principle of economic or social rationality, authority) comprise the components of a structured set that represents *organization*. The resultant structure provides the basic problem-solving framework of a system such as the EU.

The basic, relatively stable structures of the EU (for example, role, normative, authority, communication structures) serve as the primary base for organizational problem solving in at least three important ways. First, they provide a base on which a member, or group of members, can rely in performing organizational tasks and carrying out programs and activities for solving

Figure A-1. Structure and Organization.

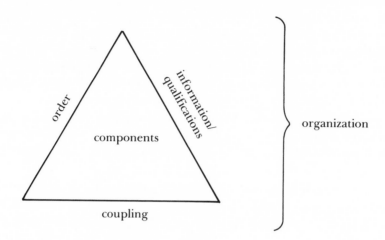

particular problems. Second, they provide a base for selecting among or switching between programs for dealing with particular problems. Third, the structures serve as a base for developing, elaborating, and initiating new programs for solving problems.

Structures and Performance Programs

In their efforts to solve the problems of coordination, allocation, and the like, EU members in effect select and implement various "performance programs" (March and Simon, 1958). Such programs may vary substantially in their degree of specificity and completeness, in complexity and rationality, and also in the extent to which they allow discretion to the performers. Generally, performance programs may specify activities (means) and/or may specify objectives (ends); "the further the program goes in the latter direction, the more discretion it allows for the person implementing the program to supply the means-ends connection" (March and Simon, 1958, p. 147).

Related decision issues may be categorized in terms of the relative certainty characterizing ends, or outcome preferences, and means-ends or cause/effect relations (Thompson and others, 1959; Thompson, 1967, p. 134). Performance programs will be likely to specify means when beliefs about cause/effect relations are relatively certain (that is, under conditions of relatively high rationality); they will be likely to specify ends when beliefs regarding such relations are uncertain. Some programs, of course, may specify both ends and means. This will be likely when there is relative certainty concerning both ends and means-ends relations.

March and Simon (1958) view performance programs as an important (though least stable) aspect of an organization's structure. Within our framework, such programs are viewed as *second-order* structures because they are less basic and less stable than the *first-order* role, authority, normative, and communication structures of an organization. Similarly, the activities in which members or groups of members engage in implementing performance programs are viewed as *third-order* structures. The third-order structures build upon second-order structures, and both the second- and third-order structures rely on the basic first-order structures of the system.

Assuming that an organization has a repertoire of performance programs, it will be able to solve problems by selecting appropriate programs in reacting to specific situations (March and Simon, 1958). The rules used to select programs, called "switching rules" by March and Simon, may be highly specified or may offer members discretion in the selection of performance programs. Thompson's (1967) distinction between decision issues which involve certainty versus uncertainty regarding outcome preferences also is relevant here. Specified switching rules are likely to be used when preferences regarding outcomes are relatively clear or certain; less specified or more discretionary switching procedures are likely to be used when preferences about outcomes are relatively uncertain.

Though various factors will affect the adequacy of problem solving within the EU, problem-solving adequacy will in large part depend upon the structural bases available in the organization. Some of the basic structures of the system may be specialized, in the sense that they serve as a base for the resolution of specific problems. Others, such as the role or authority structure, tend to be multipurpose structures. In general, the ability of the system to solve a problem in a particular area depends, at least in part, on the availability of an appropriate program which is consistent with the existing basic structures. (It also depends, of course, on the performance potential of the system.)

Performance programs that specify activities are probably carried out most effectively in systems which already have highly specified role structures. Members of a system structured in this manner, for example, may be able to implement a program for achieving coordination which clearly specifies and standardizes their interdependent efforts. This same system, in the absence of other structural bases, may be unable to effectively implement programs which specify objectives rather than activities. In situations of extensive reciprocal interdependence (Thompson, 1967), where feedback and mutual adjustment are needed to achieve the coordination objective, highly specified roles do not provide an adequate base. In such situations, members are usually required (or forced) to exercise discretion both in estimating means-ends relations and in carrying out the actual problem-solving activities. The normative structure of the system therefore is likely to be a more critical base for implementing this type of performance program than is the role structure.*

The organization's structures also provide a base on which system members can rely for selecting among, or switching between, performance programs. The nature of the first-order structures for the most part dictates the kinds of switching procedures used by the system and influences the efficacy of these procedures. A system that is highly structured in terms of roles, for example, can often use standardized procedures for selecting among alternative programs. Systems which are less structured in terms of roles but more reliant on norms, on the other hand, may have to depend upon the discretion of members for selecting the programs. Such discretionary selections will depend both upon the

---

*For a discussion of the role structure of a specialized patient unit, see Georgopoulos and Christman (1970); for a discussion of the normative structure of organizations, see Georgopoulos (1965).

existing structures and on the members' knowledge, experience, and criteria of rationality (economic, social, or clinical). Selected programs in part will reflect the members' own preferences and priorities, their expectations that particular programs can be performed in view of the available bases, and their expectations that particular programs can solve particular problems.

Generally, the stable structural arrangements and associated patterns of relationships among the components of an organizational system such as the EU are relevant to the selection of performance programs in two ways: (1) the structures may provide a base for the use of rules and regulations for program selection or a base for the discretionary selection of programs; and (2) the selection of programs, whether by specified regulation or by discretionary decision, will be made in consideration of the available bases on which members can rely to implement the programs.

The first-order structures of an organization are also relevant to, and eventually also a reflection of, the arrangements (among the components of the system) which are associated with the development and elaboration of performance programs (March and Simon, 1958). In a sense, these structures correspond to the basic learning capabilities of the system. As performance programs and activities are implemented in an organization, members become more adept at assessing the extent to which specific activities have effectively solved the relevant problems as intended. Such experience, when supported and reinforced by appropriate structures, can be used by the members to select programs in the future and, equally important, to develop more appropriate performance programs. In the long run, the problem-solving effectiveness of the system depends on the availability of first-order structures that can be used to generate new and/or more appropriate performance programs and activities.

Structures and Problem-Solving Efficacy

Organizational structures, or at least subsets of these structures, will also have implications for the *type* of problem solving which is likely to take place within an EU. Both programmed and nonprogrammed approaches and various types of problem solving may be used, including promotive, preventive, regulatory, and corrective problem solving (Georgopoulos and Mann, 1962; Georgopoulos, 1972). The different types of problem solving are based on different assumptions concerning the second- and third-order structures (that is, the available performance programs and associated activities) of the system. *Regulatory* problem solving, which involves the use of formalized arrangements to resolve problems, is based on the assumption that the existing structures in the system are relatively sound; the intent is to maintain the "status quo" through regulation of behavior that respects the existing structures. *Corrective* problem solving, which involves reacting to problems after they have occurred in order to remedy the problem, is based on a similar assumption; the intent is to resolve problems by correcting deviations, errors, and aberrations without tampering with the basic structures. *Preventive* problem solving, on the other hand, assumes that regulation and correction are insufficient and that available programs and activities are not entirely satisfactory; this type of problem solving therefore involves anticipatory behavior and efforts aimed at avoiding (or reducing the magnitude of) the problem before it occurs. Finally, *promotive* problem solving attempts to generate improved or more perfect solutions than those prevailing and is based on the assumption that existing second- and third-order structures, and even first-order structures, are questionable and may need to be revised or replaced.

While the various types of problem solving are based on different assumptions regarding second- and third-order structures, the efficacy of each type of problem solving may be dependent more upon the first-order structures of the system than upon either second- or third-order structures. In other words, the efficacy of problem solving is ultimately a function of the system's basic structures. Specifically, the efficacy of promotive problem solving depends upon the availability of structures for the discretionary developing, instituting, and revising of *performance programs* on the part of members (this presumes relatively flexible structures and high equifinality). The efficacy of preventive problem solving depends on the availability of structural bases on which members can rely to select, in a discretionary manner, programs and activities that can help to avoid problems (this also presumes structural flexibility and anticipatory behavior). The efficacy of regulatory problem solving is related to the availability of bases that support the implementation of rules and regulations for the selection of problem-relevant performance programs (this presumes sufficient structural continuity in the system). This does not mean that all regulatory problem solving is nondiscretionary; some regulatory behavior may be based on traditions and general norms that allow a degree of discretion. Finally, the efficacy of corrective problem solving depends on the availability of structural bases on which members can rely for selecting and implementing remedial solutions to problems after they have occurred.

The first-order structures of the system also have implications for the efficacy of different *modes* of problem solving. Problem solving, and the solutions to problems, generally may be either programmed or nonprogrammed (March and Simon, 1958; Georgopoulos and Mann, 1962). *Programmed* solutions are realized through the selection of performance programs that specify activities/means. Adequate performance of such activities, however, still depends upon the availability of appropriate bases, such as a highly specified role structure. *Nonprogrammed* solutions, on the other hand, may be attained through the selection of programs that specify ends or objectives. Although these programs may specify means as well as ends, the activities (means) are less clearly and less completely specified, also less emphasized, than the objectives. This suggests that standardization does not work; instead, feedback and spontaneous adjustments on the part of the performers are necessary for the members to respond to each other's discretionary activities (Georgopoulos and Mann, 1962; Thompson, 1967). The efficacy of this mode of problem solving is therefore dependent upon the availability of bases, such as the normative structure of the system, which are consistent with high levels of communication and flexibility.

Particular types and modes of problem solving may be more or less appropriate for the various problem situations faced by EUs. With some modification, Thompson's matrix (1967, p. 134), which proposes four types of decision issues, can be used to specify "appropriate" types and modes of problem solving in the present framework. The matrix involves two dimensions: (1) certainty/uncertainty regarding cause/effect relations or preferences for means and (2) certainty/uncertainty regarding outcome preferences or ends (see Figure A-2).

Under conditions of relative certainty in terms of both outcome preferences and cause/effect relations, according to Thompson, decision issues can be approached via a "computational" strategy. This strategy relies on planning and technical decision making. It would generally correspond either to regulatory-programmed problem solving (that is, both the performance program and the activities are specified in advance) or corrective-programmed problem solving. A judgmental or "professional" strategy is appropriate for issues which are clear in terms of outcome preferences but unclear as to cause/effect relations (or in terms of the means/activities which will achieve the ends). This strategy would generally correspond either to corrective-nonprogrammed or to regulatory-programmed problem solving. A "political" or compromise strategy is called for if the cause/effect relationships are certain but the outcome preferences are not. The dominant type of problem solving in this case would be preventive-programmed or, perhaps, regulatory-programmed that involves some discretion on the part of performers.

In terms of our model, the preventive-nonprogrammed approach to problem solving would be appropriate for situations in which there is uncertainty regarding both means and ends. This approach would involve use of both political and judgmental strategies, and combinations of practical-administrative and professional-expert decisions. (To the extent that one of these strategies is used prior to the other, the problem situation would be "pushed" to another cell of the matrix; for example, the initial use of the political strategy would imply a movement toward certainty regarding outcome preferences, and regulatory-nonprogrammed problem solving would subsequently be used.) Promotive problem solving would be another dominant type under these uncertain conditions and would imply the development and implementation of relatively innovative or radical solutions. If neither a preventive-nonprogrammed nor a

Figure A-2. Dominant Types and Modes of Problem Solving: Expected Typical Patterns.

	Relative Certainty (Stability, Agreement) Regarding Outcome Preferences or Ends	
	Certainty	Uncertainty
Relative Certainty (Agreement) Regarding Cause/Effect or Means/Ends Relations — Certainty	**I** *Strategy:* "Computational" *Decision Form:* Technical planning *Dominant Mode:* Programmed *Dominant Type:* Regulatory or Corrective	**III** *Strategy:* "Political" *Decision Form:* Administrative-practical *Dominant Mode:* Programmed *Dominant Type:* Preventive or discretionary Regulatory
Uncertainty	**II** *Strategy:* "Judgmental" *Decision Form:* Professional, expert opinion *Dominant Mode:* Nonprogrammed *Dominant Type:* Corrective or Regulatory	**IV** *Strategy:* "Inspirational" *Decision Form:* Combination of administrative and professional *Dominant Mode:* Nonprogrammed *Dominant Type:* Preventive or Promotive (also trial-and-error behavior and nondecision)

Note: Figure A-2 represents a modification and extension of J. D. Thompson's model for the analysis of decision issues in terms of decision strategy and form based on the dimension of certainty/agreement regarding means/ends (see Thompson and others, 1959; Thompson, 1967).

promotive-nonprogrammed approach is taken, trial-and-error problem solving may be necessary. The trial-and-error approach may correspond to "crisis management." Such an approach would be also likely when problems within any of the other three cells of the matrix were not being solved by the more appropriate strategies. Finally, under conditions of high uncertainty regarding both means and ends, "resolution" might take the form of *nondecision*. In effect, the system defaults and fails to deal with the problem. Such failure (assuming the problem persists) is likely to have dysfunctional consequences for the system (for example, strain), including the possibility of a crisis and a tendency to "entropy" (Baker, 1973; Katz and Kahn, 1966) or disorganization.

The present framework, with minor modifications, can also be used to understand problem solving within each of the major problem areas. (In the above matrix, the concepts of stability and agreement may be substituted for the concept of certainty, and those of instability and disagreement may be substituted for that of uncertainty.) The problem of adaptation, for example, may be analyzed by reference to the stability of the external affairs of the EU system, if the certainty/uncertainty dimension regarding outcome preferences were replaced by the concept of stability/ instability of preferences for adaptation outcomes.

Similarly, the relevance of various approaches to solving resource allocation problems could be analyzed by reference to the stability/instability of available resources and to the agreement/ disagreement regarding the distribution of these resources among system components. Finally, the relevance/appropriateness of the various approaches to solving the coordination problem may be analyzed by reference to the stability/instability and other characteristics of the patterns of interdependence among performers in the system and the relative certainty regarding the activities to be performed in order to resolve the coordination problems.

Interrelations Among Problem Areas and
Consequences of Problem Solving

Significant interrelationships among the major problem areas are logically inevitable, with respect to both problem generation and problem resolution, because of the pervasive interdependence that characterizes organizations. Because of interdependence, change in one aspect or part of the system has consequences for the rest: difficulties in a particular area have implications for the nature of the problems that the system will encounter in the other areas; similarly, the resolution of difficulties in one area has implications for problem resolution in the rest. The specific consequences may be strong or weak, direct or indirect, immediate or delayed, and so on, depending upon the magnitude of the difficulty and efficacy of solution reached, and depending upon the specific problem areas examined. (The general consequences of problem solving are discussed in the next section.)

Interdependence is not the only reason for the expected interrelationships among problem areas. The other basic properties of the system are also involved, particularly with regard to the generation of problems. It was noted earlier that the problems of adaptation, resource allocation, coordination, integration, strain, and maintenance partly have their origins in the system's properties. It was also noted that particular properties are associated with specific problems. However, since the different properties are interrelated, so are the problems encountered in the different areas. Thus, certain problems can arise simultaneously in different areas because they are the result of different but interrelated properties. For example, the system properties of external constancy and internal continuity are interrelated and, as such, may simultaneously give rise to problems of adaptation and maintenance. In addition, of course, certain problems may arise simultaneously in different areas because they originate in one and the same system property. For example, problems of both integration and resource allocation can arise as the system tends toward increased differentiation.

Just as the problems in the various areas are interrelated at the point of their generation, they are also interrelated at the point of their resolution. First, other things being equal, successful problem solving in one area may generalize into other areas due to interdependence. Second, the problem areas may be interrelated, in respect to the extent to which they are ameliorated, because there are certain similarities in the ways in which the various problems are solved (as discussed earlier). Adequate problem solving generally presupposes some recognition and acceptance of the problem, selection (not necessarily systematic or always deliberate) of a performance program relevant to the problem, and the implementation of activities implied by the program(s) selected. The efficacy of implementing programs intended to solve different problems—regardless of the area to which the problem belongs—in turn depends upon the availability of appropriate structural bases. To the extent that performance programs and activities relevant to different problem areas rely on the same or similar bases, some consistency in the adequacy of problem solving across problem areas also may be expected. Furthermore, a particular first-order structure, such as the role structure, in the system may serve as the base for generating multipurpose performance programs, that is, programs for resolving problems in more than one area. To the extent that this is the case, adequate problem solving in one area should correlate to some degree with adequate problem solving in other areas.

Third, problem solving in one area may directly facilitate *or* hinder problem solving in another area. Other things being equal, for example, adequate resolution of the integration problem will probably facilitate the amelioration of coordination and adaptation problems. Integration is especially important as a facilitator to coordination and adaptation problem solving when nonprogrammed solutions are appropriate. Nonprogrammed solutions are more likely to be pursued by system members when integration is perceived to be adequate, and when integration is adequate, nonprogrammed activities are more likely to be performed effectively. However, adequate problem solving in one area may also exacerbate the difficulties encountered in another area. For example, the differential allocation of resources, authority, information, and the like to various groups and members may increase differentiation and make the problem of integration more difficult to solve. Similarly, successful resolution of the maintenance problem may hinder, counteract, or cancel out solutions to the adaptation problem or exacerbate the problem of strain.

Fourth, whether adequate or inadequate, the resolution of problems in certain areas may *generate* problems in other areas. It was noted earlier that the problem of strain may be a derived or second-order problem. Strain can arise not only as a result of basic system properties (for example, organization-environmental interdependence) but also as a result of inadequate problem solving in other areas (for example, coordination). Further, strain can arise as a result of simultaneously solving problems in the other major areas. Simultaneous efforts aimed at solving an adaptation problem and a maintenance problem imply the performance of activities which may be inconsistent: activities related to adaptation require some structural flexibility, for example, while those related to maintenance require stability. The concurrent or sequential carrying out of antithetical activities will generate strain—a second-order problem which must be solved by the system.

Finally, the adequacy of problem solving in one area may be either positively or negatively related to the adequacy of problem solving in the other areas as a result of the criteria of rationality that are applied in resolving problems. In an EU, problems may be dealt with in terms of economic, social, and/or clinical criteria of rationality.* (This implies that as many as three different four-cell matrices, such as illustrated in Figure A-2, may be relevant to each problem area, depending on how many of the different criteria of rationality are used.) The criteria of rationality used to resolve problems in a particular area may have either positive or negative consequences for problem solving in other areas. For example, if economic rationality criteria are used when handling resource allocation problems, the integration and strain problems may become more difficult to resolve. If social and/or clinical rationality criteria are applied in allocating resources, on the other hand, the solution of integration and strain problems

*We define rationality as the principle of making decisions according to known, or presumed, cause-and-effect relations or means-ends relations. Such relations may involve economic, social-psychological, or clinical/service considerations. The corresponding three kinds of rationality need not be congruent or mutually compatible (see Georgopoulos, 1982).

may be facilitated at the same time. For example, integration may be enhanced and strain may be reduced because the outcomes of allocation based on such a process are more acceptable to members (for example, allow members discretion), and the way in which resources are distributed may make the outcome of resource allocation more satisfactory to the members.

Overall, with regard to problem-solving adequacy, the interrelationships across problem areas are expected to be positive. Although some negative relationships could result due to opposing forces or incompatible requirements such as those mentioned in the preceding discussion, it seems that such inverse relationships will be relatively infrequent, generally being counteracted and offset by positive forces. At the same time, the interrelationships among the various problem areas are not expected to be equally strong or uniformly high or low. Depending upon the areas compared, the correlation patterns will vary, as will the magnitude of the corresponding correlations. (The differential strength of such interrelationships is supported by the data reported by Georgopoulos and Matejko, 1967.) The generally positive nature of problem-solving interrelationships across the various areas is illustrated in Figure A-3.

Figure A-3. Interrelationships Among Problem Areas.

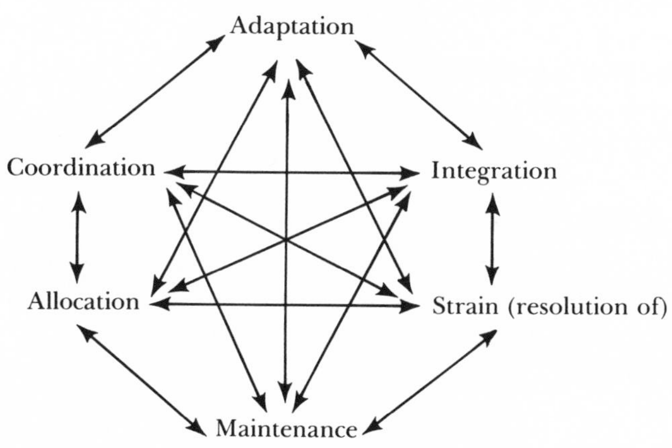

Consequences of Problem Solving

Problem solving on the part of EU members, or groups of members, will have at least four major consequences. First, the efficacy of problem solving within a given area will imply both adequate resolution (albeit temporary) of the particular problem and enhancement of the system property most associated with the problem. For example, efficacious problem solving in the area of coordination will imply both more adequate coordination than previously and increased facilitative interdependence in the system. Second, as already pointed out, problem solving in one area may facilitate or hinder problem solving in other areas. Third, over the long run, problem solving in the major areas discussed may imply changes in the basic, first-order structures of the system. Fourth, and most important, adequate problem solving will promote and correlate positively with the overall organizational effectiveness of the system. As the first two consequences have been already discussed, the following discussion will focus on the latter two consequences.

Consequences for the Structural Arrangements of the System. First-order structures, such as the role structure, have been distinguished from second-order structures (performance programs) and third-order structures (performance activities). First-order structures provide a base on which system members can rely for selecting and carrying out performance programs and the activities dictated by the particular programs. Compared to the first-order structures of the system, performance programs are relatively unstable structures (March and Simon, 1958), and activities are even more unstable and temporary than the corresponding performance programs. If such activities recur with some regularity, however, over time they can become institutionalized and incorporated into performance programs (that is, second-order structures) and eventually even lead to modification of the system's first-order structures.*

---

*It may be noted at this point that much of what "leadership" entails is coextensive with performance activities (third-order structures), the specification of such activities in performance programs (second-order

If the activities in question are specified by existing performance programs (that is, by the second-order structures of the system), then to some extent they are patterned and "structured" to begin with—they constitute third-order structures. More important, those of the specified activities which prove successful in resolving some major problem are likely to be invoked again when dealing with similar difficulties in the future. After this process is repeated a number of times, the particular activities will not only become a stable and integral aspect of the performance program(s) which dictated them initially but also may be institutionalized and incorporated into the roles of the members, thus becoming a part of a basic first-order structure. In other words, existing roles in the system may be revised, redefined, or expanded as a result of institutionalizing performance activities that initially constituted third-order structures.

If, on the other hand, the activities in question were not specified by some performance program but instead were "selected" on a discretionary basis or were tried during the process of program implementation, then they would probably be specified in future performance programs (and thus become third-order structures) to the extent that they proved efficacious. The same applies to *informal* discretionary activities:* if they recur and prove efficacious, they will be used again in solving problems and thus become third-order structures that in the future are specified by particular performance programs (second-order structures). Subsequently, of course, such activities also may lead eventually to modification of the basic first-order structures of the system through the above-outlined process.

Our treatment of organizational structure, it might be noted, is different from though not incompatible with that of other

---

structures), and/or the selection and monitoring of performance programs and activities.

*Performance programs may stipulate or mandate specific activities or may merely call for relevant discretionary activities. Performers may, in addition, engage in informal discretionary activities, that is, activities outside any program specification, in the process of solving a problem.

organization system theorists. For example, following Allport (1962), Katz and Kahn define organizational structure in terms of interrelated sets of events "which return upon themselves to complete and renew a cycle of activities" (1966, p. 21). Such activities are viewed within our framework as relatively unstable aspects of structure, which are based on the more stable second-order structures and basic first-order structures of the system. Nevertheless, some of these activities—those which recur over time, prove efficacious, and become institutionalized—can have important implications for the vertical and horizontal ordering of the system's components, and therefore consequences for the basic structural arrangements of the system. Alterations in the basic structure of the system may be the result. Such alterations, however, could have either positive or negative consequences. For example, they could be dysfunctional if they occasioned goal displacement or organizational rigidities (Gouldner, 1954; Merton, 1957) in the process. Additionally, structures evolving from the institutionalization of recurring performance activities could be single-purpose or special-purpose structures that might not facilitate problem solving in other areas. On the other hand, some of them might be multipurpose structures and thus promote problem solving in more than one problem area.

Consequences for System Effectiveness. Finally, the effectiveness of an organization such as an EU is mainly a function of the problem-solving behavior of the system in the major problem areas discussed. Here, the EU has been viewed and treated as a complex work-performing and problem-solving system (although, strictly speaking, the EU is a *sub*system of an even more complex system—its parent hospital). The organizational problems to be solved by hospital EUs have been described, as have the basic properties and structures of the system, together with the interrelationships among structures, problems, and properties.

Special emphasis has been placed upon the consequences and implications of the system's structures for problem solving, mainly because the relevance of the nature of the work to be done and of the qualifications of components to problem solving is considerably more obvious and more familiar than is the relevance of system properties. It should be obvious, for example, that the competence of the performers (a major qualification of the system's components) is a critical determinant of the quantity and quality of work that gets done. Other "qualifications," such as member motivation and involvement, commitment to organizational values and objectives, participation in decision making and problem solving, and other similar psychological characteristics, are likewise important as "independent variables" in relation to work performance and problem solving. Similarly, the nature of work to be done—in terms of its human and technical requirements or such things as task complexity, specialization, professionalization, variability, uncertainty, routinization, functional interdependence, and general homogeneity/heterogeneity of inputs and outputs—has important implications for both work performance and problem solving.

The relevance of the system's structures and properties to problem solving has been discussed in great detail in the preceding pages. Very briefly, the organization's structures were seen as the basic problem-solving framework of the system, and the basic properties of the system (along with the nature of work to be done and the qualifications of the performers) were seen as the sources of the major organizational problems that the system encounters along its input-transformation-output work cycle. Thus, structures, properties, and problems were all carefully considered and related to one another theoretically.

Here, the principal objective was to develop a working conceptual-theoretical framework for the study and understanding of the EU as a complex work-performing and problem-solving system. In our view, such a framework is essential to assessing the overall organizational effectiveness of EUs. Effectiveness was viewed as a joint outcome of the clinical, economic, and social efficiency of the organization (these three kinds of efficiency, which need not be mutually reinforcing or capable of compensating for one another, correspond to the three kinds of rationality that were discussed in relation to problem solving). In turn, the overall efficiency of an EU in each of these three areas is expected to be a joint (and probably unequally weighted) function of the problem-solving outcomes achieved by the system in the major problem areas discussed. Schematically, our

Figure A-4. Outline of the Research Model.

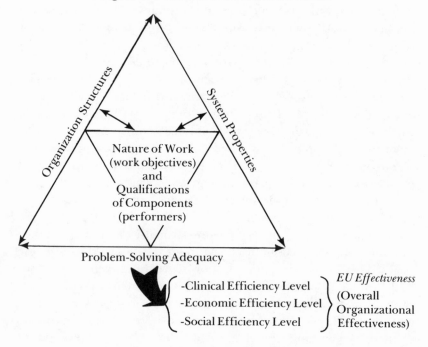

theoretical expectations concerning system effectiveness are outlined in Figure A-4.

Concluding Note

Further elaboration of this research model, as applied and implemented in the present study of hospital emergency services, is presented throughout this book. The model is depicted more fully in Figure 1-1 of the book. The specific hypotheses tested in the study concern relationships among some of the variables specified by this model, and especially relationships between organizational structure and problem solving, on the one hand, and emergency unit effectiveness, on the other. These hypotheses and the empirical findings pertaining to them, in turn, provide additional elaboration of the research model (see Chapters Eight, Nine, and Ten).

Study Sample:
Design and Sampling Error

The population of organizations for this study consisted of 436 nongovernmental, not-for-profit hospitals for short-term care which have emergency departments and bed capacities for inpatient care in the range of 100 to 499 beds. The hospitals were located in six states of the North Central Region: Michigan, Ohio, Indiana, Illinois, Wisconsin, and Minnesota.

Research interest focuses on some aspects of hospital emergency department services that are assumed to be independent of the number of beds in the parent hospital for inpatient care. Nevertheless, for purposes of sampling and analysis, the hospitals were assigned to three size groups according to the total number of beds (including beds for extended as well as short-term care) reported in the 1976 edition of the *Guide to the Health Care Field* (American Hospital Association, 1976). The three size groups were 100–199 beds, 200–299 beds, and 300–499 beds. These groups contain roughly equal numbers of hospitals.

The Standard Metropolitan Statistical Area (SMSA) (Executive Office of the President, Office of Management and Budget, 1975) classification was used to approximate an urban-rural

Note: This technical account incorporates material from two memoranda about the sample of the study written by staff of the Sampling Section of the Survey Research Center, under the direction of Irene Hess. The Sampling Section drew the sample and later performed the sampling error computations discussed here.

categorization. Hospitals in any part of an SMSA were so classified; all other hospitals were assigned to the non-SMSA class.

Using the probability sampling technique of controlled selection (Goodman and Kish, 1950; Groves and Hess, 1975), a sample of forty-four hospitals was selected, with equal probability after stratification by geographical location, size group, and SMSA class. Two considerations prompted the choice of equal selection probabilities: (1) there were no data specific to emergency services, and none were to be collected prior to the interviewing phase of the study; and (2) approximately equal numbers of sample hospitals from the three size groups were desired, so that each group could be analyzed separately. The distributions of the population and of the sample are displayed in Table B-1.

A fourth stratification variable, hospital control, had two classes: (1) church-related and (2) all other not-for-profit hospitals. In the population, there are 140 hospitals in the first class and 296 in the second. To simplify the selection of 44 hospitals from seventy-two potential groups (six states, three size groups, two SMSA classes, two control groups), the fourth variable was less strictly controlled than were the first three. As shown in Table B-2, 16 church-related hospitals and 28 other not-for-profit hospitals were selected for the sample, a minor departure from the expected sample size of 14.2 and 29.9.

The research design required that all emergency department medical and nursing staffs be included in the study. There was no sampling of staff. Therefore, sampling was at one stage only: the selection of hospitals with an emergency unit (EU) or department. The research design specified a sample of approximately 10 percent. In consultation with the research staff, we chose to fix the sample size at 44, implying a sampling rate of 44:436 (or 1:9.909).

The research staff requested that four stratification variables be considered: size group, state, urbanization, and control (or ownership). The first three variables have three, six, and two classes, resulting in thirty-six subgroups or cells in the cross-tabulations. Distributing forty-four selections across thirty-six cells is already a thinly spread sample without increasing the cells to seventy-two by adding the fourth stratification variable with two classes. Further, the available computer program for controlled selection (Goodman and Kish, 1950; Groves and Hess, 1975) could accept no more than three control variables. To make forty-four selections from seventy-two cells using a manual procedure would have been an excessively time-consuming and difficult operation. Therefore, we elected to use the computer to generate the controlled sample selection. It was our understanding that of the four stratification variables, the first three were to be given priority; this was done, as can be seen in Table B-1.

Two other decisions were necessary before the sample selection could proceed: What selection probability was to be assigned to each hospital? How were measures of sampling variability to be calculated?

Equal selection probabilities, initially proposed by the research staff, appeared to be the best choice after considering the following factors:

- Because no measure of emergency service for each hospital was available, equal selection seemed as reasonable as (if not more reasonable than) probabilities proportionate to number of beds for inpatient care.
- Since the population was defined to be relatively homogeneous and the range in bed capacity was restricted to 100–499 beds, we could not argue strongly for varying selection probabilities by size groups.
- Because the nature of the research required no sampling within emergency departments, the analysis could be simplified if weights (to correct for disproportionate sampling) were not introduced.
- Another possibility, also rejected, was the formation of explicit strata or homogeneous groups of hospitals. We could not form 44 strata of equal size from a population of 436 hospitals when size was defined as the number of hospitals. Approximately equal-sized strata would have been sufficient if sampling continued through additional stages; but with only one stage of sampling, selection probabilities would have remained unequal.

Although probability selection would seem to guarantee that estimates of sampling variability could be calculated from the

Table B-1. Distributions of the Population and Sample of General Hospitals for Short-Term Care, by State, Size Group, and SMSA Class.

	All Groups			Group 1 (100–199 beds)			Group 2 (200–299 beds)			Group 3 (300–499 beds)		
Classification	Total	SMSA	Non-SMSA	Total	SMSA	Non-SMSA	Total	SMSA	Non-SMSA	Total	SMSA	Non-SMSA
1	2	3	4	5	6	7	8	9	10	11	12	13
All States												
Population	436	312	124	165	92	73	129	87	42	142	133	9
Sample size												
Expected	44.00	31.49	12.51	16.65	9.28	7.37	13.01	8.78	4.23	14.34	13.43	0.91
Actual	44	31	13	17	9	8	13	9	4	14	13	1
Michigan												
Population	76	58	18	30	17	13	23	18	5	23	23	0
Sample size												
Expected	7.67	5.85	1.82	3.03	1.71	1.32	2.32	1.82	.50	2.32	2.32	0
Actual	7	5	2	3	1	2	2	2	0	2	2	0
Ohio												
Population	99	72	27	35	22	13	33	22	11	31	28	3
Sample size												
Expected	9.99	7.27	2.72	3.53	2.22	1.31	3.33	2.22	1.11	3.13	2.83	.03
Actual	10	7	3	3	2	1	4	2	2	3	3	0

Indiana												
Population	36	24	12	11	4	7	6	2	4	19	18	1
Sample size												
Expected	3.63	2.42	1.21	1.11	.40	.71	.60	.20	.40	1.92	1.82	.10
Actual	4	3	1	2	1	1	0	0	0	2	2	0
Illinois												
Population	130	105	25	42	28	14	44	34	10	44	43	
Sample size												
Expected	13.12	10.60	2.52	4.24	2.83	1.41	4.44	3.43	1.01	4.44	4.34	
Actual	14	11	3	4	2	2	5	4	1	5	5	
Wisconsin												
Population	63	34	29	28	12	16	18	8	10	17	14	3
Sample size												
Expected	6.36	3.43	2.93	2.82	1.21	1.61	1.82	.81	1.01	1.72	1.41	.31
Actual	6	3	3	3	2	1	1	0	1	2	1	1
Minnesota												
Population	32	19	13	19	9	10	5	3	2	8	7	1
Sample size												
Expected	3.23	1.92	1.31	1.92	.91	1.01	.50	.30	.20	.81	.71	.10
Actual	3	2	1	2	1	1	1	1	0	0	0	0

Note: The population is restricted to nongovernment, not-for-profit hospitals with emergency units.
Source: American Hospital Association, 1976.

sample, that condition may be only approximately met with some sample designs. We considered two procedures; the second procedure was eventually chosen.

> *Procedure 1.* Allocating 22 primary selections to the 36 cells of the cross-tabulations; then selecting not one but two hospitals from each cell designed for a primary selection. We would then use a paired selection model to calculate sampling errors (Kish and Hess, 1949). Actually, it would be necessary to sacrifice some of the stratification by combining cells to ensure that every cell retained in the selection process had a minimum of two hospitals.

> *Procedure 2.* Allocating 44 selections to the 36 cells and using a successive difference model to calculate approximately measures of sampling variability, although these measures do not reflect the refinements that we believe the stratification gives to the sample data (Kish and Hess, 1949).

Table B-1 shows the cross-tabulations of the population by size group, state, and SMSA class, the expected sample size from each cell, and the actual number of sample hospitals from each. The expected sample size is recorded to two decimal places. The whole number to the left of the decimal is the minimum sample size, and the fraction on the right of the decimal may be interpreted as the probability of obtaining one more than the minimum number from a cell. For example, the expected sample size from Michigan is 7.67; the minimum sample is 7, and the probability of one more selection is .67. The actual number of sample hospitals from Michigan turned out to be 7.

The expected sample sizes from the 36 cells and their marginals, given the sampling rate of 1:9.909, comprise the input to the computer, which then generated 100 possible samples, not necessarily all different, each satisfying the 36 expectations and the marginals. Collectively, the 100 samples satisfied the probabilities for the minimum and the maximum samples from each cell of Table B-1. In the case of Michigan, 67 of the 100 samples had 8 selections from Michigan and 33 had 7. Similarly, 63 of the 100 samples had 4 selections from Indiana and 37 had 3.

From the 100 samples generated by the computer, one was chosen to be the sample of hospitals for the study of emergency department services. The actual sample was the third of each set of three lines in Table B-1.

There remained the task of identifying sample hospitals from each cell having one or more sampling selections. Notice that within each cell the sample satisfies controls by state, size group, and SMSA class. We next introduced some stratification by ownership, subject to the restrictions of the ownership distributions within the designated cells. As sampling continued independently within cells having two or more selections, a modest geographical control was added (for example, Chicago SMSA versus the other SMSAs in Illinois). When only one selection was to be made from a cell, a control on ownership across those cells was introduced. Of the 44 sample hospitals, 16 are church-operated, only a slight departure from an expectation of 140/9.909 or 14.12, which could become either 14 or 15 when the number was rounded. One should not expect that, for all characteristics of interest, the sample would conform to the population as closely as it did for variables used as controls.

With the exception that the hospital participation rate turned out to be somewhat lower than expected, the sample was executed as designed. In Table B-2, the distributions of the total sample (participating and nonparticipating hospitals) are shown. When nearly a third of the sample is withdrawn on a "subjective" basis, such as nonresponse, the remainder is no longer a strict probability sample. What population did the remainder represent? How were sample data to be interpreted? Should nonparticipating hospitals have been replaced with subjectively selected hospitals? Should data from participating hospitals have been weighted to adjust for nonresponse? How could measures of sampling variability have been estimated from sample data? How were estimates of sampling errors affected by the bias of nonresponse? There were no clear answers to these questions. During the data collection period, the research staff chose to make no substitutions for nonparticipating hospitals; furthermore, analysis plans did not include weight adjustments for nonresponding hospitals. Yet some measures of sampling variability were desired for estimated means of the form

$$\overline{m} = \frac{\sum\limits_{i=1}^{30} m_i}{\sum\limits_{i=1}^{30} n_i} \quad , \text{where} \quad m_i = \frac{Y_i}{X_i} = \frac{\sum\limits_{j} Y_{ij}}{\sum\limits_{j} X_{ij}}$$

The subscript j identifies an individual staff member, and Y_i and X_i include all elements (staff members) in the study population within the ith emergency unit; no sampling is involved within sampled units. For example, Y_{ij} might be an attitudinal scale value for the X_{ij} respondent in the EU of the ith hospital. $\sum\limits_{j} Y_{ij}$ would be the sum of the scale values and $\sum\limits_{j} X_{ij}$ the total number of respondents in the ith hospital; m_i is then the mean scale value for the ith hospital, of which there were $\sum\limits_{i} n_i = 30$ participating in the study.

The sample of 44 emergency departments may be regarded as sample selections from 44 strata, one selection per stratum. Although when only one primary selection is made from a stratum there are no exact formulas for the calculation of measures of sampling variability, sampling errors may still be approximated using a successive difference model of the type appropriate for the selection of systematic samples (Kish and Hess, 1949, pp. 429–430). However, with data from only 30 of the 44 sample selections, a requirement that each of the 44 strata be represented in the sample can no longer be met. Uncertain of the effects of nonresponse, calculations were made for estimated means of particular interest to the research staff, using two different procedures: (1) only 30 strata in the population were assumed and the sampling errors were calculated using the successive difference model and (2) the 44 strata were retained, assuming the 14 nonparticipating hospitals had means of zero, and then proceeding with the successive difference calculations. The calculations resulting from these two procedures, presented in Table B-3, are quite similar. In each case, the denominator or base of the ratio is the number of hospitals reporting data. In Procedure 2, the 14 nonparticipating hospitals make a nonzero contribution to the variance calculation but leave the mean unaffected.

Table B-2. Distribution of the Sample of General Hospitals for Short-Term Care by Participation in Data Collection, Control, Size Group, and SMSA Class.

	All Groups			Group 1 (100–199 beds)			Group 2 (200–299 beds)			Group 3 (300–499 beds)		
Classification	Total	SMSA	Non-SMSA	Total	SMSA	Non-SMSA	Total	SMSA	Non-SMSA	Total	SMSA	Non-SMSA
1	2	3	4	5	6	7	8	9	10	11	12	13
All classes												
Number	44	31	13	17	9	8	13	9	4	14	13	1
Percent	100.0	70.5	29.5	38.6	20.5	18.2	29.5	20.5	9.1	31.8	29.5	2.3
Church-related												
Number	16	10	6	5	2	3	5	3	2	6	5	1
Percent	36.3	22.7	13.6	11.4	4.5	6.8	11.4	6.8	4.5	13.6	11.4	2.3
Other not-for-profit												
Number	28	21	7	12	7	5	8	6	2	8	8	0
Percent	63.6	47.7	15.9	27.2	15.9	11.4	18.2	13.6	4.5	18.2	18.2	0
Participating												
Number	30	21	9	12	7	5	9	6	3	9	8	1
Percent	68.2	47.7	20.5	27.2	15.9	11.4	20.5	13.6	6.8	20.5	18.2	2.3
Church-related												
Number	10	6	4	3	1	2	3	2	1	4	3	1
Percent	22.7	13.6	9.1	6.8	2.3	4.5	6.8	4.5	2.3	9.1	6.8	2.3
Other not-for-profit												
Number	20	15	5	9	6	3	6	4	2	5	5	0
Percent	45.5	34.1	11.4	20.5	13.6	6.8	13.6	9.1	4.5	11.4	11.4	0
Nonparticipating												
Number	14	10	4	5	2	3	4	3	1	5	5	0
Percent	31.8	22.7	9.1	11.4	4.5	6.8	9.1	6.8	2.3	11.4	11.4	0
Church-related												
Number	6	4	2	2	1	1	2	1	1	2	2	0
Percent	13.6	9.1	4.5	4.5	2.3	2.3	4.5	2.3	2.3	4.5	4.5	0
Other not-for-profit												
Number	8	6	2	3	1	2	2	2	0	3	3	0
Percent	18.2	13.6	4.5	6.8	2.3	4.5	4.5	4.5	0	6.8	6.8	0

Table B-3. Estimated Means and Approximate Sampling Errors Calculated by Two Procedures.

Variable Number[a]	Estimated Mean	Base of Mean	Procedure 1[b]		Procedure 2[b]	
			Standard Error of Mean	$\left[\dfrac{Var\,(M)}{SRV\,(M)}\right]^{1/2}$[c]	Standard Error of Mean	$\left[\dfrac{Var\,(M)}{SRV\,(M)}\right]^{1/2}$[c]
1	2	3	4	5	6	7
230	2.07	30	.093	1.0203	.088	.9713
231	2.48	30	.099	.9887	.100	.9987
406	2.36	30	.055	.8673	.053	.8312
311	68.76	30	4.404	.9211	4.221	.8828
217	124.10	30	8.711	.8511	9.860	.9633
322	2.55	30	.127	1.1579	.115	1.0531
238	2.00	30	.048	1.1938	.045	1.1322
141	16.46	30	2.320	.9120	2.602	1.0231
110	348.28	30	32.906	.7679	38.510	.8986
219	238.87	30	16.729	.7483	19.627	.8779
409	2.70	30	.096	1.0171	.098	1.0353
414	3.11	30	.082	.9615	.078	.9190
383	2.46	30	.067	.8914	.069	.9223
386	2.39	30	.164	1.0313	.164	1.0287
136	6.42	30	.441	.8545	.505	.9787
137	8.81	30	.655	.9542	.663	.9684
100	4.37	30	.520	.9483	.517	.9431
101	2.21	29	.379	.8364	.433	.9564
102	6.93	30	.818	.8289	.868	.8797

Notes:
[a]See Table B-4 for descriptions of variables.
[b]Procedure 1 assumes a probability sample of 30 hospitals. Procedure 2 assumes a probability sample of 44 hospitals with means of zero assigned to the 14 nonparticipating hospitals.
[c]SRV denotes simple random variance, assuming the estimated mean and sample size reported for the sample.

Table B-4. Description of Estimated Means in Table B-3.

Variable Number	Description	Data Source	Type of Estimate
230	If, in the next two months, patient visits were to *increase by 10%–15%* but the quality of patient care were to remain at its current level, how well could the present staff of this Emergency Unit handle the increased patient volume? (1) Handle without any difficulties; (2) Some minor difficulties; (3) Moderate difficulties; (4) Great difficulties; (5) Very great difficulties; (6) Could not handle it at all.	Medical doctors' questionnaires	Mean scale
231	Same as 230.	Registered Nurses' questionnaires	Mean scale
406	On the basis of your experience and information, how would you rate the *quality of nursing care* that patients generally receive in the Emergency Unit? (1) Outstanding; (2) Excellent; (3) Very good; (4) Good; (5) Fair; (6) Rather poor; (7) Poor.	MDs' questionnaires	Mean scale
311	Currently, does the Emergency Unit have any written agreements ("transfer protocols") or informal agreements with other institutions for *sending particular patients to other hospitals* or emergency facilities?	MDs' interviews	Percent "Yes" responses
217	Ordinarily, about how many *hours a week do you work in this Emergency Unit?*	MDs' questionnaires	Total number of hours for all MDs
322	At the present time, *what kind of reputation* does this Emergency Unit have in the community outside? (1) Excellent; (2) Very good; (3) Good; (4) Fair; (5) Rather poor.	RNs' interviews	Mean scale
238	Overall, how well do the *different jobs and activities around the patient fit together* in the Emergency Unit? (1) Extremely well; (2) Very well; (3) Fairly well; (4) Not so well; (5) Not well at all.	RNs' interviews	Mean scale

Table B-4. Description of Estimated Means in Table B-3, Cont'd.

Variable Number	Description	Data Source	Type of Estimate
141	Does the Emergency Unit tend to concentrate on (or to specialize in) the treatment of any *particular kinds of patients?*	RNs' interviews	Percent "Yes" responses
110	What was the total *number of patient visits* to the Emergency Unit during the *most recent week* for which data are available?	Organizational records	Mean
219	Please provide the name and *number of hours worked* in the Emergency Unit for *each RN* (including the Supervisor of Nursing or Head Nurse) who worked there during the most recent week for which data are available.	Organizational records	Mean
409	Please consider the patients in the categories specified who visited this Emergency Unit over the past four–six weeks. On the average, how well were these patients managed from a medical standpoint? [Acute psychiatric illness—suicide (depression), acute psychoses] (1) Excellent; (2) Very good; (3) Good; (4) Fair; (5) Rather poor; (6) There were no such patients.	MDs' questionnaires	Mean scale
414	Same as 409.	RNs' questionnaires	Mean scale
383	Again, thinking of the same procedures, are most of them *appropriate* from the standpoint of enabling the staff to provide care at the *lowest cost possible?* (1) All or almost all very appropriate; (2) Large majority very appropriate; (3) Majority very appropriate; (4) About half very appropriate; (5) Fewer than half very appropriate.	MDs' questionnaires	Mean scale
386	On the whole, in the Emergency Unit, *how well performed* (or how well carried out) are the *medical treatment and nursing care procedures* from the standpoint of providing patient care at the lowest cost possible? (1) Extremely well performed; (2) Very well; (3) Fairly well; (4) Not so well; (5) Not performed well at all.	RNs' questionnaires	Mean scale

Table B-4. Description of Estimated Means in Table B-3, Cont'd.

Variable Number	Description	Data Source	Type of Estimate
136	Over the past four weeks, about what percent of the patients visiting the Emergency Unit arrived in what you would judge to be a "life-threatening" condition?	MDs' questionnaires	Mean percent
137	Same as 136.	RNs' questionnaires	Mean percent
100	Number of treatment rooms in Emergency Unit	Organizational records	Mean number
101	Number of other rooms available for Emergency Unit	Organizational records	Mean number
102	Number of beds in Emergency Unit	Organizational records	Mean number

Other variance calculation methods could be designed (reproducing data from similar hospitals to substitute for nonparticipating hospitals or weighing participating hospitals to compensate for nonresponse), but the purpose of the preceding exercise was an attempt to relate the variance calculations to the estimated means as computed by the analysts.

Table B-3, columns 5 and 7, show how the calculated variances compare with variances from simple random samples of the same number of participating hospitals. Most of the comparisons are close to but less than one, and only a few exceed one (moderately). This indicates that if the sample is regarded as a proper probability sample, then the precision of estimates is higher than those that would be obtained from a simple random sample of the same size. This finding was not unexpected, since the stratification should result in some gains. In general, it seems justifiable to conclude that variance calculations made under assumptions of simple random sampling of hospitals would produce estimates of sampling variances that are reasonable approximations to those that would have been obtained if the sample had been completed as designed. For estimates other than simple ratios, variance calculations were not explored.

Characteristics of Respondents and Local Populations

This appendix describes some of the characteristics of the individuals who provided data for the study. First, background data are presented about the several groups of respondents, including (1) those working in the emergency unit—physicians (MDs), registered nurses (RNs), and licensed practical nurses (LPNs); (2) those working in the parent hospital—hospital administrators (HAs) and hospital physicians (HMDs); and (3) community respondents (CRs). Information is provided about the length of association with their respective institutions, their main fields of interest or professional specialization, and other factors that may have a bearing on their attitudes and perspectives. For a variety of descriptive findings based on both attitudinal and nonattitudinal data provided by respondents, see Chapter Three; see also Georgopoulos, Cooke, and Associates (1980).

The patients (PATs) who completed questionnaires for the study are described in terms of the number of years they have lived in their respective communities, their age and sex, and their education and family income. Information about the patients' reasons for visiting the particular EU, as well as their usual sources of medical care, is also included.

Note: The material presented in Appendix C was published in substantially the same form in the appendix to Georgopoulos, Cooke, and Associates (1980) and is reproduced here with permission of the Institute for Social Research, publisher.

Also presented are certain data from U.S. Census reports regarding the local populations of the cities and towns in which the EUs studied are located. These data show the percentage of families with incomes below the "poverty level," the percentage of the city's population classified as minority population, and the median school years completed by persons twenty-five years old or older.

In examining the data included in this appendix, the reader should note that the percentages and mean scores shown in the various tables (with the exception of Table C-10) represent the percentage or average score for *individual* respondents rather than the mean or mean percentage score of hospitals or emergency units. The total number of respondents from all EUs combined, in each case, is indicated near the top of the columns in each table. The number of respondents for each of the various groupings of EUs shown in Table 2-2 may be greater than the corresponding number in the tables of this appendix because some individuals did not provide the relevant background information.

Selected Characteristics of Particular Respondents

The first three tables show, for particular groups of respondents, their length of professional experience, length of association with their respective hospitals, and length of time that they have been working in their emergency units.

Length of Professional Experience

Based on data obtained from questionnaires to each group of respondents, Table C-1 focuses on the professional work experience of EU MDs and RNs, and of the selected physicians (HMDs) from the parent hospitals of the emergency units. On the average, HMDs have been practicing medicine longer than the physicians (MDs) working in the EU; the former average 19.6 years of professional experience and the latter 12.3 years. The RNs (full and part time combined) in the same EUs average 13.1 years of professional experience.

Table C-1. Length of Professional Experience for Selected Groups of Respondents.

	Average Number of Years That		
Respondents Associated with	*RNs Have Been Working in Nursing*[a]	*MDs Have Been Practicing Medicine*[b]	*HMDs Have Been Practicing Medicine*[b]
All Emergency Units (EUs) in the Study	13.1	12.3	19.6
Sample	(N = 270)	(N = 211)	(N = 215)
EUs with:			
Low patient volume	14.1	12.7	16.8
Medium patient volume	12.2	9.3	19.6
High patient volume	13.0	14.4	21.2
EUs in:			
Church-operated hospitals	12.4	14.5	19.5
Osteopathic hospitals	12.9	3.9	14.2
All other hospitals	13.4	12.1	20.6
EUs Located in:			
SMSA (urban) areas	13.4	11.0	19.4
Non-SMSA areas	12.1	15.5	20.1
EUs in Hospitals Having:			
Medical teaching affiliations	12.6	11.9	19.5
No medical teaching affiliations	13.8	12.7	19.8
EUs in Hospitals Having:			
Emergency personnel training programs	13.2	13.0	18.8
No training programs	13.0	11.5	20.5

Notes: The results for each group of respondents are based on data about all of the individual respondents in the group from all institutions combined in each case. In other words, the numbers shown pertain to the membership of each group and are *not* institutional averages.

[a]Average number of years was computed from the responses of registered nurses (RNs) from the various EUs to the following question: "How long have you been working as a nurse?"

[b]Average number of years was computed from the responses of EU physicians (MDs), and selected hospital physicians (HMDs), to the following question: "How long have you been practicing medicine?"

The MDs in EUs with a medium patient volume have been practicing medicine for a shorter period of time than those in either low- or high-patient-volume EUs; this is even more pronounced for the MDs in osteopathic than in other institutions.

A similar pattern characterizes the HMDs, who, unlike the MDs, have been practicing medicine for a shorter period of time in hospitals whose EUs have a low, compared to either a medium or a high, patient volume. The RNs in the total sample, and also in most of the EU groupings, have been practicing nursing somewhat longer than the MDs have been practicing medicine. In three groupings, however, the reverse applies: in EUs with a high patient volume, in church-operated institutions, and in nonurban-area EUs.

Length of Association with Present Hospital

Information about the number of years that respondents have been associated with their present hospitals is provided in Table C-2. The HMDs, averaging 13.7 years, generally have been associated with their present hospitals longer than the hospital administrators (HAs) (12.0 years), the licensed practical nurses (LPNs) working full time in the EU (8.4 years), the RNs (7.8 years), or the MDs (7.2 years). Exceptions to this pattern are the HAs in nonurban-area hospitals and in hospitals without medical teaching affiliations, who, on the average, have been associated with their present institution slightly longer than the HMDs. It is rather interesting that, of all these groups, the emergency unit MDs and RNs have had the shortest association with their present hospitals.

The data also show that physicians working in low- and high-patient-volume EUs have been associated with their respective hospitals longer than have their colleagues in medium-volume units. Further, they and the HAs in nonurban areas have been associated with their present institutions longer than their counterparts in urban-area hospitals have. LPNs who work full time in EUs with a low patient volume generally have been with their present hospitals considerably fewer years (only 3.7 years) than have those who work in EUs with a medium or high patient volume (9.9 and 9.0 years, respectively). The length of association of RNs with their respective hospitals, which averages 7.8 years, does not vary significantly across the different groupings of EUs.

Table C-2. Length of Association with Their Respective Institutions for Selected Groups of Respondents.

Respondents Associated with	*Average Number of Years Associated with the Present Hospital for*				
	HAs	*HMDs*	*MDs*	*RNs*	*LPNs*[a]
All Emergency Units (EUs) in the Study Sample	12.0 (N = 68)	13.7 (N = 215)	7.2 (N = 211)	7.8 (N = 272)	8.4 (N = 47)
EUs with:					
Low patient volume	10.9	11.6	8.3	7.3	3.7
Medium patient volume	10.7	13.6	5.1	8.1	9.9
High patient volume	14.0	14.9	7.7	8.1	9.0
EUs in:					
Church-operated hospitals	10.1	12.0	9.5	7.5	9.7
Osteopathic hospitals	9.7	12.0	3.3	6.8	5.4
All other hospitals	13.3	14.5	6.3	8.2	8.7
EUs Located in:					
SMSA (urban) areas	10.5	13.8	6.0	7.6	8.2
Non-SMSA areas	16.3	13.4	10.3	8.5	9.4
EUs in Hospitals Having:					
Medical teaching affiliations	10.7	13.7	6.6	7.7	9.2
No medical teaching affiliations	14.2	13.6	7.8	8.0	6.2
EUs in Hospitals Having:					
Emergency personnel training programs	11.2	13.6	7.7	7.8	9.0
No training programs	13.0	13.8	6.7	7.8	7.9

Notes: The results for each group are based on data about all of the individual respondents in the group from all institutions combined in each case. Accordingly, the numbers of years shown pertain to the membership of each group and are *not* institutional averages. Average numbers of years were computed from the responses of the members of each group to the following question: "How long have you been working in (associated with) this hospital?"

[a]The LPN group includes only LPNs working full time; however, not all EUs had full-time LPNs.

Length of Association with the Emergency Unit

Table C-3 shows the percentage of MDs and RNs who have worked in their respective EUs for (1) less than one year and (2) four years or more. Overall, approximately 26 percent of the MDs and 26 percent of the RNs have worked in their present units for less than one year, but slightly more than 40 percent of them, in each case, have worked there for at least four years. Similarly (not

Table C-3. Length of Association with Their Respective Emergency Units for the Physicians (MDs) and Registered Nurses (RNs) Who Work There.

| Respondents Associated with | Percentage of Group Members Working in the Emergency Unit for | | | |
| | Less Than One Year | | Four Years or More | |
	MDs	RNs	MDs	RNs
All Emergency Units (EUs) in the Study Sample	26.4% (N = 208)	26.5% (N = 268)	43.3% (N = 208)	41.8% (N = 268)
EUs with:				
Low patient volume	24.7	32.1	46.9	38.5
Medium patient volume	29.5	25.3	32.8	42.7
High patient volume	25.8	23.5	48.5	43.5
EUs in:				
Church-operated hospitals	23.3	32.0	52.1	38.7
Osteopathic hospitals	29.4	21.4	29.4	32.1
All other hospitals	28.0	24.8	39.8	44.8
EUs Located in:				
SMSA (urban) areas	26.0	26.5	40.0	40.3
Non-SMSA areas	27.6	26.4	51.8	45.8
EUs in Hospitals Having:				
Medical teaching affiliations	25.2	22.9	46.8	40.1
No medical teaching affiliations	27.8	31.5	39.2	44.1
EUs in Hospitals Having:				
Emergency personnel training programs	23.1	24.3	45.2	43.9
No training programs	29.8	29.2	41.3	39.2

Note: The percentage figures shown for each group are based on data about all the individual respondents in the group from all institutions combined in each case. Accordingly, they pertain to the membership of each group and are *not* institutional averages. The percentages were computed from the responses of MDs and RNs to the following question: "How long have you been working in this Emergency Unit?"

shown in the table), 23 percent of the full-time LPNs have worked in their respective EUs less than one year, while 43 percent have worked for four years or more. A number of differences across EU groupings with respect to these patterns may also be seen in Table C-3.

Professional Specialization

Emergency unit MDs and RNs were also asked to indicate their major field of interest or specialty (data are not presented in table form). Of the RNs, 51 percent mentioned "emergency nursing" or "emergency medicine" in response to this question. The balance indicated surgery and/or operating room specialties (11 percent), intensive care or cardiac care (9 percent), supervision or administrative nursing (7 percent), and various other fields that together account for about 21 percent of all the RNs. These patterns differ somewhat across EU groupings. Most notably, a larger proportion of RNs in EUs with a high patient volume mention emergency nursing (59 percent) compared to the overall average of 51 percent, in contrast to their counterparts in EUs with a low patient volume (34 percent). Additionally, there is a larger percentage of supervisory/administrative and also surgery/operating room nurses, but a smaller percentage of nurses specializing in trauma, in church-operated units than in non-church-operated (excluding osteopathic) units. Also, proportionately more of the EU nurses are in supervision and administration in hospitals without medical teaching affiliations, and without emergency personnel training programs, than in hospitals with such affiliations or programs.

Compared to the large percentage of RNs who mentioned emergency nursing as their special field, a relatively small percentage of the MDs working in the units specified "emergency medicine." Of a total of 212 MDs responding to this question, only 12 percent indicated emergency medicine as their specialty. However, an additional 21 percent indicated surgery (including general surgery and "trauma medicine") or orthopedics as their field. It is also interesting to note, however, that 25 percent of all the MDs specified family practice or family medicine as their specialty—the largest percentage of responses received from any single medical specialty/field. An additional 17 percent of the MDs mentioned internal medicine or cardiology. Of the remaining, 9 percent indicated "general practice," 6 percent pediatrics, 3 percent obstetrics/gynecology, and the balance (a total of 7 percent) indicated other fields.

The percentage of MDs specializing in emergency medicine varies greatly across EU groupings. A much higher percentage of the MDs in osteopathic hospitals indicate emergency medicine (29 percent), for example, than of the MDs in other non-church-operated institutions (13 percent) or in church-operated institutions (5 percent). Similarly, a higher percentage of the MDs in urban-area units (14 percent) specialize in emergency medicine than in nonurban-area units (5 percent). The same is true of MDs in hospitals with medical teaching affiliations (18 percent) than without such affiliations (4 percent), and in hospitals with emergency personnel training programs (16 percent) than without such programs (8 percent). Finally, the higher the patient volume of the units, the greater the percentage of MDs who specialize in emergency medicine.

Membership in Certain Professional Associations

Emergency unit MDs and RNs were also asked whether they are currently members of the American College of Emergency Physicians (ACEP) or the Emergency Department Nurses Association (EDNA), respectively. About 22 percent of the RNs indicated that they are members of EDNA, and 25 percent of the MDs indicated that they are members of ACEP (data not shown in table form). A greater percentage of the MDs, and of the RNs, working in EUs with a high, compared to low, patient volume report membership in these associations. RNs in osteopathic hospital units are less likely to belong to EDNA than are those working in the units of other hospitals; and MDs in church-operated units are less likely to belong to ACEP than are those in non-church-operated units. Further, a much larger percentage of MDs in hospitals with medical teaching affiliations, and with emergency personnel training programs, belong to ACEP compared to MDs in hospitals without such affiliations or programs. A similar though weaker pattern characterizes the RNs with respect to membership in EDNA.

Demographic Characteristics

Respondents working in the EUs studied, as well as the hospital administrators, were asked to provide information about their age. In general, the administrators are the oldest group, followed by the emergency unit MDs, the RNs, and then the LPNs who work full time in the units. (The administrators group includes the chief executive officer of each hospital, the next highest administrative officer, if any, who has responsibility for the EU, and the hospital's director of nursing.) More specifically, 44 percent of the administrators, 20 percent of the physicians, 16 percent of the registered nurses, and 9 percent of the practical nurses are fifty years of age or older. Incidentally, 94 percent of the physicians working in the EUs are male, while 98 percent of the RNs are female.

Characteristics of EU Patients Who Participated in the Study

The tables in this section provide background data about the patients (PATs) who completed questionnaires for the study, including demographic data and information about the patients' reasons for visiting the EUs, and about the patients' usual sources of medical care. Participating patients included those over fifteen years of age who visited the EUs at any time from 8:00 A.M. Friday until 12:00 P.M. Saturday of the week during which each particular hospital was scheduled for on-site data collection, excluding those who were unable to, or who preferred not to, consent. In reviewing the data in this section (particularly in Tables C-5 and C-6), the reader should keep in mind the group of patients involved.

The first table in the series, Table C-4, concerns the length of time the PATs have lived in their present communities. Specifically, the table shows the percentage of PATs who have lived in their present communities for (1) two years or less and (2) more than ten years. Overall, more than half (57 percent) of the PATs have lived in their present communities for over ten years, and only about 20 percent of them have lived there less than two

**Table C-4. Length of Time Patient Respondents (PATs) Have Lived
in Their Present Communities.**

	Percentage of Patients Who Have Lived in Their Respective Communities for	
Respondents Associated with	*Two Years or Less*	*More Than Ten Years*
All Emergency Units (EUs) in the Study	18.8%	56.7%
Sample[a]	(N = 388)	(N = 388)
EUs with:		
Low patient volume	17.8	57.0
Medium patient volume	20.5	55.4
High patient volume	18.3	57.4
EUs in:		
Church-operated hospitals	15.1	54.7
Osteopathic hospitals	20.0	51.1
All other hospitals	19.3	57.9
EUs Located in:		
SMSA (urban) areas	20.7	53.9
Non-SMSA areas	15.2	62.1
EUs in Hospitals Having:		
Medical teaching affiliations	19.6	54.2
No medical teaching affiliations	17.6	60.8
EUs in Hospitals Having:		
Emergency personnel training programs	18.6	56.4
No training programs	19.0	57.1

Notes: The percentage figures shown are based on data about all of the PATs from all institutions combined in each case. Accordingly, they pertain to the collectivity of patients and are *not* institutional averages. The percentages were computed from the responses of PATs to the following question: "How long have you lived in the community in which you now live?"

[a]Two of the hospitals in the study sample did not allow patient participation, and their EU PATs are therefore not included.

years. Moreover, there are no major differences across EU groupings with respect to the length of time that, on the average, patients have been living in their present communities. However, somewhat more of the patients in the urban-area units, compared to other units, have lived in their respective communities for two years or less. And somewhat fewer of the patients in osteopathic

**Table C-5. Percentage of Respondents from Each Specified Group
with the Sex and Age Characteristics Shown.**

Respondents Associated with	Percentage of CRs and Percentage of PATs Who Are Female		Percentage of PATs Who Are	
			16–25 Years Old	*65 Years or Older*
	CRs	*PATs*		
All Emergency Units (EUs) in the Study	10.0%	52.1%	36.1%	9.5%
Sample	(N = 201)	(N = 386)	(N = 388)	(N = 388)
EUs with:				
Low patient volume	11.4	38.5	44.3	7.6
Medium patient volume	14.3	65.8	31.3	15.2
High patient volume	5.3	49.7	35.5	7.1
EUs in:				
Church-operated hospitals	8.3	36.5	35.8	7.5
Osteopathic hospitals	18.8	75.6	37.8	8.9
All other hospitals	9.6	51.2	35.9	10.0
EUs Located in:				
SMSA (urban) areas	8.2	57.6	37.1	8.6
Non-SMSA areas	13.4	41.2	34.1	11.4
EUs in Hospitals Having:				
Medical teaching affiliations	8.1	54.8	34.2	9.6
No medical teaching affiliations	12.2	47.6	39.2	9.5
EUs in Hospitals Having:				
Emergency personnel training programs	4.7	48.8	36.8	8.3
No training programs	15.8	55.7	35.3	10.9

Note: The percentage figures shown are based on information reported by the respondents themselves—the patients (PATs) or the selected community respondents (CRs). They pertain to the collectivity of respondents from all institutions combined in each case, and are *not* institutional averages. (Two of the hospitals in the study sample did not allow patient participation, and their EU patients are therefore not included.)

hospitals, urban-area hospitals, and hospitals with teaching affiliations (compared to the other institutions in each case) have lived in their present community longer than ten years.

Table C-5 shows the sex and age distributions of the PATs who completed questionnaires for the study. The same table also shows the sex distribution of the selected community respondents

(CRs) who participated in the research. On the average, only 10 percent of the CRs are female, though the figure is somewhat higher for certain EU groupings (including EUs with a medium patient volume, the EUs of osteopathic hospitals, and the EUs of hospitals without training programs). As would be expected, on the other hand, a much larger percentage of the patients—namely, 52 percent—are female. The percentage of patients who are female is particularly high for EUs with a medium patient volume and EUs in osteopathic hospitals. Overall, 36.1 percent of the PATs are between sixteen and twenty-five years of age, while 9.5 percent are sixty-five years old or older. Proportionately, more of the PATs in EUs with a low, compared to either a medium or a high, patient volume are sixteen to twenty-five years old. And more of the patients in EUs with a medium, compared to a low or high, patient volume are sixty-five years old or older.

Information about the formal education of PATs is summarized in Table C-6. One-third of the patients have completed high school (but have not attended college), and an additional 25 percent have attended at least some college. The remaining patients have had less than a full high school education. Because a considerable number of PATs (12 percent) are between the ages of sixteen and eighteen, and an even higher number (36 percent) are between sixteen and twenty-five, many have not yet completed their formal education. There are no significant differences across EU groupings in the proportion of patients who have at least completed high school (around 59 percent on the average). However, the percentage of patients who have had at least some college education is higher for church-operated than for osteopathic EUs. It is also somewhat higher for urban- compared to nonurban-area units, and for the units of hospitals that have, compared to those that do not have, emergency personnel training programs.

Table C-7 provides data about the family income of patient respondents. It shows the percentage of PATs with family incomes (1) under $6,000 a year and (2) $20,000 a year or more (at the time of fieldwork). Overall, about 21 percent of the 351 patients who provided this information report a total family income of less than $6,000, and almost an equal proportion (22 percent) report a

**Table C-6. Percentage of EU Patients (PATs) with Specified
Levels of Formal Education.**

| | Percentage of Patients Who Have | |
| | Had at Least Some College Education | Completed High School Only |
Respondents Associated with		
All Emergency Units (EUs) in the Study	25.5%	33.0%
Sample	(N = 385)	(N = 385)
EUs with:		
Low patient volume	25.4	35.4
Medium patient volume	22.5	34.2
High patient volume	27.2	31.3
EUs in:		
Church-operated hospitals	32.0	30.2
Osteopathic hospitals	20.0	42.2
All other hospitals	25.1	32.1
EUs Located in:		
SMSA (urban) areas	27.4	32.5
Non-SMSA areas	21.6	33.8
EUs in Hospitals Having:		
Medical teaching affiliations	25.5	32.2
No medical teaching affiliations	25.3	34.2
EUs in Hospitals Having:		
Emergency personnel training programs	28.7	31.7
No training programs	21.9	34.4

Note: The percentage figures shown are based on the answers of patient respondents (PATs) to the following questionnaire item: "How much formal education have you had? (Check the *highest* completed.)" The response alternatives were (1) Grade school education only, (2) Some high school, (3) Completed high school, (4) Some college, (5) Completed college, (6) Completed more than four years of college, and (7) Other. The percentages pertain to the collectivity of patient respondents from all institutions combined in each case, and are *not* institutional averages.

family income of $20,000 or more. Proportionately, fewer of the patients in EUs with a low, compared to either a medium or a high, patient volume report a low family income, and the same is true for patients in church-operated compared to non-church-operated institutions. Conversely, a higher proportion of the patients in hospitals which are non-church-operated (excluding

**Table C-7. Percentage of Patient Respondents (PATs) Reporting
Particular Levels of Total Family Income.**

Respondents Associated with	Percentage of Patients Reporting a Family Income of	
	Less than $6,000	$20,000 or More
All Emergency Units (EUs) in the Study Sample	21.1% (N = 351)	22.2% (N = 351)
EUs with:		
Low patient volume	12.3	23.3
Medium patient volume	25.0	19.8
High patient volume	22.5	23.0
EUs in:		
Church-operated hospitals	10.5	16.7
Osteopathic hospitals	29.3	14.6
All other hospitals	21.7	24.4
EUs Located in:		
SMSA (urban) areas	20.6	27.9
Non-SMSA areas	22.1	11.0
EUs in Hospitals Having:		
Medical teaching affiliations	21.9	23.4
No medical teaching affiliations	19.7	20.5
EUs in Hospitals Having:		
Emergency personnel training programs	21.0	24.6
No training programs	21.3	19.4

Note: The percentages shown are based on the answers of patient respondents (PATs) to the following questionnaire item: "What was your *total family income* before taxes in 1976?" The response alternatives ranged from "(1) less than $2,000" to "(9) $30,000 or more." (Of all the patients in the study sample, 9.5 percent did not answer the question and are therefore excluded. Also excluded are patients from the two study hospitals that did not allow patient participation.) The percentages shown pertain to the collectivity of patient respondents from all institutions combined in each case and are *not* institutional averages.

osteopathic institutions) report a high family income compared to patients in both osteopathic and church-operated institutions. And, similarly, a larger proportion of the patients visiting urban, compared to nonurban, EUs report a high family income.

Patients' Reasons for Visiting the Emergency Unit

Each patient who participated in the study was asked the following question: "Why did you go to this particular emergency room instead of some other emergency room?" The question provided eleven different response alternatives, as noted in Table C-8. Overall, the reason most frequently selected by the patients was "This emergency room was the nearest one to go to" (selected by 31 percent of the PATs). The second and third most frequently selected reasons were "I (or my family) had used this emergency room before" (25 percent) and "I knew that the hospital is a good one" (10 percent). These three reasons together account for the responses of two-thirds of all the patients who completed questionnaires for the study.

The data also show, however, that patient responses to the above question differ from the general pattern for some of the EU groupings. For example, patients visiting EUs with a medium patient volume, and EUs in osteopathic hospitals, were much less likely than others to select "This emergency room was the nearest one to go to." Patients going to the units of osteopathic hospitals, and to medium-patient-volume units, were particularly likely to give as their reason "I (or my family) had used this emergency room before." This is also true of patients visiting emergency units in urban compared to nonurban areas, and units of hospitals with medical teaching affiliations compared to those without such affiliations.

The fourth most frequently selected reason was "My doctor told me to go there" (8 percent). And the fifth most frequently given reason was "This was the only available place to go for care" (selected by 6 percent of the patients). However, this last reason was given more often by patients who visited EUs with a low patient volume (15 percent), EUs in nonurban areas (11 percent), and EUs in hospitals without medical teaching affiliations (11 percent).

Patients' Usual Source(s) of Medical Care

Patient respondents were also asked: "When you or a member of your family needs medical attention, where do you

Table C-8. Percentage of Patients (PATs) Giving Particular Reasons for Visiting the Emergency Unit.

Hospital Emergency Units	Total Number of Patients	Three Reasons Most Frequently Selected by Patients, and the Percentage of Patients Selecting Them		
		First	Second	Third
All EUs in the Study Sample (N = 28 Hospital EUs)	387	This EU was the nearest (31.5%)	Had used this EU before (25.1%)	The hospital is a good one (10.3%)
EUs with:				
Low patient volume (N = 9)	79	This EU was the nearest (38.0%)	Had used this EU before (20.3%)	It was the only available place (15.2%)
Medium patient volume (N = 10)	111	Had used this EU before (31.5%)	This EU was the nearest (15.3%)	The hospital is a good one (12.6%)
High patient volume (N = 9)	197	This EU was the nearest (38.1%)	Had used this EU before (23.4%)	The hospital is a good one (10.2%)
EUs in:				
Church-operated hospitals (N = 8)	53	This EU was the nearest (37.7%)	Had used this EU before (17.0%)	My doctor told me to go to this EU (11.3%)
Osteopathic hospitals (N = 3)	45	Had used this EU before (46.7%)	My doctor told me to go to this EU (13.3%)	The hospital is a good one (8.9%)
All other hospitals (N = 17)	289	This EU was the nearest (34.3%)	Had used this EU before (23.2%)	The hospital is a good one (11.1%)

EUs Located in:				
SMSA (urban) areas (N = 19)	256	This EU was the nearest (30.1%)	Had used this EU before (28.5%)	The hospital is a good one (11.3%)
Non-SMSA areas (N = 9)	131	This EU was the nearest (34.4%)	Had used this EU before (18.3%)	It was the only available place (11.5%)
EUs in Hospitals Having:				
Medical teaching affiliations (N = 16)	239	Had used this EU before (28.9%)	This EU was the nearest (27.2%)	The hospital is a good one (13.4%)
No medical teaching affiliations (N = 12)	148	This EU was the nearest (38.5%)	Had used this EU before (18.9%)	It was the only available place (11.5%)
EUs in Hospitals Having:				
Emergency personnel training programs (N = 13)	204	This EU was the nearest (35.3%)	Had used this EU before (26.5%)	The hospital is a good one (11.3%)
No training programs (N = 15)	183	This EU was the nearest (27.3%)	Had used this EU before (23.5%)	The hospital is a good one (9.3%)

Note: The results shown are based on the responses of recent patients (PATs) from the various EUs to the following question: "Why did you go to this particular emergency room instead of some other emergency room? What would you say was the *main reason?*" The response alternatives were (1) I (or my family) had used this emergency room before, (2) I thought this would be a good emergency room, (3) I knew that the *hospital* is a good one, (4) This emergency room was the nearest one to go to, (5) This was the only available place to go for care, (6) They just took me there, (7) My visit there was scheduled in advance, (8) My doctor told me to go there, (9) I wanted to see a particular doctor who worked there, (10) I was sent there from another emergency room or hospital, and (11) Some other reason. The percentages enclosed in parentheses are based on the corresponding "total number of patients" indicated. Emergency unit patients from two of the study hospitals that did not allow patient participation are not included.

Table C-9. Percentage of Emergency Unit Patients (PATs) Indicating Particular Sources as Their "Usual" Sources for Medical Care.

Hospital Emergency Units	Total Number of Patients	The Three Sources Most Frequently Indicated by the Patients and the Percentage of Patients Selecting Them		
		First	Second	Third
All EUs in the Study Sample (N = 28 Hospital EUs)	381	Our regular family doctor (76.1%)	A hospital emergency room (8.4%)	A doctor other than regular family doctor (6.3%); A clinic not in a hospital (6.3%)
EUs with:				
Low patient volume (N = 9)	79	Our regular family doctor (81.0%)	A clinic not in a hospital (8.9%)	A doctor other than regular family doctor (5.1%)
Medium patient volume (N = 10)	110	Our regular family doctor (70.0%)	A clinic not in a hospital (10.0%)	A doctor other than regular family doctor (7.3%)
High patient volume (N = 9)	192	Our regular family doctor (77.6%)	A hospital emergency room (11.5%)	A doctor other than regular family doctor (6.3%)
EUs in:				
Church-operated hospitals (N = 8)	53	Our regular family doctor (73.6%)	A clinic not in a hospital (13.2%)	A doctor other than regular family doctor (5.7%); A hospital emergency room (5.7%)
Osteopathic hospitals (N = 3)	44	Our regular family doctor (84.1%)	A doctor other than regular family doctor (6.8%)	A clinic not in a hospital (4.5%)

	N			
All other hospitals (N = 17)	284	Our regular family doctor (75.4%)	A hospital emergency room (9.9%)	A doctor other than regular family doctor (6.3%)
EUs located in:				
SMSA (urban) areas (N = 19)	252	Our regular family doctor (75.0%)	A doctor other than regular family doctor (8.3%)	A hospital emergency room (6.7%); A clinic not in a hospital (6.7%)
Non-SMSA areas (N = 9)	129	Our regular family doctor (78.3%)	A hospital emergency room (11.6%)	A clinic not in a hospital (5.4%)
EUs in Hospitals Having:				
Medical teaching affiliations (N = 16)	234	Our regular family doctor (72.2%)	A hospital emergency room (9.4%)	A doctor other than regular family doctor (7.7%)
No medical teaching affiliations (N = 12)	147	Our regular family doctor (82.3%)	A hospital emergency room (6.8%)	A clinic not in a hospital (4.8%)
EUs in Hospitals Having:				
Emergency personnel training programs (N = 13)	200	Our regular family doctor (78.5%)	A hospital emergency room (9.0%)	A doctor other than regular family doctor (7.0%)
No training programs (N = 15)	181	Our regular family doctor (73.5%)	A clinic not in a hospital (8.3%)	A hospital emergency room (7.7%)

Note: The results shown are based on the responses of recent patients (PATs) from the various EUs to the following question: "When you or a member of your family needs medical attention, where do you *usually* go for care?" The response alternatives were (1) To our regular family doctor, (2) To a private doctor's office but not a regular family doctor, (3) To a clinic which is *not* located in a hospital, (4) To a hospital clinic (or outpatient department), (5) To a hospital emergency room, and (6) To some other care facility. The percentages enclosed in parentheses are based on the corresponding total number of patients indicated. Emergency unit patients from two of the study hospitals that did not allow patient participation are not included.

usually go for care?" Table C-9 presents the findings, which are rather surprising. Overall, 76 percent of the patients report that they usually go "to our regular family doctor" for care. A distant second choice was "a hospital emergency room" (selected by 8 percent of the patients). The third and fourth most frequently chosen medical sources (with equal frequency) are "a private doctor's office but not a regular family doctor" (6 percent) and "a clinic that is not located in a hospital" (also 6 percent).

Patients visiting emergency units with a high patient volume were more likely to report going to a hospital emergency room and much less likely to report going to a clinic that is not located in a hospital than were patients visiting EUs with a medium or low patient volume. Patients visiting the EUs of urban-area hospitals were less likely to report going to a hospital emergency room than were patients visiting nonurban-area EUs. In contrast, the former were more likely to report going to a private doctor's office but not a regular family doctor than were the latter.

Population Characteristics of the Cities in Which the Emergency Units Are Located

The final table in this appendix, Table C-10, provides some background data from relevant U.S. Census reports published after the 1970 population census. These data indicate some of the population characteristics of the cities or towns in which the EUs studied are located. (Compared to the other data in this appendix, these data are considerably less recent and probably also less interesting; nevertheless, they may be useful as supplementary information.) The specific characteristics included are median level of formal education, the proportion of the population classified as minority population, and the proportion of families with income below the "poverty level."

These population characteristics, of course, do not necessarily reflect the characteristics of the patients treated by the EUs, or those of the patients who participated in the study, because hospitals serve patients from outside the cities as well. Furthermore, the data in Table C-10 may differ from corresponding data

Table C-10. Selected Characteristics of the Population of the Cities in Which the Study Hospitals Are Located, Based on U.S. Census Data.

Cities Where the Hospital Emergency Units (EUs) Involved Are Located		Median School Years Completed by Persons 25 Years or Older	Percentage of Population Classified as Minority Population	Percentage of Families with Income Below "Poverty Level"
All Cities in Which the EUs in the Study Sample Are Located (N = 30 Hospital EUs)	Mean:	12.1	6.8%	6.4%
	Range:	(10.5–14.5)	(0.1%–34.4%)	(1.2%–15.3%)
Cities Where Located, for EUs with:				
Low patient volume (N = 10)		12.2	1.4	5.3
Medium patient volume (N = 10)		11.9	11.8	7.4
High patient volume (N = 10)		12.2	7.2	6.5
Cities Where Located, for EUs in:				
Church-operated hospitals (N = 9)		11.9	7.3	6.5
Osteopathic hospitals (N = 3)		12.5	5.3	4.2
All other hospitals (N = 18)		12.1	6.8	6.8
Cities Where Located, for EUs in:				
SMSA (urban) areas (N = 21)		12.2	8.8	5.8
Non-SMSA areas (N = 9)		11.8	2.2	7.9
Cities Where Located, for EUs in Hospitals with:				
Medical teaching affiliations (N = 17)		12.2	8.6	6.6
No medical teaching affiliations (N = 13)		12.0	4.4	6.3
Cities Where Located, for EUs in Hospitals with:				
Emergency personnel training programs (N = 15)		12.2	4.9	6.0
No training programs (N = 15)		12.0	8.7	6.9

Note: The background information presented in this table is in all cases based on data from relevant U.S. Census reports published after the 1970 census.

provided by the patient respondents, because the latter information is more current and pertains to the particular group of patients involved. Nevertheless, the data in Table C-10 may be useful for comparing, at least in a gross way, the different community environments within which the various emergency units operate.

The first column in Table C-10 shows, for the populations indicated, the median school years completed by persons twenty-five years old or older. For all the cities/towns combined (and properly averaged), the median number of school years completed is 12.1 years. However, the range across the individual cities/towns involved is substantial for this measure, from a median of only 10.5 school years (reflecting some high school education) to a median of 14.5 years (reflecting 2.5 years of college). On the other hand, the range of mean scores for cities in which particular groups of EUs are located is very small (from 11.8 to 12.5 median school years), there being no significant differences among the EU groupings specified.

The cities in which the various EUs are located also differ greatly with respect to the percentage of the population classified as minority population. Only 0.1 percent of the population of one of the cities, for example, is so classified, compared to 34.4 percent of the population of another city. The average figure for all the cities is 6.8 percent. There are also some differences among groups of cities in which particular groups of EUs are located. For example, the cities in which EUs with a medium patient volume are located have a higher percentage of minority population than do those in which EUs with a low patient volume are located. The percentage of the population classified as minority is also higher for cities/towns in urban (SMSA) areas than non-SMSA areas.

Finally, Table C-10 shows the percentage of families with incomes below the "poverty level" for the cities in which the EUs studied are located. This ranges from a low of 1.2 percent to a high of 15.3 percent, depending upon the particular group of cities considered, and averages 6.4 percent for all of the cities/towns involved. The figure is relatively low for cities in which osteopathic hospital EUs, and also EUs with a low patient volume, are located.

References

Allport, F. H. *Institutional Behavior*. Chapel Hill: University of North Carolina Press, 1933.

Allport, G. W. "The Open System in Personality Theory." *Journal of Abnormal and Social Psychology*, 1962, *61*, 301–311.

Alpert, J. J., and others. "Types of Families That Use an Emergency Clinic." *Medical Care*, 1969, *7*, 55–61.

American Hospital Association. *American Hospital Association Guide to the Health Care Field, 1976 Edition*. Chicago: American Hospital Association, 1976.

Argote, L. M. "Input Uncertainty and Organizational Problem Solving in Hospital Emergency Service Units." Unpublished doctoral dissertation, Department of Psychology, University of Michigan, 1979.

Argote, L. M. "Input Uncertainty and Organizational Coordination in Hospital Emergency Units." *Administrative Science Quarterly*, 1982, *27*, 420–434.

Ashby, W. R. *Design for a Brain*. (2nd ed.) New York: Wiley, 1960.

Avery, R. H., and others. *Quality of Medical Care Assessment Using Outcome Measures: Eight Disease-Specific Applications*. Vol. II (R-2021/2-HEW). Santa Monica, Calif.: Rand Corporation, 1976.

Baker, F. "Introduction: Organizations as Open Systems." In F. Baker (ed.), *Organizational Systems: General Systems Ap-*

proaches to Complex Organizations. Homewood, Ill.: Irwin, 1973.

Baker, S. P., and others. "Cumulative Illness Rating Scale." *Journal of the American Geriatrics Society,* 1968, *16,* 622.

Bakke, E. W. "Concept of the Social Organization." In M. Hare (ed.), *Modern Organization Theory.* New York: Wiley, 1959.

Bales, R. F. "The Equilibrium Problem in Small Groups." In T. Parsons, R. F. Bales, and E. A. Shils (eds.), *Working Papers in the Theory of Action.* New York: Free Press, 1953.

Becker, S. W., and Neuhauser, D. *The Efficient Organization.* New York: Wiley, 1975.

Berkowitz, N.H., and others. "Patient Care as a Criterion Problem." *Journal of Health and Human (Social) Behavior,* 1962, *3* (3), 171–176.

Blalock, H. M., Jr., and Blalock, A. M. "Toward a Clarification of System Analysis in the Social Sciences." *Philosophy of Science,* 1959, *26,* 84–92.

Brook, R. H., and Appel, F. A. "Quality of Care Assessment: Choosing a Method for Peer Review." *New England Journal of Medicine,* 1973, *288* (25), 1323–1329.

Brook, R. H., and Stevenson, R. L. "Effectiveness of Patient Care in an Emergency Room." *New England Journal of Medicine,* 1970, *283* (17), 904–908.

Cameron, K., and Whetten, D. (eds.). *Organizational Effectiveness: A Comparison of Multiple Models.* Orlando, Fla.: Academic Press, 1983.

Campbell, A., Converse, P. E., and Rodgers, W. L. *The Quality of American Life.* New York: Russell Sage Foundation, 1976.

Cheng, J. "Organizational Coordination, Integration, Interdependence, and Their Relevance to Research Unit Effectiveness: A Comparative Study." Unpublished doctoral dissertation, Department of Organizational Behavior and Industrial Relations, School of Business, University of Michigan, 1977.

Coffee, R. M. *Patients in Public General Hospitals: Who Pays, How Sick?* Hospital Cost and Utilization Project Research Note 2, Hospital Studies Program, DHHS Publication no. [PHS] 83-3344. Washington, D.C.: National Center for Health Services Research, 1983.

Cooke, R. A., and Rousseau, D. M. "Problems of Complex Systems: A Model of System Problem Solving Applied to Schools." *Educational Administration Quarterly,* 1981, *17* (3), 15-41.

Coser, L. *The Functions of Social Conflict.* New York: Free Press, 1956.

D'Aunno, T. "Correlates of Resource Availability in Hospital Emergency Units." Unpublished doctoral dissertation, Department of Psychology, University of Michigan, 1984.

Denton, J. C., and others. "Predicting Judged Quality of Patient Care in General Hospitals." *Health Services Research,* 1967, *2,* 26-33.

Donabedian, A. "Evaluating the Quality of Medical Care." *Milbank Memorial Fund Quarterly* (Part 2), 1966, *44,* 166-206.

Etzioni, A. *Modern Organizations.* Englewood Cliffs, N.J.: Prentice-Hall, 1964.

Etzioni, A., and Dubow, F. L. (eds.). *Comparative Perspectives: Theories and Methods.* Boston: Little, Brown, 1970.

Evan, W. M. "Organization Theory and Organizational Effectiveness: An Exploratory Analysis." *Organization and Administrative Science,* 1976, *7,* 15-28.

Executive Office of the President, Office of Management and Budget. *Standard Metropolitan Statistical Areas 1975.* (Rev. ed.) Washington, D.C.: U.S. Government Printing Office, 1975.

Feibleman, J., and Friend, J. W. "The Structure and Function of Organization." *Philosophical Review,* 1945, *54,* 19-44.

Feldstein, M. *Economic Analysis of Health Services Efficiency.* Chicago: Markham, 1967.

Feller, I., and Crane, K. "National Burn Information Exchange." *Surgical Clinics of North America,* 1970, *50* (6), 1425-1436.

Feller, I., Flora, J. D., Jr., and Bawol, R. "Baseline Results of Therapy for Burned Patients." *Journal of the American Medical Association,* 1976, *236* (17), 1943-1947.

Flood, A. B., Scott, W. R., Ewy, W., and Forrest, W. H., Jr. "Effectiveness in Professional Organizations: The Impact of Surgeons and Surgical Staff Characteristics on the Quality of Care in Hospitals." *Health Services Research,* 1982, *17,* 341-366.

Forrest, W. H., Scott, W. R., and Brown, B. M. "Comparison of Hospitals with Regard to Outcomes of Surgery." *Health Services Research*, 1976, *11* (2), 112–127.

Frazier, W. H., and Brand, D. A. "Quality Assessment and the Art of Medicine: The Anatomy of Laceration Care." *Medical Care*, 1979, *17*, 480–490.

Geis, G., Chappell, D., and Cohen, F. G. *Hospital Care for Rape Victims: Results of a Nationwide Survey*. Forcible Rape Series no. 1. Seattle: Battelle Law and Justice Study Center, March 1975.

Georgopoulos, B. S. "Normative Structure Variables and Organizational Behavior: A Comparative Study." *Human Relations*, 1965, *18*, 155–169.

Georgopoulos, B. S. "The Hospital as an Organization and Problem-Solving System." In B. S. Georgopoulos (ed.), *Organization Research on Health Institutions*. Ann Arbor: Institute for Social Research, University of Michigan, 1972.

Georgopoulos, B. S. *Hospital Organization Research: Review and Source Book*. Philadelphia: Saunders, 1975.

Georgopoulos, B. S. "An Open-System Approach to Evaluating the Effectiveness of Hospital Emergency Departments." *Emergency Medical Services*, 1978, 7 (6), 118–119.

Georgopoulos, B. S. "Organizational Rationality, Medicine, and the Use of New Knowledge in American Hospitals." *Hospital and Health Services Administration*, 1982, 27 (3), 34–56.

Georgopoulos, B. S. "Organization Structure and the Performance of Hospital Emergency Services." *Annals of Emergency Medicine*, 1985, *14* (7), 677–684.

Georgopoulos, B. S., and Christman, L. "The Clinical Nurse Specialist: A Role Model." *American Journal of Nursing*, 1970, *70*, 1030–1039.

Georgopoulos, B. S., and Cooke, R. A. *Conceptual-Theoretical Framework for the Organizational Study of Hospital Emergency Services*. ISR Working Paper Series, Article 8011. Ann Arbor: Institute for Social Research, University of Michigan, 1979.

Georgopoulos, B. S., Cooke, R. A., and Associates. *A Comparative Study of the Organization and Performance of Hospital Emer-*

gency Services: Selected Descriptive Findings and the Research Instruments. Ann Arbor: Institute for Social Research, University of Michigan, 1980.

Georgopoulos, B. S., and Mann, F. C. *The Community General Hospital.* New York: Macmillan, 1962.

Georgopoulos, B. S., and Matejko, A. "The American General Hospital as a Complex Social System." *Health Services Research,* 1967, *2,* 76–112.

Georgopoulos, B. S., and Tannenbaum, A. S. "A Study of Organizational Effectiveness." *American Sociological Review,* 1957, *22,* 534–540.

Georgopoulos, B. S., and Wieland, G. F. "Nationwide Study of Coordination and Patient Care in Voluntary Hospitals." Ann Arbor: Institute for Social Research, University of Michigan, 1964.

Ghorpade, J. *Assessment of Organizational Effectiveness: Issues, Analysis, and Readings.* Pacific Palisades, Calif.: Goodyear, 1971.

Gibson, G. "EMS Evaluation: Criteria for Standards and Research Design." *Health Services Research,* 1976, *11* (2), 105–111.

Gibson, G. "EMS Research: Methodology Development or Substantive Applications?" *Health Services Research,* 1977, *12* (1), 44–55.

Gibson, G., Bugbee, G., and Anderson, O. W. *Emergency Medical Services in the Chicago Area.* Chicago: Center for Health Administration Studies, University of Chicago, 1970.

Gibson, G., Pickar, E. R., and Wagner, J. L. "Evaluative Measures and Data Collection Methods for Emergency Medical Services Systems." *Public Health Reports,* 1977, *92* (4), 312–321.

Gonnella, J. S., and Goran, M. J. "Quality of Patient Care—A Measurement Change: The Staging Concept." *Medical Care,* 1975, *13,* 467–473.

Goodman, P. S., Pennings, J. M., and Associates. *New Perspectives on Organizational Effectiveness.* San Francisco: Jossey-Bass, 1977.

Goodman, R., and Kish, L. "Controlled Selection—A Technique in Probability Sampling." *Journal of the American Statistical Association,* 1950, *45,* 350–372.

Goss, M.E.W., and Reed, J. I. "Evaluating the Quality of Hospital Care Through Severity-Adjusted Death Rates: Some Pitfalls." *Medical Care*, 1974, *12*, 202-213.

Gouldner, A. W. *Patterns of Industrial Bureaucracy.* New York: Free Press, 1954.

Greenfield, S., and others. "Comparison of a Criteria Map to a Criteria List in Quality of Care Assessment for Patients with Chest Pain: The Relation of Each to Outcome." *Medical Care,* 1981, *19*, 255-272.

Groves, R. M., and Hess, I. "An Algorithm for Controlled Selection." In I. Hess, D. C. Riedel, and T. B. Fitzpatrick (eds.), *Probability Sampling of Hospitals and Patients.* (2nd ed.) Ann Arbor: Health Administration Press, University of Michigan, 1975.

Gunter, M. J., and Ricci, E. M. *Hospital Planning for Emergency Medical Services: Organizational Issues and Interrelationships.* Pittsburgh: Health Operations Research Group, University of Pittsburgh, 1974.

Hage, J. *Communication and Organizational Control: Cybernetics in Health and Welfare Settings.* New York: Wiley-Interscience, 1974.

Haussman, R.K.D., Hegyvary, S. T., and Newman, J. F. *Monitoring Quality of Nursing Care.* Part 2: *Assessment and Study of Correlates.* DHEW Pub. No. (HRA) 76-7. Washington, D.C.: Department of Health and Human Services, 1976.

Holt, R. T., and Turner, J. E. (eds.). *The Methodology of Comparative Research.* New York: Free Press, 1970.

Johnson, E. A. "Thinking Conceptually About Hospital Efficiency." *Hospital and Health Services Administration,* 1981, *26,* 12-26.

Johnson, W. L., and Rosenfeld, L. S. "Indices of Performance in Ambulatory Care Services." *Medical Care,* 1969, *7,* 250-260.

Kanter, R. M. "Organizational Performance: Recent Developments in Measurement." *Annual Review of Sociology,* 1981, *7,* 321-349.

Katz, D., and Georgopoulos, B. S. "Organizations in a Changing World." *Journal of Applied Behavioral Science,* 1971, *7* (3), 324-370.

Katz, D., and Kahn, R. L. *The Social Psychology of Organizations.* New York: Wiley, 1966.

Katz, D., and Kahn, R. L. *The Social Psychology of Organizations.* (2nd ed.) New York: Wiley, 1978.

Kessner, D. M., Kalk, C., and Singer, J. "Assessing Health Quality—The Case for Tracers." *New England Journal of Medicine,* 1973, *288,* 189–194.

Kish, L., and Hess, I. "On Variances of Ratios and Their Differences in Multi-Stage Samples." *Journal of the American Statistical Association,* 1949, *54,* 416–446.

Klein, M. W., and others. "Problems of Measuring Patient Care in the Outpatient Department." *Journal of Health and Human Behavior,* 1961, *2* (2), 138–144.

Kresky, B. "Evaluation of Patient Care in Emergency Departments." In E. F. Pascarelli (ed.), *Hospital-Based Ambulatory Care.* East Norwalk, Conn.: Appleton-Century-Crofts, 1982.

Krischer, J. P. "Indexes of Severity: Underlying Concepts." *Health Services Research,* 1976, *11* (2), 143–157.

Lammers, C. J., and Hickson, D. J. (eds.). *Organizations Alike and Unlike: International and Interinstitutional Studies in the Sociology of Organizations.* London: Routledge & Kegan Paul, 1979.

Lave, J. R., Lave, L. B., and Silverman, L. P. "Hospital Cost Estimation Controlling for Case Mix." *Applied Economics,* 1972, *4* (3), 165–180.

Lave, J. R., and Leinhardt, S. "The Delivery of Ambulatory Care to the Poor: A Literature Review." *Management Science,* 1972, *19,* 78–79.

Lave, L. B. "Consumer Use of Emergency and Other Acute Care Services." Paper presented at Conference on Consumer Incentives in Health Care, Georgetown University, Washington, D.C., 1973.

Lavenhar, M. A., and others. "Social Class and Medical Care: Indices of Non-Urgency in Use of Hospital Emergency Services." *Medical Care,* 1968, *6,* 368–380.

Lawrence, R. *Emergency Room Physician Staffing Patterns.* New Haven, Conn.: Yale University, 1969.

Lewis, C. E., and others. "Activities, Events and Outcomes in Ambulatory Patient Care." *New England Journal of Medicine,* 1969, *280* (12), 645–649.

Likert, R. *The Human Organization.* New York: McGraw-Hill, 1967.

Lincoln, J. R., and Zeitz, G. "Organization Properties from Aggregate Data: Separating Individual and Structural Effects." *American Sociological Review,* 1980, *45* (3), 391–408.

Linn, B. S., Linn, M. W., and Gurel, L. "Cumulative Illness Rating Scale." *Journal of the American Geriatrics Society,* 1968, *16*, 622.

Longest, B. B. "Relationships Between Coordination, Efficiency, and Quality of Care in General Hospitals." *Hospital Administration,* 1974, *19*, 65–86.

MacKenzie, K. D. *A Theory of Group Structures.* Vol. 1. New York: Gordon & Breach, 1976.

March, J. G., and Simon, H. A. *Organizations.* New York: Wiley, 1958.

Merton, R. K. *Social Theory and Social Structure.* (2nd ed.) New York: Free Press, 1957.

Miller, J. G. "Living Systems: Basic Concepts." *Behavioral Science,* 1965, *10* (3), 193–237.

Miller, J. G. "The Nature of Living Systems." *Behavioral Science,* 1971, *16*, 278–301.

Miller, J. G. *Living Systems.* New York: McGraw-Hill, 1978.

Mintzberg, H. *The Structuring of Organizations.* Englewood Cliffs, N.J.: Prentice-Hall, 1979.

Money, W. H., Gilfillan, D. P., and Duncan, R. "A Comparative Study of Multiunit Health Care Organizations." In S. M. Shortell and M. Brown (eds.), *Organizational Research in Hospitals.* Chicago: Blue Cross Association, 1976.

Morehead, M. A. "The Medical Audit as an Operational Tool." *American Journal of Public Health,* 1967, *57* (9), 1643–1657.

Mott, P. E. *The Characteristics of Effective Organizations.* New York: Harper & Row, 1972.

National Center for Health Services Research. *Emergency Medical Services Research Methodology Workshop 2.* Research Proceedings Series. Washington, D.C.: National Center for Health Services Research, 1979.

National Center for Health Services Research. *Emergency Medical Services Systems Research Project Abstracts, 1979*. Research Management Series. Washington, D.C.: National Center for Health Services Research, 1980.

Neuhauser, D. *The Relationship of Administrative Activities and Hospital Performance*. Research Series 28. Chicago: Center for Health Administration Studies, University of Chicago, 1971.

Parsons, T. "Some Ingredients of a General Theory of Formal Organization." In A. W. Halpin (ed.), *Administrative Theory in Education*. New York: Macmillan, 1958.

Parsons, T., Bales, R. F., and Shils, E. A. (eds.). *Working Papers in the Theory of Action*. New York: Free Press, 1953.

Parsons, T., and Shils, E. A. *Toward a General Theory of Action*. Cambridge, Mass.: Harvard University Press, 1952.

Pascarelli, E. F. (ed.). *Hospital-Based Ambulatory Care*. East Norwalk, Conn.: Appleton-Century-Crofts, 1982.

Payne, B. C., and Lyons, T. F. *Methods of Evaluating and Improving Medical Care Quality*. Vol. 1: *Episode of Illness Study*. Ann Arbor: University of Michigan Press, 1972.

Payne, B. C., and others. *The Quality of Medical Care: Evaluation and Improvement*. Chicago: Hospital Research and Educational Trust, 1976.

Perkins, A. L. "Participative Management in Organizations: Problem Solving and Decision Making Groups." Unpublished doctoral dissertation, Department of Psychology, University of Michigan, 1983.

Perrow, C. A. *Complex Organizations: A Critical Essay*. Glenview, Ill.: Scott, Foresman, 1972.

Peterson, M. F. "Problem-Appropriate Leadership in Hospital Emergency Units and Its Relation to Selected Organizational Variables." Unpublished doctoral dissertation, Department of Psychology, University of Michigan, 1979.

Peterson, M. F. "Attitudinal Differences Among Shifts: What Do They Reflect?" *Academy of Management Journal*, 1985, *28* (3), 723-732.

Peterson, O. "Medical Care—Its Social and Organizational Aspects: Evaluation of Quality of Medical Care." *New England Journal of Medicine,* 1963, *269,* 1238-1245.

Pickle, H., and Friedlander, F. "Seven Societal Criteria of Organizational Success." *Personnel Psychology,* 1967, *20,* 165-178.

Price, J. L. *Organizational Effectiveness: An Inventory of Propositions.* Homewood, Ill.: Irwin-Dorsey, 1968.

Price, J. L. "The Study of Organizational Effectiveness." *Sociological Quarterly,* 1972, *13,* 3-15; 1973, *14,* 271-278.

Przeworski, A., and Teune, H. *The Logic of Comparative Social Inquiry.* New York: Wiley-Interscience, 1970.

Rhee, S. "Factors Determining the Quality of Physician Performance in Patient Care." *Medical Care,* 1976, *14* (9), 733-750.

Richardson, F. "Peer Review of Medical Care." *Medical Care,* 1972, *10,* 29-39.

Richardson, W. C. "Measuring the Urban Poor's Use of Physicians' Services in Response to Illness Episodes." *Medical Care,* 1970, *8,* 132-142.

Robinson, G. D., and others. "Use of Hospital Emergency Service by Children and Adolescents for Primary Care." *Canadian Medical Association Journal,* 1969, *101,* 69-73.

Roemer, M. I., Moustafa, A. T., and Hopkins, C. E. "A Proposed Hospital Quality Index: Hospital Death Rates Adjusted for Case Severity." *Health Services Research,* 1968, *3,* 96-118.

Roth, J. A. "Utilization of the Hospital Emergency Department." *Journal of Health and Social Behavior,* 1971, *12,* 312-320.

Sanazaro, P. J., and Williamson, J. W. "Physician Performance and Its Effects on Patients: A Classification Based on Reports by Internists, Surgeons, Pediatricians, and Obstetricians." *Medical Care,* 1970, *8* (4), 299-308.

Scheuch, E. K. "Cross-National Comparisons Using Aggregate Data." In A. Etzioni and F. L. Dubow (eds.), *Comparative Perspectives: Theories and Methods.* Boston: Little, Brown, 1970.

Scott, W. R., Forrest, W. H., and Brown, B. M. "Hospital Structure and Postoperative Mortality and Morbidity." In S. M. Shortell and M. Brown (eds.), *Organizational Research in Hospitals.* Chicago: Blue Cross Association, 1976.

Scott, W. R., and Shortell, S. M. "Organizational Performance: Managing for Efficiency and Effectiveness." In S. M. Shortell and A. D. Kaluzny (eds.), *Health Care Management: A Text in Organization Theory and Behavior.* New York: Wiley Medical, 1983.

Seashore, S. E. "A Framework for an Integrated Model of Organizational Effectiveness." In K. Cameron and D. Whetten (eds.), *Organizational Effectiveness: A Comparison of Multiple Models.* Orlando, Fla.: Academic Press, 1983.

Seashore, S. E., Indik, B. P., and Georgopoulos, B. S. "Relationships Among Criteria of Job Performance." *Journal of Applied Psychology,* 1960, *44,* 195-202.

Semmlow, J. L., and Cone, R. "Utility of the Injury Severity Score: A Confirmation." *Health Services Research,* 1976, *11* (1), 45-52.

Shapiro, S. "End-Result Measurements of Quality of Medical Care." *Milbank Memorial Fund Quarterly,* 1967, *45* (2), 7-30.

Shortell, S. M. "Organization Theory and Health Services Delivery." In S. M. Shortell and M. Brown (eds.), *Organizational Research in Hospitals.* Chicago: Blue Cross Association, 1976.

Shortell, S. M., Becker, S. W., and Neuhauser, D. "The Effects of Management Practice on Quality of Care." In S. M. Shortell and M. Brown (eds.), *Organizational Research in Hospitals.* Chicago: Blue Cross Association, 1976.

Shortell, S. M., and Brown, M. (eds.). *Organizational Research in Hospitals.* Chicago: Blue Cross Association, 1976.

Shortell, S. M., and Kaluzny, A. D. (eds.). *Health Care Management: A Text in Organization Theory and Behavior.* New York: Wiley Medical, 1983.

Shuman, L. J., Wolfe, H., and Hardwick, C. P. "A Predictive Hospital Reimbursement and Evaluation Model." *Inquiry: A Review of Current Research in Hospital and Medical Economics,* 1972, *9,* 17-33.

Steers, R. M. "Problems in the Measurement of Organizational Effectiveness." *Administrative Science Quarterly,* 1975, *20,* 546-558.

Steers, R. M. "When Is an Organization Effective? A Process Approach to Understanding Effectiveness." *Organizational Dynamics,* 1976, *5* (2), 50–63.

Stoddard, W. D., II. *Hospital Emergency Services: Toward More Effective Utilization of Resources and Provision of Care.* Research monograph. Ames: University of Iowa, 1969.

Sutton, R. I., and Ford, L. H. "Problem-Solving Adequacy in Hospital Sub-Units." *Human Relations,* 1982, *35* (8), 675–701.

Thompson, J. D. *Organizations in Action.* New York: McGraw-Hill, 1967.

Thompson, J. D., and others. *Comparative Studies in Administration.* Pittsburgh: University of Pittsburgh Press, 1959.

Thompson, V. *Modern Organization.* New York: Knopf, 1961.

Uhlaner, L. "Management of the Coordination Problem in Hospital Emergency Units." Unpublished doctoral dissertation, Department of Psychology, University of Michigan, 1980.

Uzun, N. E. "A Study of Hospital Emergency Units Adapting to Their Social Environments: An Interorganizational Cooperation Perspective." Unpublished doctoral dissertation, Department of Psychology, University of Michigan, 1980.

von Bertalanffy, L. "General Systems Theory." *Yearbook of Society for General Systems Research,* 1956, *1,* 1–10.

Weinerman, E. R., and Edwards, H. R. "Changing Patterns in Hospital Emergency Service." *Hospitals,* 1964, *38* (22), 55 f.

Weiss, P. "Animal Behavior as System Reaction." *Yearbook of Society for General Systems Research,* 1959, *4,* 1–44.

Welch, M. S. "Rape and the Trauma of Inadequate Care." *Prism,* 1975, *3,* 17–21, 61.

Wieland, G. F. "Complexity and Coordination in Organizations." Unpublished doctoral dissertation, Department of Psychology, University of Michigan, 1965.

Wieland, G. F. (ed.). *Improving Health Care Management: Organization Development and Organization Change.* Ann Arbor: Health Administration Press, University of Michigan, 1981.

Williamson, J. W. "Evaluating Quality of Patient Care: A Strategy Relating Outcome and Process Assessment." *Journal of the American Medical Association,* 1971, *218* (4), 564–569.

Wold, H. "Systems Under Indirect Observation Using PLS." In C. Fornell (ed.), *A Second Generation of Multivariate Analysis.* Vol. 1. New York: Praeger, 1983.

Yuchtman, E., and Seashore, S. E. "A System Resource Approach to Organizational Effectiveness." *American Sociological Review,* 1967, *32,* 891–903.

Zey-Ferrell, M. *Dimensions of Organizations.* Santa Monica, Calif.: Goodyear, 1979.

Index